GARDEN FOR LIFE

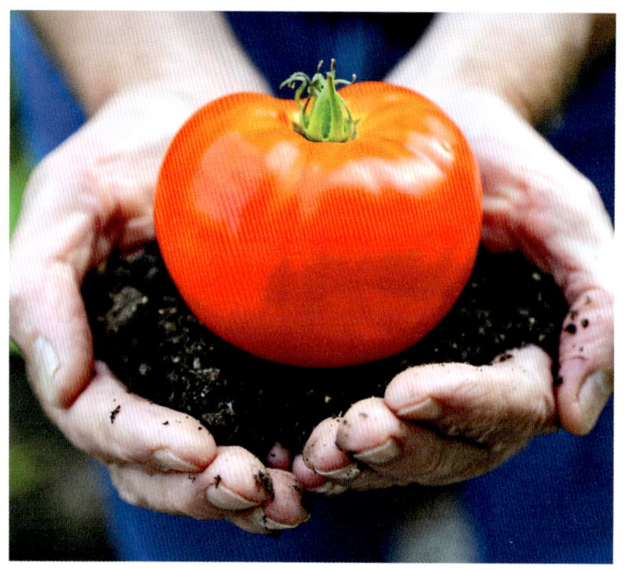

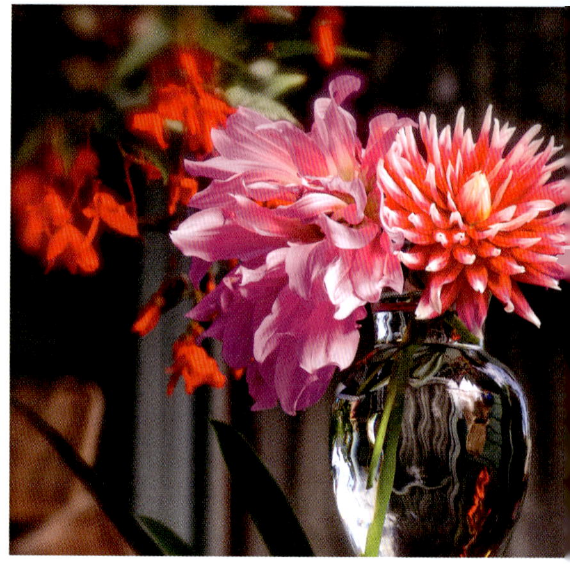

Also by Rhonda Fleming Hayes

Pollinator Friendly Gardening:
Gardening for Bees, Butterflies,
and Other Pollinators
(Voyageur Press, 2016)

PRAISE FOR *GARDEN FOR LIFE*

"This is a delightful book, full of gorgeous photographs and many good ideas. It will give older gardeners plenty of inspiration and confidence."

—Barbara Damrosch,
author of *A Life in the Garden* and *The Garden Primer*

"I couldn't put this book down. The wealth of information in *Garden for Life* truly encompasses all the aspects one should consider when gardening at any age. It captures the spirit and common thoughts, experiences, and generosity all gardeners share, and Rhonda's charming way of addressing how to create, maintain, and manage a garden as one ages is very impressive. I truly loved reading it."

—Madeline de Vries Hooper,
creator, executive producer, and host, *GardenFit*

"*Garden for Life* is the book to keep handy and dip into often. A very enjoyable, heartwarming guide packed with wisdom, tried-and-trusted methods, and incredibly useful tips for enjoying your garden in later life."

—Kathryn Bradley-Hole, author of
The Naturally Beautiful Garden and *English Gardens*

"In *Garden for Life*, Hayes uses her lifetime of gardening experience and wisdom to help us create a stunning yet manageable garden that continually delights."

—Niki Jabbour, author of
The Year-Round Vegetable Garden and *Growing Under Cover*

"Rhonda Fleming Hayes knows what we're all thinking: the garden isn't too big, our priorities are just shifting. *Garden for Life* is the no-nonsense, big-hearted guide that meets us exactly where we are with solutions that actually work. Forget those glossy magazines showing gardens that require three assistants and the knees of a twenty-year-old. Hayes gives us living mulch, rolling carts, and the permission to let things go wild at the edges. She's clever, helpful, and fiercely on our side. This book won't make you feel guilty about what you can't do anymore. It'll make you excited about what you still can do. Your future self will thank you for reading it."

—Shawna Coronado, author of *101 Organic Gardening Hacks*

"This book confirms what plant people know—that gardening can be hard work, but work made lighter by embracing inevitable change and the power of living with plants. Full of patience and hope for our world and our bodies in the form of warm and practical advice, *Garden for Life* helps us cultivate resilience in the gardens we gift to our human and wild communities."

—Benjamin Vogt, author of *Prairie Up* and *A New Garden Ethic*

"Rhonda Fleming Hayes has put together the perfect template for creating and caring for a garden as we age. She offers sage advice for downsizing and rethinking the garden, along with important growing tips, all presented with a gentle voice and wonderful sense of humor. *Garden for Life* is filled with beautiful photography, fun stories, and great information. It's a must for a generation of gardeners who have spent a lifetime gardening and wish to continue getting their hands dirty."

—Doug Oster, Emmy Award–winning garden host, writer, and producer

"*Garden for Life* pairs Rhonda's joyful approach to gardening with down-to-earth information that will make gardening easier and more fun, no matter what age you are."

—Jenny Rose Carey, author of *The Ultimate Flower Gardener's Guide* and *The Essential Guide to Bulbs*

"*Garden for Life* by Rhonda Fleming Hayes is a terrific resource for anyone looking to make their gardening time easier and more enjoyable. None of us are getting any younger, and the tools and techniques that Hayes provides can help us garden well into our senior years. Gardening itself is an act of hope, and I especially appreciate the content focused on inspiration and examples. This book includes the concept of passing gardening wisdom on to the next generation—something we all can benefit from."

—Kathy Jentz, host, *GardenDC* podcast; author of *Groundcover Revolution*

"Only a gardener who is deeply rooted in the lessons of our earth could have written such a book. Rhonda's intimate, hands-in-the-soil wisdom mixed with tips, science, cultivation, and inspiration makes for the perfect garden read."

—Sharon Lovejoy, author and illustrator of *Roots, Shoots, Buckets & Boots*

"Whether you're aging in place and paring back for easier care, moving to a smaller home and starting fresh, or gardening at a tabletop or patio-container scale, Rhonda Fleming Hayes offers practical lessons for keeping your hands in the dirt for years to come. Her book delivers a smart mix of safe design ideas, adaptable gardening practices, and ergonomic tools that reduce strain, lower the risk of injury, and leave room for the fun part: watching things grow."

—Pam Penick, author of *Lawn Gone!* and *Gardens of Texas*; publisher, *Digging* blog

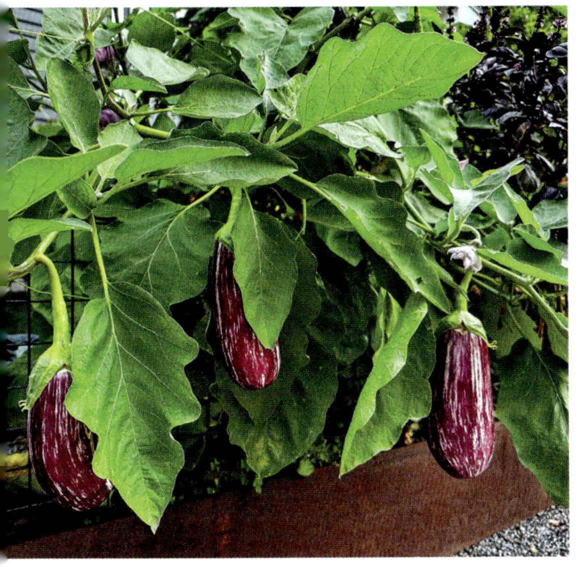
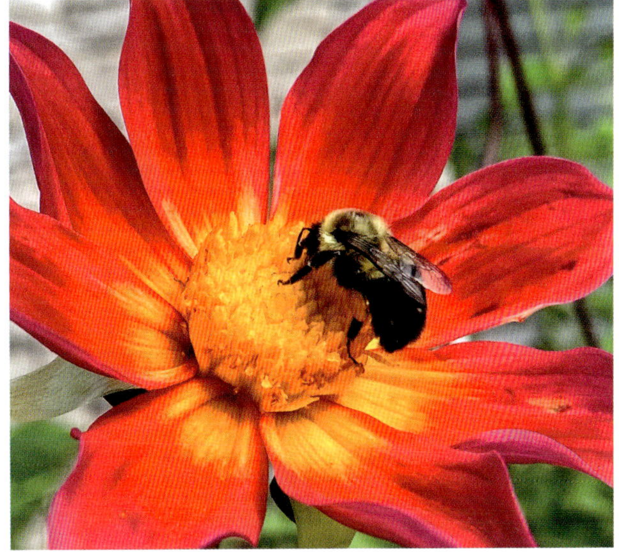

GARDEN FOR LIFE

Strategies for Easier, Greener, More Joyful Gardening as We Age

RHONDA FLEMING HAYES

Chelsea Green Publishing
White River Junction, Vermont
London, UK

First published in 2026 by Chelsea Green Publishing | PO Box 4529 | White River Junction, VT 05001 | West Wing, Somerset House, Strand | London, WC2R 1LA, UK | www.chelseagreen.com
A Division of Rizzoli International Publications, Inc. | 49 West 27th Street | New York, NY 10001 | www.rizzoliusa.com

Publisher: Charles Miers
Deputy Publisher: Matthew Derr
Project Manager: Natalie Wallace
Acquiring Editor: Anna Bliss
Developmental Editor: Phil Schmidt
Copy Editor: Buzz Poole
Proofreader: Nancy A. Crompton
Indexer: Linda Hallinger
Designer: Melissa Jacobson
Page Layout: Abrah Griggs

ISBN 978-1-64502-325-8 (paperback) | ISBN 978-1-64502-326-5 (ebook) | ISBN 978-1-64502-327-2 (audiobook)
Library of Congress Control Number: 2025051762 (print)

Our Commitment to Green Publishing
Chelsea Green sees publishing as a tool for cultural change and ecological stewardship. We strive to align our book manufacturing practices with our editorial mission and to reduce the impact of our business enterprise in the environment. We print our books using vegetable-based inks whenever possible. This book may cost slightly more because it was printed on paper supplied by Versa from well-managed, FSC®-certified forests and other controlled sources.

Authorized EU representative for product safety and compliance
Mondadori Libri S.p.A. | www.mondadori.it
via Gian Battista Vico 42 | Milan, Italy 20123

Printed in the United States of America.
10 9 8 7 6 5 4 3 2 1 26 27 28 29 30

For my grandmother, Mittie

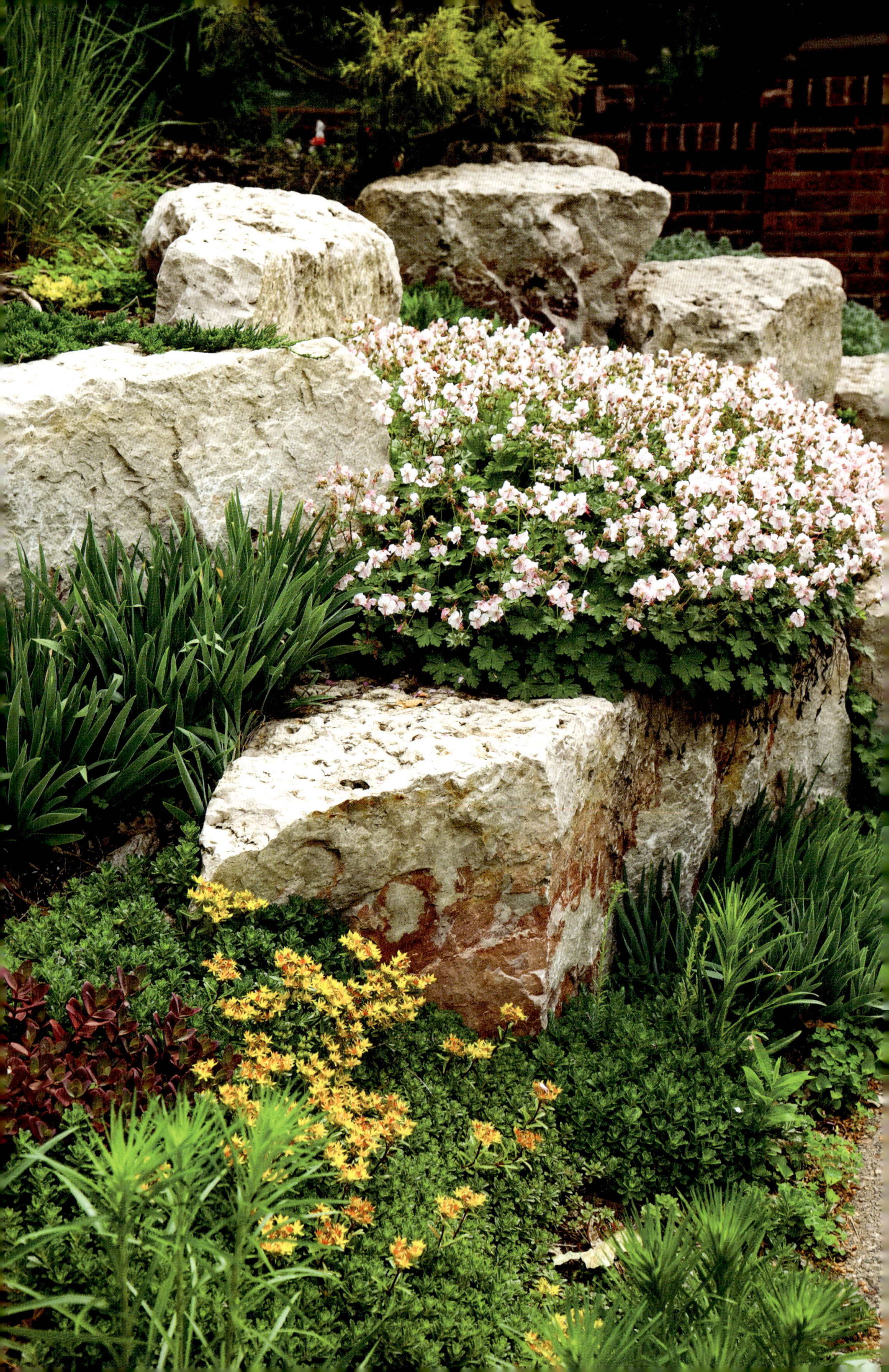

CONTENTS

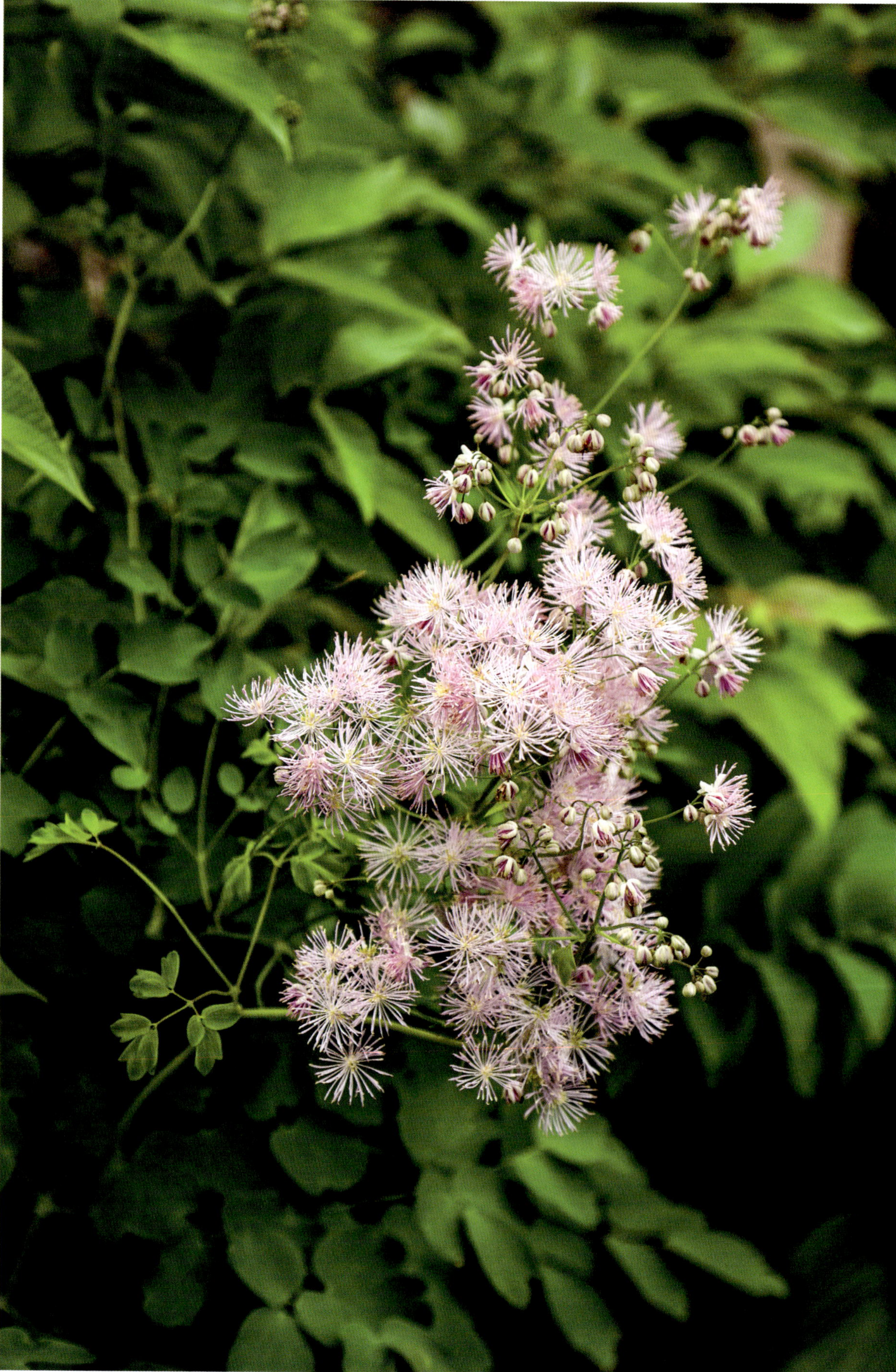

PREFACE
Pour Some Tea, and Walk with Me

Aging today looks very different from how it has for previous generations. Seniors are doing it all—golfing, swimming, tennis, hiking, biking, pickleball, and more. All of these activities undoubtedly provide healthy rewards, and yet, some would hesitate to include gardening in this list, perhaps for its lack of sporty fashion sense alone. But gardening has been described as a "full mind-body workout."

Gardening defies categories: Is it a leisure activity or is it labor? Is it a hobby, like sewing and crafting, or is it more of a lifestyle? A few years ago, when I went to the Mayo Sports Clinic with shoulder trouble, I shared the waiting room with several very tall, athletic young adults. In fact, the Minnesota Timberwolves and Minnesota Lynx training courts were right there behind the glass. I was totally serious when I told the doctor, "Gardening is my sport." And as I approach my seventh decade, I'm nowhere near ready to give it up. I don't have to convince the Mayo Clinic, though, of the benefits of gardening. They outline some of the key benefits on their website.

- Increased exercise
- Improved diet
- Time in nature
- Reduced stress
- Social benefits[1]

Older gardeners don't look like elite athletes—not even close—with our muddy knees and battered hats, and most of us are certainly not "ripped." However, we have been in it for the long haul, and multiple studies show that gardening is the number one activity for improving longevity. I'd like to open this book by explaining how gardening does exactly that.

But first it might be easier to show than tell. Join me on my morning walk through the garden. I know this is a favorite ritual for many gardeners.

Lots of you go out first thing in your pajamas (such is the pull to get out and see what's happening), and some of you don't even bother with a bathrobe! My garden is visible from the street, so I'm dressed. And before heading outside, I'm going to make a cup of tea, Irish Breakfast with lemon and honey, in my stout mug, best for the precarious places I leave it when I see something that needs tending in the garden. It's June here in Minnesota, and everything is well on its way, so I'll also bring a few colanders, my harvest containers of choice.

I go through the patio doors and down the steps by the fountain. As I pass by, I hear *plop bloop* and glimpse a green leopard frog disappearing beneath a lily pad. I pause by the broad step leading down to the kitchen garden and check on the coral-colored bedding salvia I have in containers. It was a trial seed offer, and I'm eager to see if the plant attracts hummingbirds like the larger varieties do.

The kitchen garden spans the entire south side of the house along the driveway. The gravel path crunches underfoot as I approach the first of my raised beds. I'm pleased to see there are enough peas to pick today. I lean over the trellis and harvest enough pods to fill a colander, stretching toward the center of the bed to get the last ones hiding out. It's a trick of light and shadow, and I've missed a few. On a second pass I go by feel, my fingers finding the cool weight of the pods.

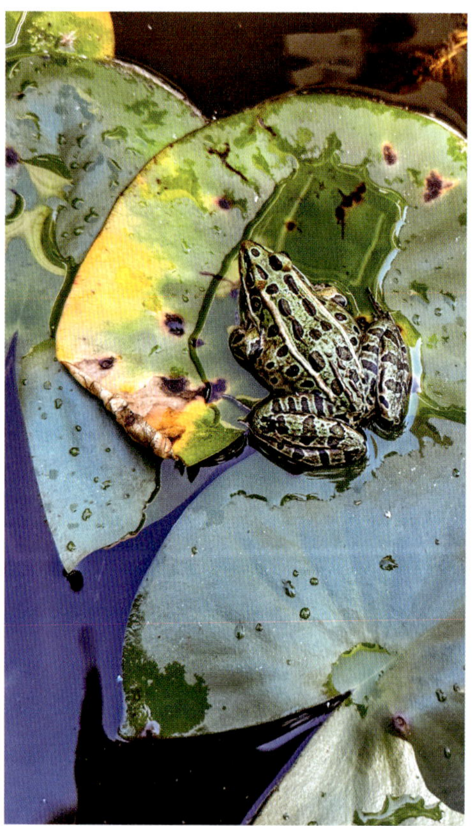

One of the frogs that visits my pond frequently.

In this year's rotation, the tomatoes are in the narrow bed against the house, where the extra warmth favors them ripening a bit early. There are lots of green ones close to turning red. I see some yellow leaves near the bottom of the plants, and I squat down and move along the row to pick off the blighted foliage.

The basil is getting bushy. I pinch out the tops one by one and add them to a colander. The sharp, sweet smell lingers on my hands, in a good way. I bend over and pull

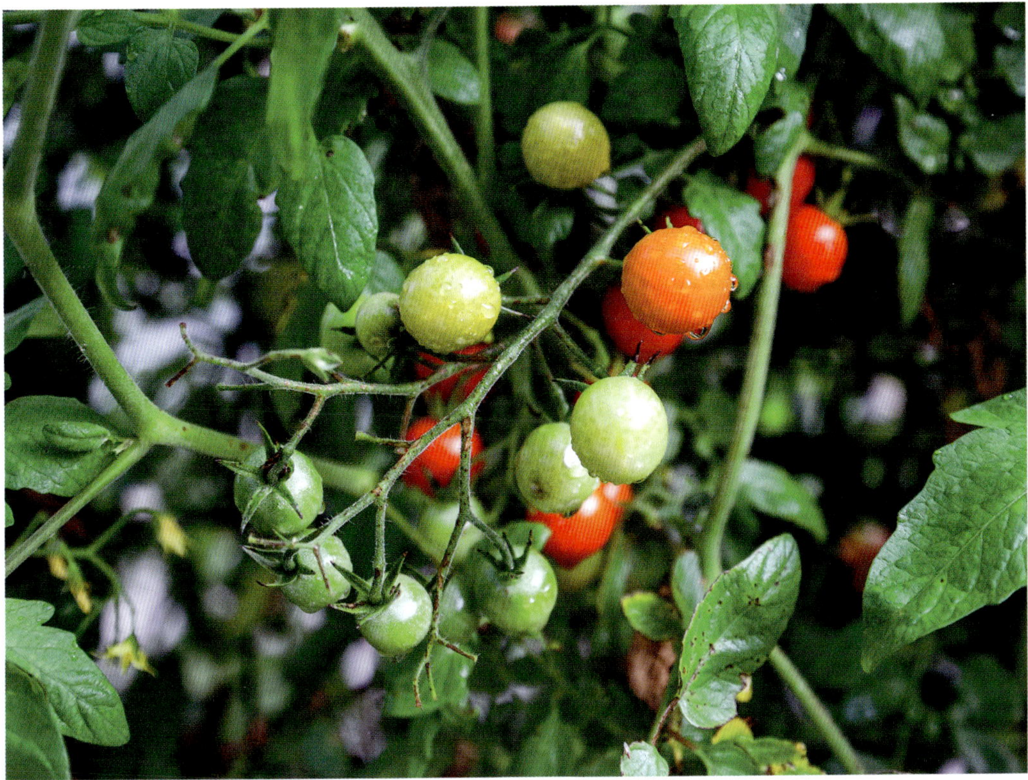

Cherry tomatoes ripening in my kitchen garden.

some weeds encroaching on the carrots. Everything else looks good, so I go around to the front yard.

While I consider the whole garden to be pollinator habitat, I've stacked the deck by the front porch with their favorites—what I call butterfly bait. When I'm working on my laptop out there, butterflies can be a great distraction. But this morning it's a bit chilly and only the bumblebees are meandering among the flowers.

Down the front walk to the sloping rock garden that faces our street, I take a step back and think about where I'd like to plant the clumping allium that I divided and dug out of the upper beds yesterday. I've been working to make this area along the sidewalk more visually cohesive and resilient, able to survive hungry rabbits, freezing temps, passing dogs, and the increasing vagaries of the weather. I really like this variety, 'Millenium,' for its fresh-looking foliage and its relatively late bloom that comes when the peak-summer flowers are waning. The orchid-color florets are always covered with bees, butterflies, and even beetles.

Surrounding the alliums I continue to "divide and multiply" different groundcovers, like sedum, ajuga, creeping phlox, cranesbill, and dwarf crested iris, so they knit together and form a weed-suppressing, living mulch. I'm very close to my goal of covering the entire area, eliminating the need for bagged mulch. Hurray!

The alliums are in a cart at the upper end of the driveway. I'll wheel them down and transplant them tomorrow while it's still cooler in the morning. I just remembered the gallon-size dwarf evergreens I bought yesterday, so I head back up the driveway and carry them back to the front, two at a time, placing them in the porch bed where I want to add more structure. More digging and planting but a good solution for that area.

One of the neighbors from down the street walks by with his dog. We say hello and both remark on the irises. Big gold and maroon blooms—inspired by the University of Minnesota, we wonder? The irises look settled and majestic nestled in the rocks at various points across the front. They were a gift, "passalong plants" from my dear gardening friend across the street. Cutting down the spent stalks is a once-a-year chore that I'll tackle in a few weeks, but for now they anchor the front landscape with their spikes of vertical foliage. I can't imagine the garden without them.

Before he walks on, the neighbor asks if I'll have cucumbers soon. I always put out a box of extras on the steps for the taking. "Soon," I tell him.

The day is getting warmer now and I see a few monarchs perusing the orange butterfly weed. I pull out my phone and record one laying her eggs on the foliage. I post the video to Instagram, #miracle. I move on, slowly up the driveway, taking time to identify all the bee species foraging on the hedge of white spirea. My original design used 'Gro-Low' sumac, but it spread way

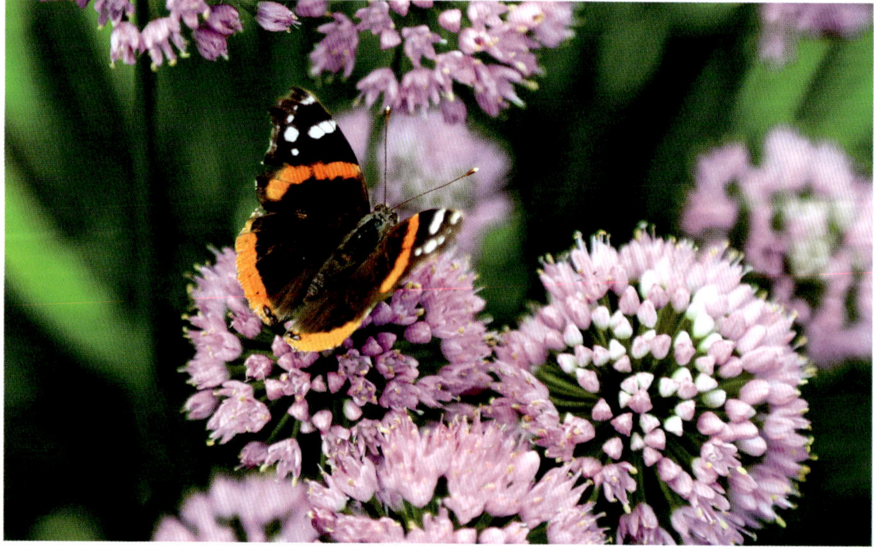

Alliums attract many pollinator species in my garden.

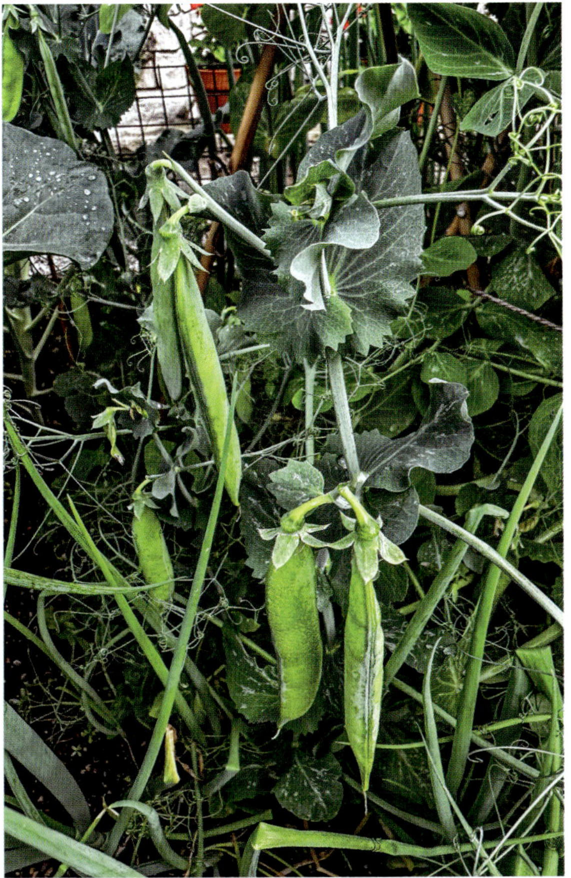

English peas, one of my favorites, growing in my kitchen garden.

beyond the narrow space it was allotted. I replaced it with 'Double Play® Blue Kazoo®' spirea, a tough, beautiful shrub with three-season interest; it also endures the missed shots from the budding soccer stars next door.

I stop and smell the roses, literally—the pink rugosa roses lining the midsection of the driveway. The fragrance hits you first, *oh so heavenly,* and then you hear them, every flower vibrating with bumblebees and emerald-green sweat bees competing for the prize inside. Farther up, the raspberry bushes are waiting until fall to do their thing.

Our backyard is not very deep. It's mostly a rain swale designed to absorb and moderate runoff. It's shady and planted with natives: Pennsylvania sedge, interrupted ferns, red-twig dogwood, and a cold-hardy redbud tree. Virginia waterleaf showed up and I let it stay. In one of the few sunny spots a serviceberry puts out a prolific harvest of purple-black fruits. I fill a smaller colander to the brim. Picking my way to the back corner of our lot, I arrive at a sunny spot where I have a secret patch of rhubarb. I pull a few ruby-red stalks to combine with the berries and head back to the patio.

Time to shell the peas I gathered. A time-consuming but meditative task, I remember how my mother loved to sit and shell black-eyed peas. Zipping open the pods and hearing the peas pop and ping into the metal bowl brings up good memories. English peas are rarely found in the grocery store. I can't wait to have them with the baby potatoes I got at the farmers market.

I collect all the colanders full of garden bounty. I find my tea where I left it on the stone wall. It's cold, but I have plans for something different: pesto and pie. It's a good day, and it's not even noon.

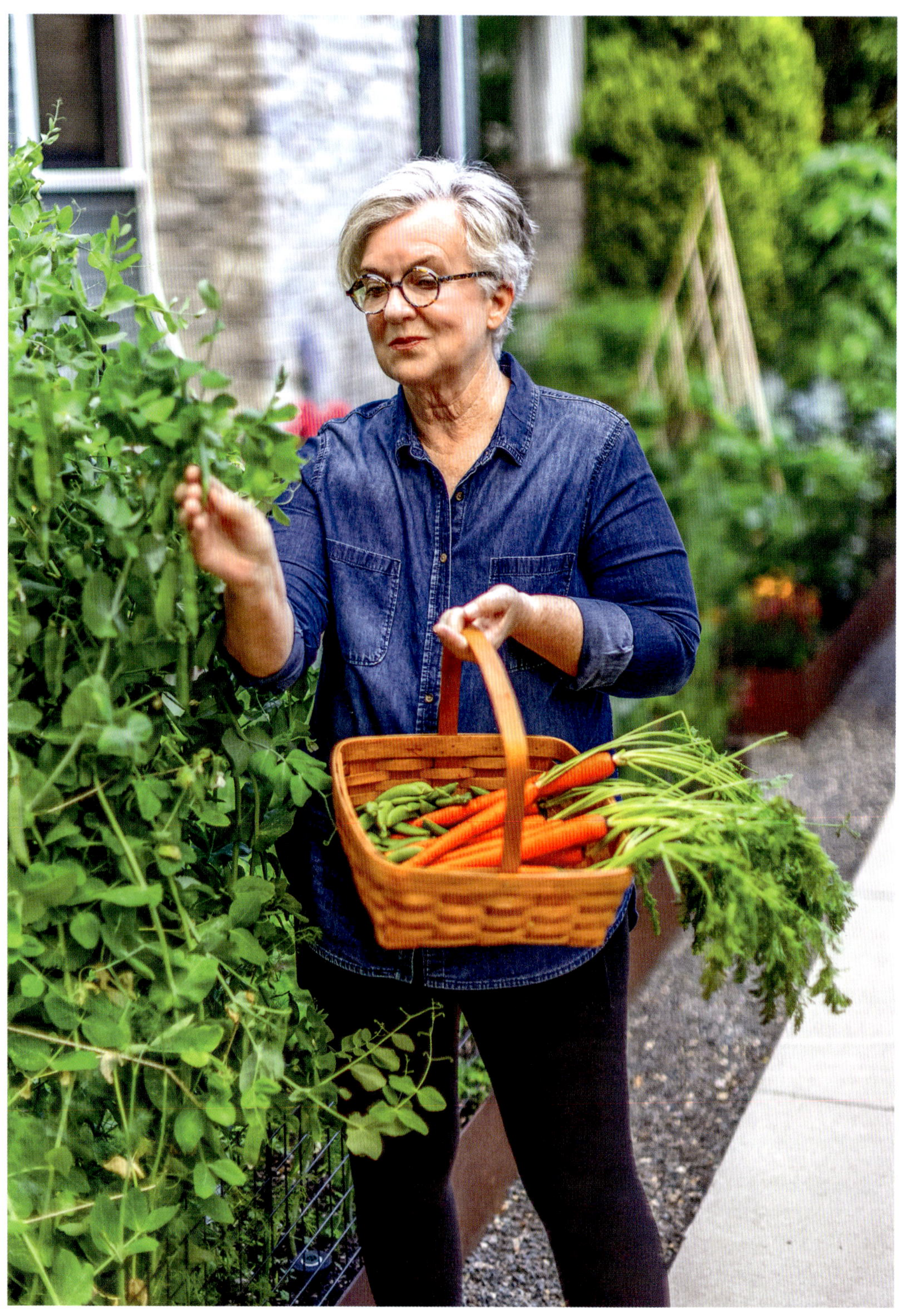

The author in her kitchen garden. *Photo courtesy of Tracy Walsh*

INTRODUCTION

Like so many of my generation, I became a gardener as a child, tagging along after my grandmother while she worked in her yard. I remember her in pink pedal-pushers and a straw hat, bent over her roses with pruners in hand. Her small patch of post-war paradise in a Southern California subdivision was worlds apart from the Mississippi farm fields where she hoed weeds and picked crops as a young girl. It was also different from the other yards in her neighborhood—filled with trees, shrubs, flowers, and fruit, she was foodscaping long before the word was invented. She plotted microclimates before that term arrived, too, planting horsetails by the leaky garden faucet and festuca grasses where the hose couldn't reach. It was all powered by lots of steer manure, her fertilizer of choice.

I remember every plant in that yard. I foraged for black raspberries and guavas. I drank fresh juice from the orange tree until my lips stung There was a large lantana bush covered in skipper butterflies that fluttered and regrouped over and over while I tried to catch them.

I'm at the age now that she was when we took a trip to the nursery, not knowing it would be the last one we would make together. The gravel crunched beneath our feet and the freeway whirred in the distance. She picked out 'John F. Kennedy,' a new hybrid tea rose with pure white petals and a spicy fragrance reminiscent of anise or licorice. Back home, she showed me how to plant it, splitting the can—no plastic pots in those days—digging the hole, throwing a small silvery fish in the hole for fertilizer, placing the rose just so, watering it in, and gently tamping the soil around it. At nine years old, I took it all to heart.

My grandmother's garden stays with me to this day. I'm so lucky to have experienced her version of gardening. For some, gardening is a set of rules and a series of chores; my grandmother passed down to me the wonder and joy of growing and tending plants. She also taught me to follow my instincts, and I inherited from her a kind of horticultural fearlessness.

In college, I grew my first garden at the back door of a rental house, filling it with strawberries, lettuces, beans, and flowers, much to the consternation of the landlord who lived next door. He finally relented and let me tear up a section of lawn to expand my efforts. Looking back, I realize his change of heart might have had something to do with the red bikini I wore to work on my tan while gardening.

After leaving California I married an engineer, a troubleshooter needed at a moment's notice, someone "subject to transfer," and we embarked on a life together as corporate nomads. As a "trailing spouse" (that was the official term, but it sounds like a Pothos plant, huh?), I attempted to make sense of what I called borrowed gardens, sometimes for barely a season. In Tennessee, I planted an apple tree but never saw it bloom. One winter in Illinois, I puttered with houseplants in the glass conservatory of our 1874 Victorian. And I planted daffodil bulbs in Iowa, but we had to move before they emerged.

Overseas in England for a few years, I mostly gawked at all the stunning gardens and stored up inspiration. There were other moves in between. Back in the States, my British-inspired kitchen garden in Kansas was met with mixed reviews—growing food in the front yard was a little too progressive for some of the neighbors, while others shouted encouragement as they passed by.

Kansas offered a baptism by fire, of sorts: searing heat, wild winds, and the occasional tornado tested my gardening skills. Seeking advice for managing this challenging environment led to me becoming an Extension Master Gardener. I knew at once I had found my tribe in this congenial group of volunteers. The education component was invaluable, and sharing it with people was so gratifying. When we relocated to Minnesota, I joined up again and was recertified, so I would know the gardening ropes in the often frozen, snowy zone 4. What a terrific way to find fellow gardeners, and your footing, when you're new in town.

Adapting to all those gardens—gardens of all climates, shapes, sizes, and designs—was frustrating, but, funny enough, it allowed me to "try them on." So, when we finally built our forever home and garden (although never say never) in a charming neighborhood by one of Minneapolis' urban lakes, I had a much better idea of what I wished for in a garden. More important, I had an idea of what I could handle, as I was starting to feel more aches and pains after a bout of digging or weeding.

Over the years of my coming up as a gardener, a new buzzword turned up and developed: sustainability. This term came with lots of definitions, according to what world it applied to, as well as actions, behaviors, and marketing. But in the gardening world it is summed up best as using gardening practices that enhance rather than harm the environment, working along with nature instead of against it. Additionally, a sustainable garden must consider the health and abilities of the gardener.

A Balancing Act

Sustainable gardening is a balancing act. My advice for maintaining a healthy garden is to do less, do your homework, and, in some cases, do nothing. Ironically, there are many times when I'm too busy writing about gardening to garden; yet, somehow the garden survives. And often it's better for being left alone.

I'm a big believer in the good bug-bad bug school of gardening. You need a delicate balance of bad bugs to feed the good bugs. After all, every bug is living its life and doing its best to get along in the world. Sustainable gardening is all about working in tandem with nature, and I'm all for letting Mother Nature do the heavy lifting. This applies to more than just bugs. I try to create an environment that allows me to team up with birds, frogs, and other wildlife to make the garden hospitable to them and enjoyable for me.

Often when a gardener finds pest damage, the default reaction is panic or guilt. But I advise you to slow down and consider this: Those circular bites in your rose or redbud leaves are from leafcutter bees using the soft foliage to line their nests. The denuded dill is what's left of the black swallowtail caterpillar's dinner. Congratulations, you've got habitat!

I had been thinking in those very terms as I toiled in and tended those borrowed gardens. Through the years, I learned what I wanted and didn't want in my home landscape. Among the many things I discovered: Mowing an acre of lawn on a riding tractor is fun the first few times, but the high decibels and smelly fumes were not good for me or the planet; a water feature brings life and wildlife to the garden; weeding on a steep, rocky slope is tempting fate; raised beds are a blessing; feed your soil and the rest will follow.

I had thought long and hard about my forever garden by the time I met with a landscape architect who I first saw on social media. I had designed bits and pieces while adapting to those borrowed gardens of the past, but this was different: a blank slate! This was an opportunity to design and install an entire landscape, and I didn't want to take any chances. He and I collaborated to create a garden that satisfied my wish list while being manageable for my gardening future.

I love to share my garden, so I knew I wanted a front-facing garden where casual conversations with passersby might evolve into meaningful connections. I wanted a pollinator-friendly landscape (my first book, *Pollinator Friendly Gardening*, was already taking shape in my mind.) I shifted the future house on the lot to make room for a kitchen garden on the sunny south side. The landscape architect suggested Corten steel for raised beds; these save me lots of bending and kneeling and also allow me to control soil,

A Word on Pest Controls

When confronted with pest damage, before you do anything to intervene, take a moment and determine the damage threshold. Is the damage potentially fatal to an irreplaceable plant or tree? Is it harmful to a food crop for one season, or is it merely cosmetic?

Identify the actual pest causing the damage. Don't accuse an innocent bystander, such as a spider hanging around looking for a meal. With so many examples online, it's easy to find the real culprit by searching the plant name and a description of the damage.

Once you identify the pest, learn about its life cycle. Is this a one-time hit, or do they reproduce in multiple generations throughout the growing season? What predators feed upon them?

In some cases, the fix is easy: Good bugs come to the rescue. For instance, you can interrupt the damaging work of aphids by spraying them with a strong blast of water from the garden hose. But stand by and monitor the situation for a few days; you might see the cavalry arrive in the form of antlions or ladybug larvae munching their way through the infestation of aphids.

If the problem is more serious and warrants further action, consider organically acceptable pest controls. However, even these are not without some risk; always follow the instructions carefully to ensure other wildlife are not harmed. The Organic Materials Review Institute (OMRI) is a good source for more information about organic pest controls and organic fertilizer products (see Resources).

Note: Pesticides and synthetic fertilizers are harmful to our soils and the biodiversity of our gardens and are not suitable for sustainable gardening practices. A physical barrier might provide an immediate solution in some cases—for example, placing mesh bags around ripening apples to prevent damage from apple maggots and coddling moths. Fencing might be the only deterrent for larger critters.

For long-term solutions, cultural controls will pay off. For vegetable gardens, use crop-rotation and pest-resistant varieties, plant trap crops, change planting dates, and practice good sanitation to avoid reinfestation.

Following the Master Gardener's mantra, planting the right plant in the right place and providing for adequate water, correct sun exposure, healthy soil, and good airflow will help to avoid lots of pest and disease issues. Build healthy soil by amending and feeding it with organic materials such as manure, compost, fish emulsion, blood or bone meal, liquid seaweed, and organic granular fertilizer.

amendments, water, and weeds without inputs like synthetic fertilizers or pesticides. Finally, a small pond built into the patio to bring sound, reflections, birds, and other wildlife.

As my Minneapolis garden came together, so did my career writing about gardening. One of the best parts was meeting and interviewing so many dedicated and talented gardeners and seeing their beautiful, unique creations. I noticed we all had one thing in common: We were, as the expression goes, "of a certain age." But these weren't gray-haired ladies (and men) just planting petunias. These gracefully aging gardeners were lifelong learners, curious and open to trying new things. And gardening seems to be the constant that keeps them young.

My gardening circle is full of these folks—one specializes in native ferns, one grows dye plants that become the ink in her artwork, one teaches people to use small hydroponic gardens for homegrown greens in winter. Others are working with school gardens and underserved communities. These gardeners have challenges, too: heart and mobility issues, family obligations, and more. Such is the life of all aging individuals, yet the old saying holds true: You don't give up gardening when you grow old; you grow old when you give up gardening.

This book aims to inspire gardeners, despite age and circumstance, to keep on gardening in some form or fashion for as long as possible. It hopes to reinvigorate gardeners' views on the role of their garden and the importance of their part as steward, no matter the size of their plot. I believe there's a garden and its multitude of benefits for everyone—and not every garden has to fit the traditional model. I'll help readers expand their views on what it is to garden, so they can imagine for themselves gardening experiences that don't always depend upon homeownership or supple knees.

Starting with a discussion about change—for our gardens and ourselves—I outline the many health, mental, and even spiritual benefits of gardening as we age. Gardening is considered the best activity for longevity, according to Dan Buettner, who first identified the regions known for their long lifespans in his documentary *Live to 100: Secrets of the Blue Zones*. While Buettner's claims have gained traction in the media, there are numerous studies, from the US to Finland, South Korea, and Australia, which further support the idea that gardening is one of the very top activities for longevity. I'll encourage folks to keep on gardening to reap those physical and mental rewards.

According to the AARP, nearly 75 percent of adults over the age of 65 want to "age in place" in their current homes. And the same as you can make household changes and accommodations that allow for this, you can do the same for your garden. I'll help you evaluate your garden for potential problems and offer ideas for "gardening in place" at your current residence. If it's better to downsize (but not downgrade), this book has ideas for right-sizing a new garden that keeps you outside, engaged, and active without having to do dreaded tasks.

This book will show you how the right choices in hardscape and plantings will make it easier to maintain your yard. There's a wealth of products that can help, too: ergonomic tools, planters, and elevated beds, to name a few. In addition, growing techniques can make the difference between a fun project and a back-breaking chore. I'll also share strategies for making your garden more resilient in the face of climate change.

Along the way, you will meet inspiring older gardeners and their gardens—real-life, doable gardens, not show gardens. In fact, for my photos of these gardens, I've asked my subjects not to tidy up before I arrive. Or, I yelled, "Stop!" when my husband and I were out and about and jumped out of the car—I love finding great examples of age-minded smart gardening that I can photograph from the sidewalk.

The very definition of gardening is growing and changing. You don't always have to be down on your knees in the dirt to experience the joys of nature and cultivating plants, which is why I also offer ideas and suggestions for gardening with limitations, disabilities, and mild memory loss.

As a final note, it important to reflect on our role in the timeless act of gardening. As seasoned gardeners, we possess loads of collective wisdom. It's our responsibility to share that with younger gardeners and wannabe gardeners, just as my grandmother shared her passion and knowledge with me. You don't have to be a grandparent (although I live in hope) to be the one who, pardon the pun, plants the seed and grows a new gardener.

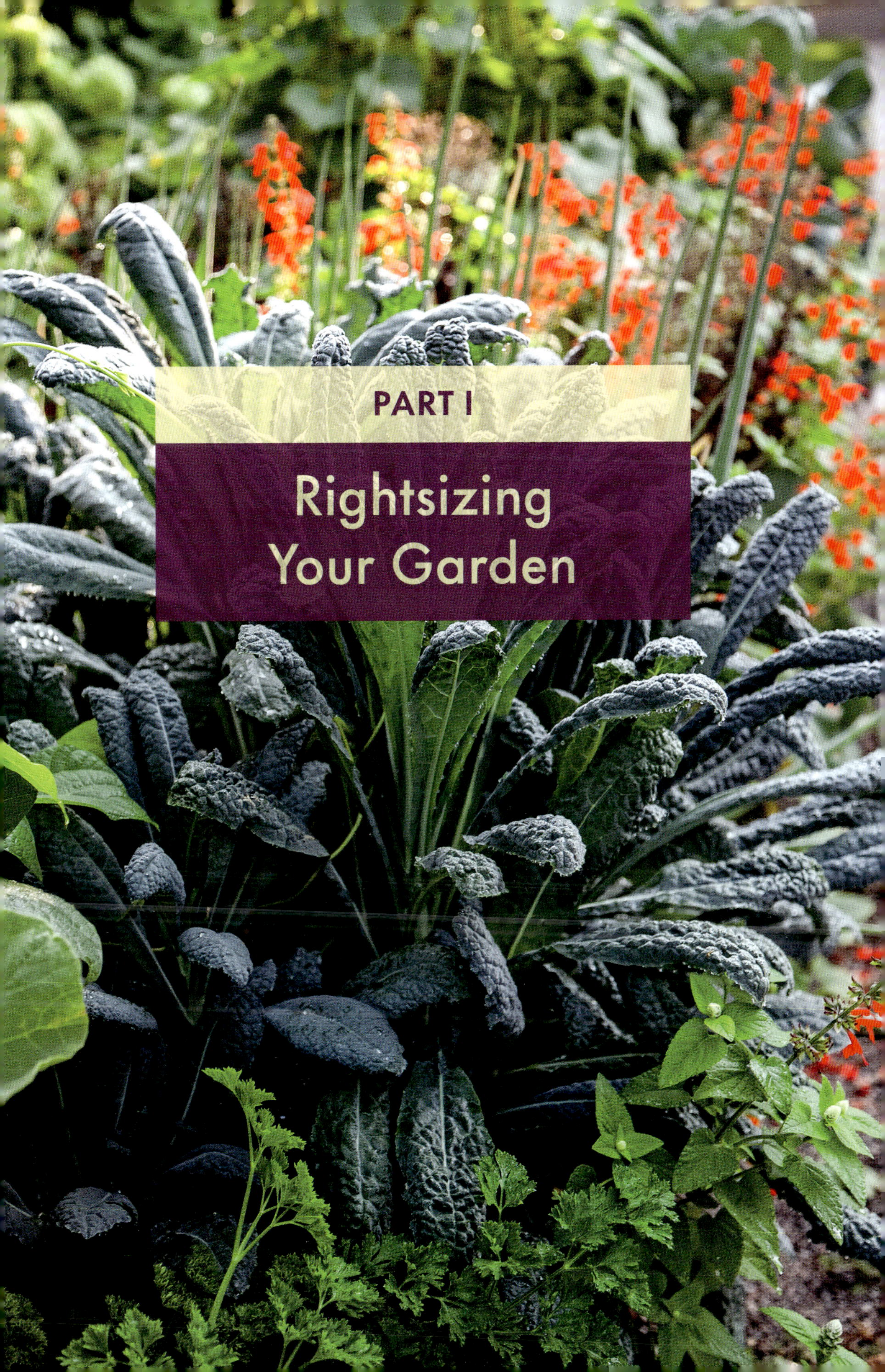

PART I

Rightsizing Your Garden

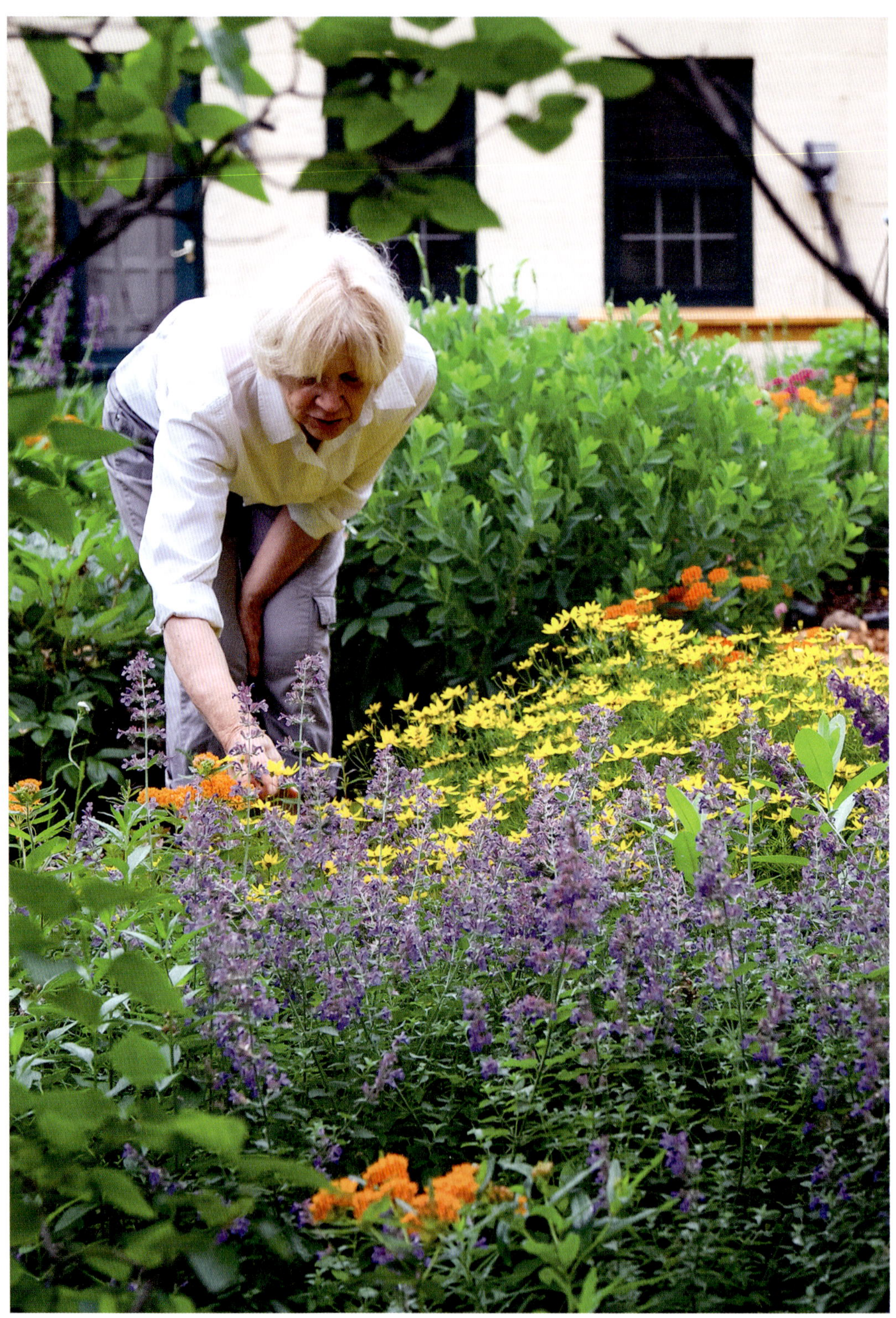

Donna Hamilton bending to check on her perennial garden.

CHAPTER 1

Changes and Positive Aging

It happens gradually—you might notice that a typical garden chore like trimming shrubs or planting bulbs takes longer or tires you out sooner. You're stiff and sore the next day, at least more than usual. When you kneel down to pull weeds you hear a pop-creak sound. There's no way around it: You are getting older. Yet, you might not think of yourself as old. As Oliver Wendell Holmes, Jr. supposedly said, "Old age is always fifteen years older than I am." It's a moving target.

We can't prevent, or slow, the years from passing, but we can influence how our bodies and minds change over time. And if there's one activity that ticks all the right boxes for positive aging, it is gardening. In this chapter, we'll look at the many health and wellness benefits of gardening, along with a bit of the science behind aging and why gardening helps.

Other things we can't prevent are natural events that test our gardens and the ongoing challenges presented by climate change. What we certainly can do is adapt—that's what gardeners do best. And we can do more than that: As stewards of our own little natural environments, we can play an important role in providing for pollinators, supporting beneficial plant species and ecosystems, and taking many more very doable steps to help move society toward a more sustainable future.

Why Gardening Is Good for You

Gardening is so good for us because it challenges and stimulates our bodies and minds. Routine gardening tasks incorporate a variety of natural movements, an ideal form of low-impact exercise. Applying our thoughts and creativity to planning and problem-solving in a garden has numerous mental and emotional benefits, and the hands-on activity of tending plants promotes both physical and mental dexterity. Gardens can be private sanctuaries that provide respite from worldly concerns, and they can encourage us to strengthen connections with neighbors and others in our communities.

NATURAL MOVEMENT

During our walk together at the beginning of this book, did you catch all my physical movements as I went through the garden? Bending, stretching, kneeling, lifting, and then the digging, pushing, and pulling I planned for the next day? They aren't very different from exercises at the gym—squats, push-ups, lunges, and the "farmer's carry" with kettlebells. But I didn't think to count reps or sets.

Exercise is one of the first defenses against the effects of aging. As we age, our muscles naturally lose mass and strength in a process called sarcopenia, and this accelerates after the age of sixty. Folks over fifty, especially postmenopausal women, suffer from osteoporosis, or loss of bone mass. Joint deterioration from osteoarthritis can start as early as our late forties and can increase with age.

Weight-bearing exercise, often referred to as resistance training—the kind that forces you to work against gravity—is the best exercise to combat the ill effects of these aging issues. We engage in many of these exercises while gardening, often without a second thought:

- Pulling weeds
- Pushing a mower
- Carrying plants and supplies
- Hauling hoses
- Digging holes
- Turning compost

Because gardening engages all the major muscle groups—arms, legs, shoulders, back, and abdomen—it also improves mobility and builds endurance. Moving from task to task improves mobility and balance, engaging the proprioceptive nerve endings that give us a sense of where our body is positioned. According to a study published in the National Library of Medicine, significantly fewer gardeners than nongardeners reported a fall in the past two years.[1]

Natural movement is mobility, and mobility improves flexibility. There is evidence that maintaining flexibility is a key part of longevity. Turns out that stretching your body, like gardeners do, stretches the years, too.

DEXTERITY

As you followed me through the garden, I used my hands to harvest pea pods, pinch out basil plants, pick blighted leaves off tomato vines, pluck berries, pull rhubarb stalks, yank out weeds, and shell peas. While gardening, your hands are moving without a thought. You are much more aware of the larger

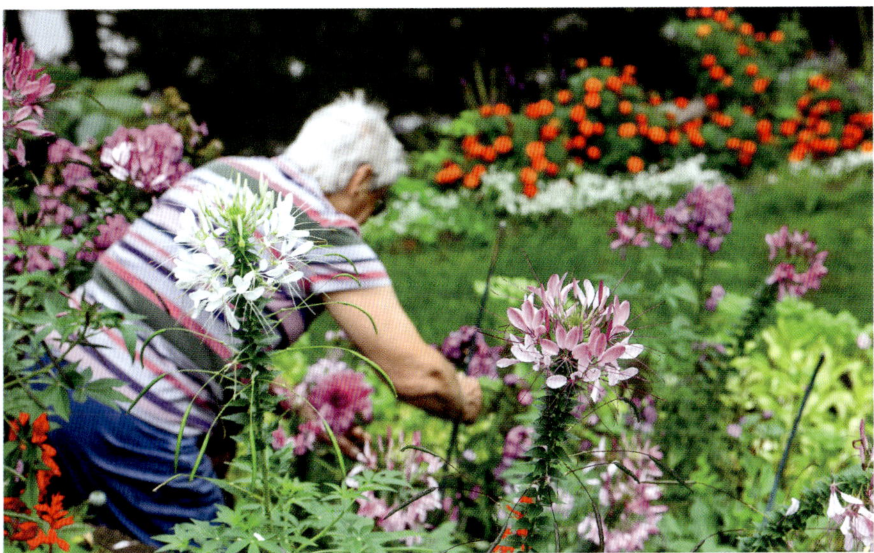

Janet Robidoux staking a cleome, one of her 400 annuals; around the time of this picture, she and her twin sister, Janice, downsized to that number from 1,000.

muscles you are using for things like digging and lifting (and sometimes they scream at you). But when you sow seeds, deadhead flowers, or snip herbs, you might not realize you're giving your hands a workout. Those precise movements increase dexterity and hand strength, which diminish with age.

It turns out that working with your hands is good for your brain, too. A large portion of your brain is dedicated to the voluntary movement of your hands. Whether it's through knitting, woodworking, painting, or sowing seeds, using fine motor skills stimulates the brain more than pushing buttons or swiping screens. Handwriting lights up the brain in ways that typing doesn't. Hands-on activities like these are associated with cognitive benefits, including improved memory and attention span.

Some researchers credit the rhythm and repetition of these activities for calming anxiety and reducing symptoms of depression, rather than the actual hand-mind connection. It might come down to this: When your hands are busy, your brain rests. Who hasn't zoned out while pulling weeds or perhaps channeled some anger into them, too?

Kelly Lambert, a professor of behavioral neuroscience at the University of Richmond who studies effort-based rewards, has another theory. She sees "the connection between the effort we put into something and the reward we get from it" and believes that working with our hands gives a sense of accomplishment. In other words, when we create a drawing or a sweater by hand it's a uniquely gratifying experience, a sort of handmade happiness. The same can be said for a garden.

EMOTIONAL REWARDS

When I'm having a bad day or the news is overwhelming, I step out to the garden. I imagine you do, too. We don't need an expert to tell us the garden will sooth our woes, if only for a moment. Yet it's intriguing to know how that occurs.

When the dentist tells you to go to your happy place, science says there's a 90 percent chance you'll imagine a scene from nature—the beach, the forest, or, for many of us, the garden. *Biophilia* literally translates to "love of life" and can be described as the desire to commune with nature and living things. Humans have a tendency to be drawn to their natural surroundings, where they find a sense of well-being and emotional connection. Witnessing nature's life force in green spaces is to feel like a part of something bigger than ourselves.

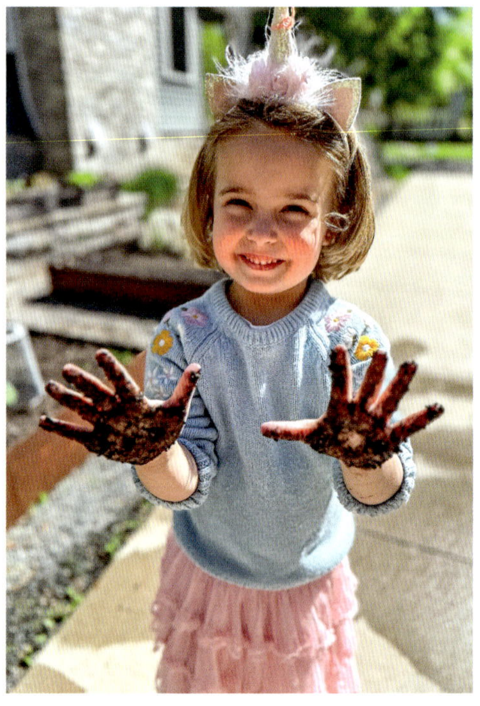

My little neighbor Nora's muddy fingers and smile prove how good soil can make you feel.

When I first saw the claim that soil was a natural antidepressant, I was skeptical. After some digging (ha!) I found the dirt. Exposure to soil microbes, specifically *Mycobacterium vaccae*, activates your brain cells to produce serotonin, the feel-good hormone. This chemical found in the soil can reduce stress and improve mood. You don't even have to dig in the dirt to reap the benefits. Simply sitting in or walking through a garden lowers cortisol, the primary stress hormone, and produces a sense of calm and well-being. I'm convinced of this every time I do my morning garden stroll.

Like everyone, I can get dragged down by the weighty burden of world events. However, I'm always an optimist in the garden. It doesn't take much to sway my mood: a perfect ruffly head of lettuce, a thriving new plant, or whenever that frog plops off the lily pad in my garden pond. Feeling optimistic in a garden seems natural, since gardening is a forward-looking pursuit. This is embodied in the gardener's mantra of "next year." Around the time I'm eating my first garden-grown salad or watching bees buzz around a new flower, I'm already thinking about what I'll do in the garden next year, whether it's repeating my results with a particular plant variety or improving upon a growing method. I'm motivated to keep growing in more ways than one.

The Japanese concept of *ikigai* refers to having a reason for living, a sense of purpose, something to get up for every day, and it is believed that this sense of purpose and value is the key to a long and happy life. Chances are you find your ikigai in the garden.

BRAIN HEALTH

When you walked through the garden with me on that glorious June morning you saw the culmination of hours and hours of planning and problem-solving. Every winter, you can be sure I'm combing through seed catalogs, looking back at photos of my past designs, recalling memorable harvests and dinners, dreaming and debating with myself, and sketching and scheming to create the next vision for my kitchen garden. This special garden is not only bountiful, it's also beautiful. We have a compressed season in Minnesota, and I have only a few chances to get it right. The rest of my landscape is more forgiving; however, I'm thinking about that, too, pondering ways to make it more sustainable and easier to maintain.

Building and tending a garden involves a series of decisions: how to help your plants thrive; sun or shade; acidic or alkaline; loam or clay; wet, dry, or somewhere in between? You consider color, shape, size, and texture when it comes to flowers and foliage. You look for advantages in microclimates. You design and think in 3D to make your landscape come to life in a way that's visually appealing, as well as sustainable. You strive for "the right plant in the right place."

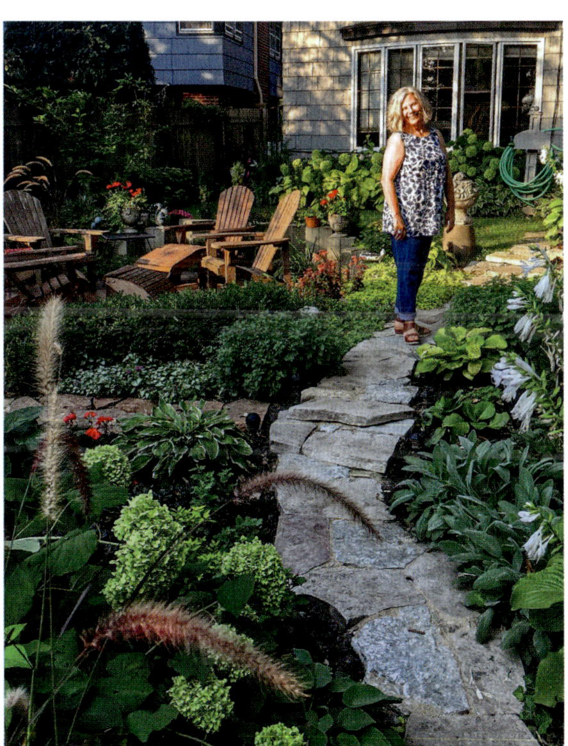
Christine Scotillo choreographs her garden.

A friend of mine, Christine Scotillo, is an incredibly talented gardener who draws on her background in dance to "choreograph" her plants to achieve stunning results—a brilliant stretch of the imagination. Brain exercises like this help to improve and preserve cognitive function.

My garden is many things for me: a sanctuary, a playground, a grocery store, a chapel. It's also a laboratory. I'm always observing, researching, and experimenting, trying out new things, watching and wondering. Isn't it funny how the garden relaxes us and stimulates us at the same time?

BETTER NUTRITION

Remember the fresh produce I harvested on that quick jaunt through my kitchen garden? There's a lot more where that came from. Depending upon the month, I'm picking leafy greens and lettuces, tomatoes and peppers, assorted root vegetables, summer favorites like corn and melons, and all manner of herbs, not to mention the fruit growing at the edges of my property.

It's no secret that homegrown produce tastes better than store-bought. A lot of that has to do with the short distance it travels from the veggie plot outside your door to the kitchen table. Food that travels long distances not only loses texture and flavor but also nutrients. It can't get any more local than your own garden.

As people age, the number and size of their taste buds decline, affecting their sense of taste. It makes sense to eat better- and brighter-tasting fruits and vegetables grown in your backyard, and to spice them up with an abundance of herbs (which would cost a fortune at the store.) In addition, the visual appeal of a colorful plate helps to stimulate appetite. Vegetables of all colors contain phytonutrients, compounds that give them their color, taste, and smell. These potent compounds help fight cancer and heart disease.

So many folks dread the question, "What's for dinner?" I turn the tables and pose the same question to my garden. It rarely fails to come up with a delicious solution. I love it when I can put together a meal without a trip to the grocery store. I admit feeling a bit smug when I walk out there with my clippers and basket, even if it's just to snip a few chives for baked potatoes. Fresh food right at your back door makes it simpler to skip fast food and highly processed meals. It makes "Meatless Monday" so much easier for those who celebrate it.

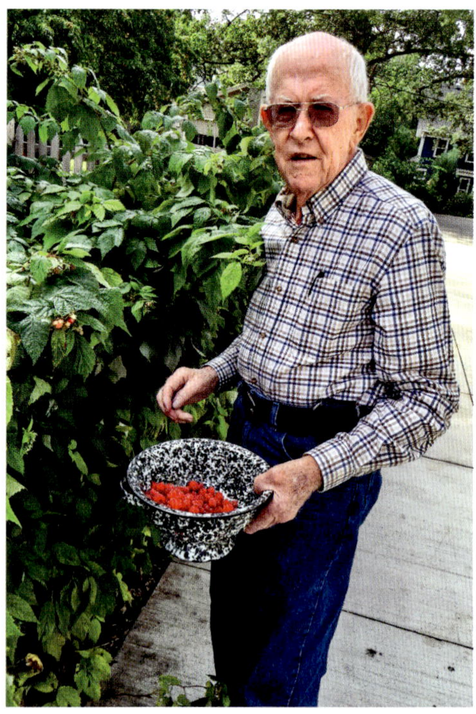

My father-in-law, Joe, picking raspberries with me.

Experts observing countries with a high number of centenarians report that gardening and the resulting "plant slant" of their diet is a major reason for their long life spans. Dan Buettner, the face of the Blue Zone phenomenon, posts on social media that gardening is a "nudge" and explains that "you plant the seed, and then you water it, weed it, and eventually eat this organic vegetable that you must like because you planted it."

Gardeners are more likely to try new foods and have a more diverse diet. Every year, I challenge myself to grow something new or new to me. Recently it was lima beans (butterbeans to those of you down South), and, lo and behold, I liked them. Fresh from the garden they were so much better than the mealy ones I'd been served elsewhere. I even made hummus from them.

SOCIAL CONNECTIONS

It is said that humans are social animals. People associate belongingness and acceptance with a sense of security. Laughing with a group of acquaintances or confiding in a close friend gives your brain a hit of dopamine and encourages you to keep seeking out social opportunities. Social connection is essential to successful aging. Friendships can lower blood pressure, reduce inflammation, and improve cardiovascular health.

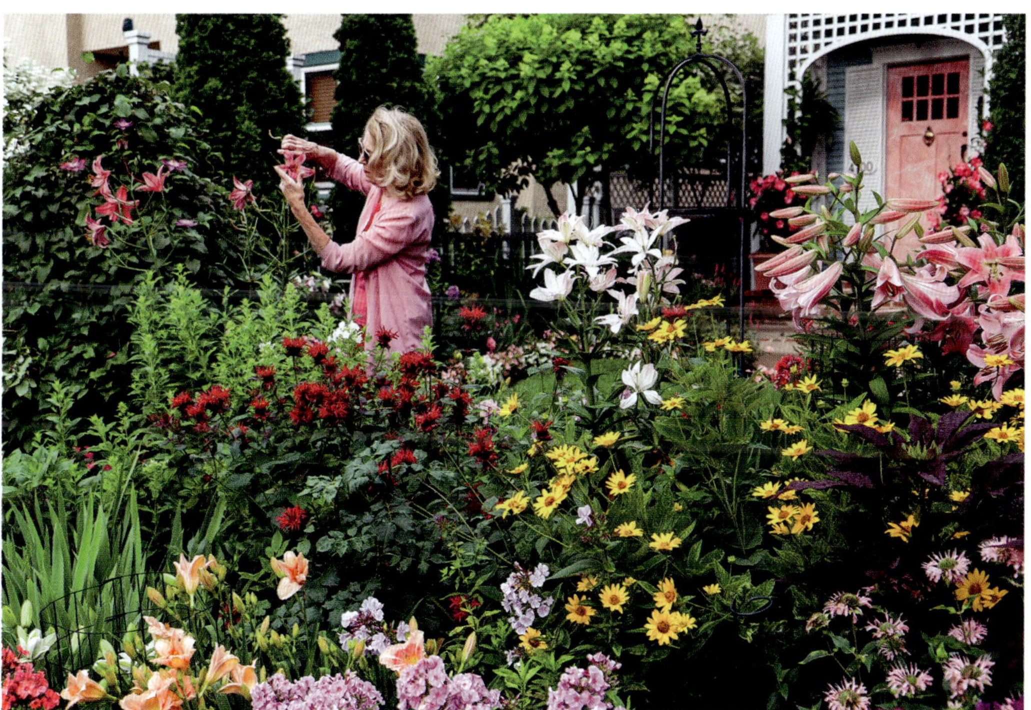

At 82, Sandra Mangel, whose motto is "Just keep going," started a garden design business. Passersby *ooh* and *ah* over her gorgeous garden.

There are a number of friendship levels: acquaintances, casual friends, work friends, close friends, and lifelong friends. And don't forget social media friends. We need all kinds. Some of those friendships depend upon shared activities, others certain locations. Close friends are the ones you choose, and lifelong friends might not be in your life every day, but you can pick up where you left off with the greatest of ease. Gardening friends can overlap all of those categories and might shift with time. Friends on social media sometimes become friends IRL ("in real life").

I find my tribe in fellow gardeners. Like many writers, I'm an introvert. I'm completely happy in my own world. I have to push myself to socialize. I can feel awkward in a group of people. I might panic at parties, but I can speak about gardening to a room of 200 people without a problem. I credit gardening as that bridge that connects me with other people. It's my safe space.

In spite of being an introvert, I really like sharing my garden with other people. I'm fortunate to live in a very walkable community. I love the unexpected, organic conversations that happen with people of all ages who pass by my garden while I'm out there weeding or planting, even if it's only to commiserate about the rabbits. The neighborhood kids raise monarchs and know they are welcome to pick milkweed foliage for their hungry, hungry caterpillars. When passersby are amazed by the masses of monarch butterflies on the meadow blazing star (*Liatris ligulistylis*) I become a sidewalk educator, evangelizing and extolling on pollinators. I treasure all of these interactions.

Gardeners often work alone in their gardens, but that shared interest gathers people together in countless ways. Seeking some garden friends? Look to plant societies, garden clubs, service days, plant swaps, garden tours, and, my favorite, Extension Master Gardeners.

FAITH AND RITUAL

Regardless of their spiritual bent, many gardeners go beyond growing pretty flowers to seek deeper meaning in their gardens. Any type of gardening takes faith: that complete trust, the expectation that a tiny seed will germinate and flourish, that an acorn will someday provide shade, that food plants will nourish a family. And then there is the other type of faith, faith in a higher power that gives one the strength to withstand personal or global turmoil. Gardeners of faith can find meaning and metaphor in the natural processes and beauty of nature.

Another form of spiritual practice is ritual. It's even found inside the word *spiritual*. Ritual is different from routine in that it is done with intentionality and is often imbued with symbolic meaning and sometimes ceremony. An example can be found in the way I prepare my kitchen garden beds each spring. I routinely add manure, compost, and organic granular fertilizer. In

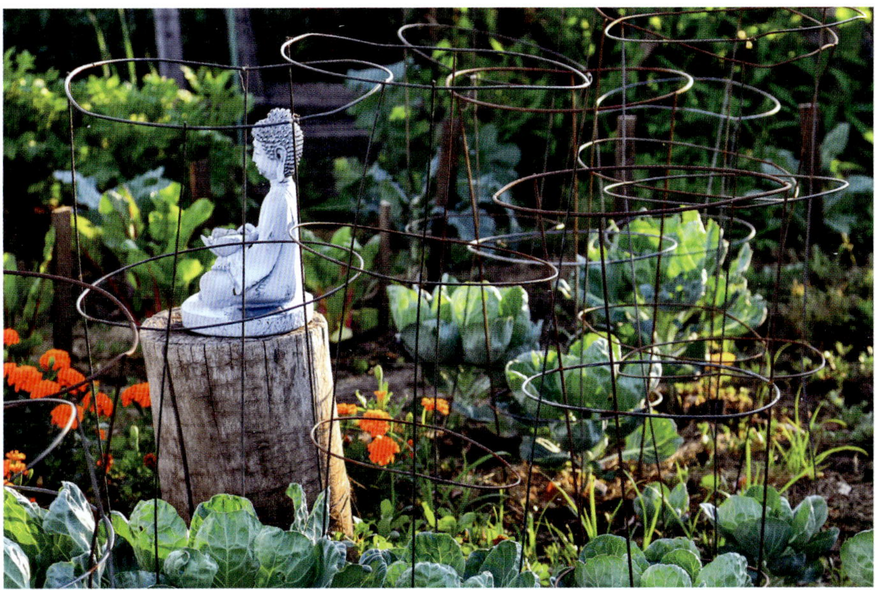

A goddess statue in Community Peace Gardens in Minneapolis.

this way, a yearly routine is tied to best practice, to productivity. After I've dug it in and turned the soil just enough, the silent thanks I add is a small ritual.

Rituals can mark religious events, family milestones, or annual gatherings. They can celebrate seasonal events in nature, like the equinox or phases of the moon. In the garden they can be enhanced with art, song, or aromatherapy, with offerings like mandalas made from garden materials, herb bundles, altars, chants, and singing. The grounding effect of ritual can be a reassuring practice that gives people predictability and consistency in times of uncertainty, which in turn lessens stress.

IMPROVES SLEEP

Daytime hours spent in your garden will help you sleep better at night. Obviously, fresh air and exercise give you that "good tired" sensation. In addition, all of that time outside increases vitamin D exposure, which helps regulate your wake-sleep cycle. Time outside in natural sunlight also helps to reset your circadian rhythms by influencing the production of hormones, such as melatonin and cortisol, which regulate sleep and wakefulness. The end result: a well-rested gardener ready for another day in paradise.

Aging as a process is biological, but also social and psychological. It can deeply affect our hopes and dreams for the future, adding further insult to the physical changes we undergo. The best way to fight ageism is to be aware of it. Once you see it, you'll be able to resist its gloomy prognostications. I caution you to be on the lookout for any negative stereotypes that

A Different View on Aging

Old doesn't look like it used to. The boomer generation, those born between 1946 and 1964, has seen to that. You are most likely the ones reading this book. While our generation has not gone quietly into old age, it is the one most singled-out for the barrage of anti-aging messages that plagues the marketplace and the media. It is hard not to think badly of your advancing years in the face of this bias.

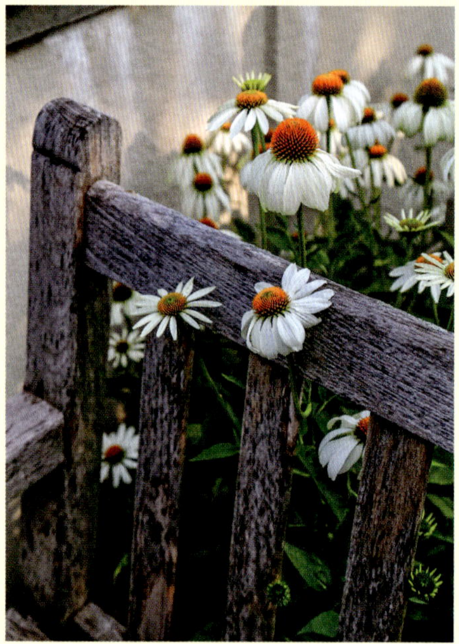

A weathered bench reminds us of terms used to describe aging.

I spent a lot of time pondering how to describe people "of a certain age" in this book. There are many options with positive connotations: older (it is what it is), mature, senior, wise, seasoned, venerable, gray. And, of course, there are plenty of less-than-complimentary descriptors: decrepit, elderly, over-the-hill, ancient, geriatric, grizzled (although I kind of like that one). I ended up using the more positive ones interchangeably, but I think "older" is the most straightforward. I like the idea of saying "growing older" because it implies growth is still possible. I also like the term "gracefully aging gardener" because I feel it imparts a sense of dignity and optimism (and I love alliteration). These and other expressions support the growing movement toward the idea of positive aging.

dampen your enthusiasm for gardening, your gardening future, and life in general. In the end, there's much to the saying "It's not how old you are. It's how you are old."

Our Lives Change

Big changes happen starting in your sixties. These developments might have you rethinking your gardening goals as your circumstances and priorities undergo a sea change. It's not only aches and pains. Transformational shifts, such as an empty nest, career changes, aging parents, marriage and divorce, illness, death of a spouse, retirement, and grandchildren, can all affect your gardening future.

Your garden might take a backseat to any of these factors. Whether it is permanent or not depends on your situation. Yet for many, gardening can be the life preserver that keeps them afloat through these changes. If you're reading or just perusing this book, you haven't given up on gardening completely; your next step could be seeing how it looks in the future.

RETIREMENT RESET

For many, retirement is a time of personal growth, an opportunity to pursue hobbies, travel, spend more time with family, and seek out new experiences. For some, retirement means a loss of identity and purpose, periods of boredom, loneliness, and depression. Financial factors play a huge part. People miss their old routine and work friends or feel aimless without the structure of schedules, meetings, and appointments. Whatever your situation, it can take time to find your rhythm.

My husband, a man with a busy mind and boundless energy, was adamant that he didn't want to wake up and wonder what to do on his first day of retirement, so he made a plan. For decades I had driven him to the airport with his bag and briefcase as he traveled the world for work. But when I drove him to the airport on that first day of his retirement, he had only a small backpack. For the next month he walked 500 miles (805 km) across Spain on the Camino de Santiago pilgrimage trail. He returned with blistered feet but felt a "reset" coming back to his family and hobbies with a new vigor. Not everyone can pick up and do that, but diving into a new activity, such as a gardening project, might be just the ticket.

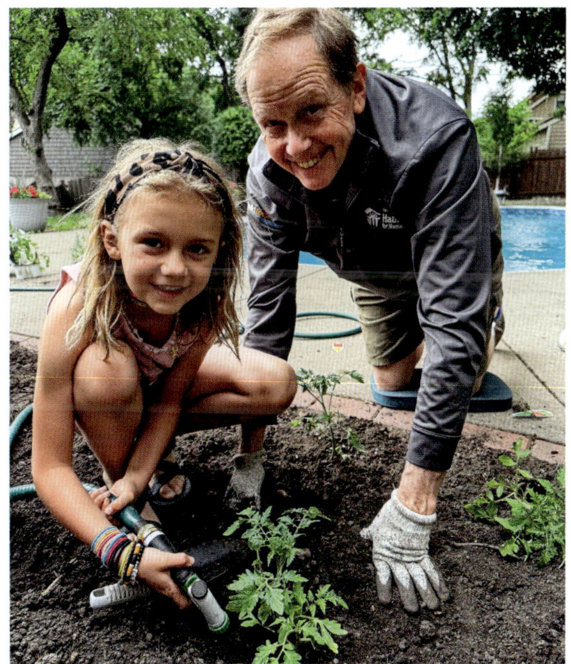

Dean Erickson gardening with his granddaughter Ida. *Photo courtesy of Donna Erickson*

GARDENING WITH GRANDCHILDREN

Grandchildren are a game changer. They are a busy group, with days full of play dates, soccer games, music recitals, swimming lessons, you name it. Modern grandparents aren't sitting around either; they are just as likely to take the grandkids on a Disney cruise or a ski trip. One of the gardeners you'll meet in this book hosts an annual "cousin camp" for her grandchildren, complete with outdoor tents and activities. According to the AARP, 80 percent of grandparents feel it is important to live near their children and grandchildren. Nowadays it's not unusual for grandparents to move for that reason.

But relocating to another city later in life requires courage and flexibility. And moving to a smaller home, condo, or apartment amid plans to spend quality time with grandkids can impact your time and energy, not to mention your space allotted for gardening. However, gardening can also play a role in making that time with family enjoyable. According to experts, it is important to find your own social life and activities apart from the grandchildren, to maintain your independence and family harmony. And don't underestimate the power of sharing the garden with the grandkids. So many of us found our passion for plants right there at our grandparents' sides.

Others might find themselves ready to transition into independent living at some type of senior residence. Many of these facilities have gardening opportunities and gardening programs designed to fit the needs of older adults. In fact, continued contact with nature should be at the top of your criteria when choosing to make such a significant move.

Gardens Change

Gardens are constantly changed by seasonal fluctuations, plant maturity, garden trends, gardeners' choices, and, in recent years, climate change. Trees are probably the most visible symbols of change; they grow up, they come down. Our neighbors love to tell the story of the tiny maple sapling they received as a promotional gift from their bank. A mere sprig in a can at the time. The story is even sweeter when told while we sit in the shade of that towering tree during impromptu happy hours.

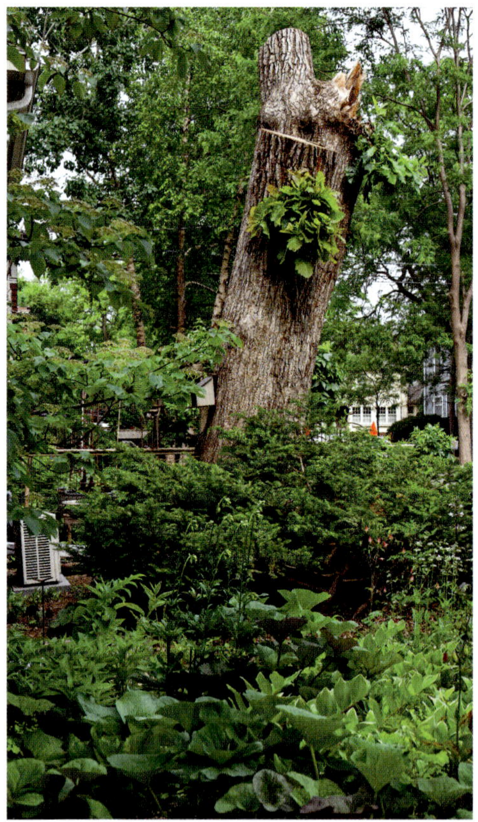

All that's left of a beautiful bur oak after a storm—a big change.

Down the street, my neighbor Broadus Miller's garden has gone through big changes. He lost several boulevard trees from storms and disease, leaving his beautiful shade gardens exposed to the southwestern sun and causing him to reconsider his plant selection. I pass by this garden all the time on dog walks, and I marvel to think he began 34 years ago with no gardening experience. The yard had only three or four plants. Starting from scratch, as he tells it, "I made mistakes along the way, lots of them, and just learned, loved it, and kept learning."

Replacing those lost trees, Broadus decided to go smaller—our block already has lots of huge trees. Now in the spring, I look forward to seeing his new pear tree and new serviceberry tree full of white flowers. At 78 he now hires help for some tasks. As for growing older, he says, "I will do as much as I can as long as my body allows it. I'll stay here as long as I can and keep the garden."

Older gardens can also suffer from tree root intrusion, soil compaction, overgrown shrubbery, poor soil quality, unwanted weeds, invasive species, and more. Hardscape could be outdated or failing. Chapter 2 discusses how to evaluate problems like these that are common in aging gardens.

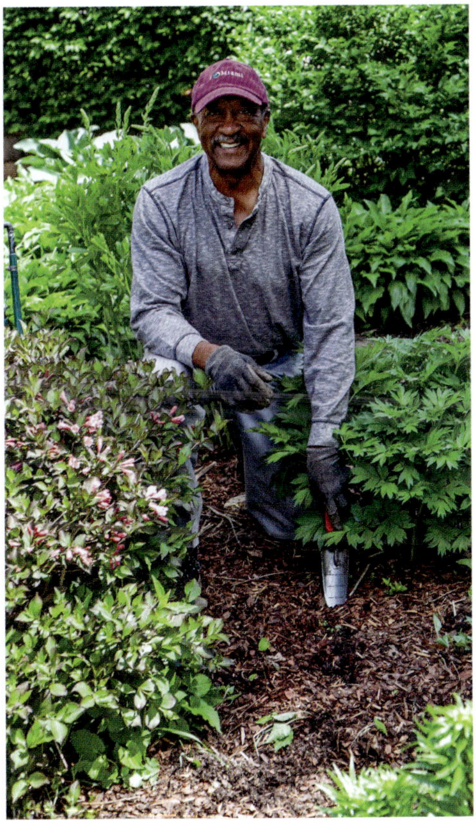

Broadus Miller grows more sun-loving plants after the loss of two large trees.

Gardening in a Changing Climate

Gardeners have seen climate change coming for quite a while. Perhaps you've already noticed effects in your garden. Some are subtle, some more sudden, many are disturbing—lilac bushes reblooming in August, a sparse peach harvest from lack of chilling hours through dormancy in winter, a scarcity of bees. These are just a few of the signs you witness as erratic weather becomes the norm rather than the exception.

The symptoms of climate change will affect everyone: rising temperatures, increased pest populations, more plant diseases, heat waves, changes in precipitation patterns, more severe

A Brief History of Gardening

It's interesting to see where today's gardens fit into the long trajectory of gardening history in the Western world. Think the concept of outdoor garden rooms is new? The Romans did that in Italy as early as the year 43 AD, creating courtyards featuring plants, fountains, statues, and seating. Jumping ahead a bit, we'll start our timeline in England. If social media influencers had existed back then, these are the gardens they would be posting from.

Late 1400s–1600: Tudor gardens are designed to impress, with intricate knot gardens and labyrinths.

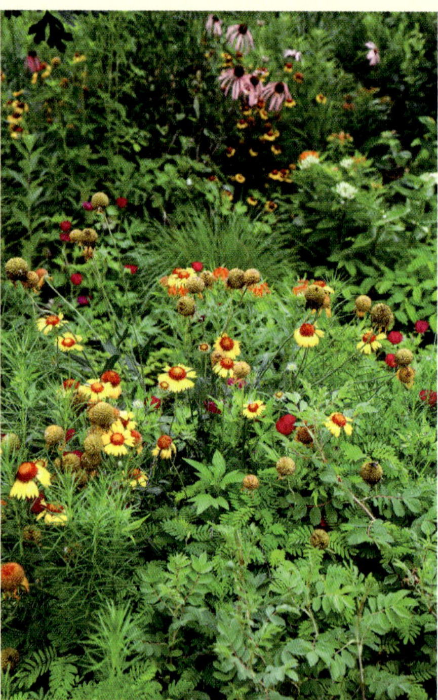

Naturalistic planting with gaillardia, coneflower, and wine cups in a St. Paul front yard.

1600–1700: Stuart era gardens are characterized by patterned plantings intended to be viewed from above on large terraces.

1700–1800: Early Georgian gardens embrace antiquities with lots of temples, statues, and grottoes in formal designs.

Late 1700s–mid 1800s: Late Georgian and Regency gardens, influenced by landscape architect Capability Brown, feature wild, natural spaces like woodlands and meadows that emphasize the "picturesque."

Meanwhile in America . . .

1700s: Early colonists plant food crops for survival, using seeds brought from England, while also learning to grow indigenous plants like tobacco, squash, and corn.

Early 1600s–1865: Slaves tend crops for landowners and grow their own gardens for food, a sense of autonomy, and pleasure.

Early 1800s: As pioneers head west, gardens are grown close to the house to protect crops and facilitate harvesting; food and medicine plants are grown in "cottage" and "kitchen" gardens.

Mid 1800s: Ornamental gardening begins in earnest.

1860: Pyrethrin, derived from chrysanthemums, is first used as a pesticide.

Late 1800s: Victorians grow lawns, plant "carpet beds," and covet exotic imported plants brought from foreign lands by intrepid

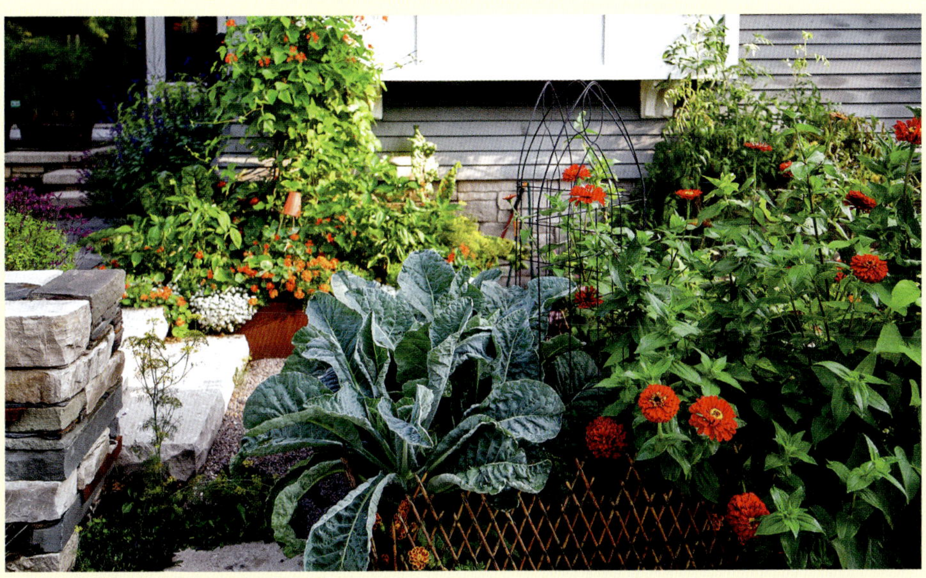

The author's kitchen garden is a mix of vegetables, herbs, and flowers.

plant hunters in the Golden Age of Botanical Exploration; greenhouses and conservatories become popular.

1858: Central Park, designed by Frederick Law Olmsted, makes nature accessible to the residents of New York City.

Early 1900s: Home gardeners go for larger lawns, perennial beds, and foundation plantings.

1943: During World War II, 20 million "victory gardens" supply 40 percent of the nation's produce.

1950s: Gardeners increase their use of pesticides; Astroturf is invented at Monsanto and given the name "ChemGrass."

1960s: With increased leisure time, gardens become an extension of the home.

1970s: Organic gardening and edible landscaping start to make inroads as Americans celebrate Earth Day for the first time on April 22, 1970.

1980s: Need for water conservation drives xeriscaping, low-maintenance gardens, and drought-tolerant landscaping.

1980s–90s: The New Perennial movement, or New Wave movement, emphasizes naturalistic planting styles, celebrating the entire life cycle of plants and embracing a more wild and ecological aesthetic; container plantings proliferate in small urban gardens.

2000s: Gardens go full circle; native plants are used to create wildlife and pollinator habitat and edible gardens incorporate vegetables, flowers, herbs, and fruits, sometimes in the front yard.

2025: Maximalist gardening, or chaos gardening, becomes a movement. (Or is it just a trend?)

storms, and extreme weather events. All of this will continue to alter growing conditions that people have depended upon for centuries. Indeed, our entire physical and societal infrastructure was developed around climatic patterns that no longer exist.

POLLINATION AND HEAT STRESS

A warming climate has already made itself known with average temperatures creeping upward every year. Heat stress affects plants in multiple ways, and the negative consequences for pollination are especially concerning. According to the University of Maryland Extension:

> *All fruiting plants have an optimal temperature range for the pollination and fertilization process. High temperatures can reduce pollen production, prevent anthers from releasing pollen, kill pollen outright, and interfere with the pollen tubes that serve as conduits for uniting sperm cells and eggs (fertilization) inside undeveloped seeds (ovules). High temperatures can even injure flowers before they open. Night temperatures are increasing at a faster rate than day temperatures as a result of climate change and seem to be most responsible for these pollination problems.*[2]

Looking at pollination problems from another angle, consider the effect on America's favorite backyard vegetable crop, the tomato:

- Prolonged daytime temperatures over 90°F (32°C) and nighttime temps above 70°F (21°C): Pollen production decreases, resulting in poor flowering and reduced fruit set.
- Prolonged daytime temperatures of 95°F (35°C): Tomatoes stop producing red pigment.
- Prolonged daytime temperatures of 100°F (38°C) and nighttime temps of 80°F (27°C): Ripening stops.

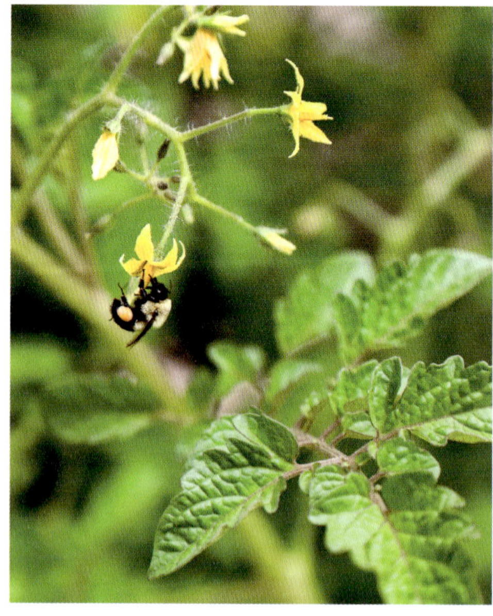

Bumblebee pollinating a tomato plant.

Poor pollination on other heat-stressed vegetables is evident in partially developed zucchini with yellow withering at the flower end and undersized cucumbers with a stunted, pointed tip. Some varieties will fare better than others. The challenge to find more resilient plants will take on more urgency.

Climate change throws ecosystems, evolved over thousands of years, out of synch. This is seen when flowers and insects that have adapted to bloom and emerge at the same time fail to do so. This can have a profound effect on species like specialist bees that collect pollen from a single plant species or a limited number of plants. That symbiotic relationship is so finely tuned that the bees' mouth parts have evolved to reach that unique nectar source. If "their" flower doesn't bloom as they emerge, they are out of luck, and that flower will remain unpollinated. Sometimes specialist bees remain dormant in their nest if that flower isn't blooming at the right time, hoping it does the next year.

Specialist bees are referred to as *oligolectic*, from the term "chosen few." For example, cellophane bees (*Colletes aberrans*) feed only on prairie clover. Sunflower mining bees (*Andrena helianthi*) feed their larvae with only the pollen of members of the *Helianthus* family, such as sunflowers, Jerusalem artichoke, and coneflowers. Thankfully, there are more generalist bees that are able to forage upon a large number of floral options. Yet, specialists are especially vulnerable and deserve our attention when planning habitat. As you can see in table 1.1, their specialty is often suggested in their name.

Table 1.1. Specialist Bees and Host Plants

Bee Species	Host Plant
Bee balm fairy bee (*Perdita gerhardi*)	spotted beebalm (*Monarda punctata*)
Bellflower resin bee (*Megachile campanulae*)	bellflower (*Campanula* family)
Eastern willow mining bee (*Andrena bisalicis*)	willow (*Salix*)
Faithful leafcutter bee (*Megachile fidelis*)	daisy (Asteraceae family)
Patellar oil-collecting bee (*Macropsis patellata*)	yellow loosestrife (*Lysimachia*)
Pickerelweed long-horned bee (*Melissodes apicatus*)*	pickerelweed (*Pontederia cordata*)
Waterleaf mining bee (*Andrena geranii*)*	Virginia waterleaf (*Hydrophyllum virginianum*)

* These bees are unique in that they collect floral oils besides pollen.

Habitat
Eunice Cajun Prairie Site
This is how many caterpillars
2 chickadee parents
have to find in 10 days for 5 babies

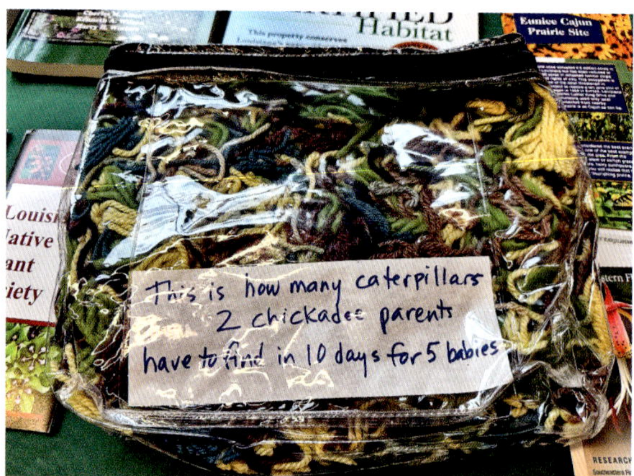

This bag of yarn pieces represents all the worms one chickadee feeds her brood in a single day.

BIRD MIGRATION

Climate change affects the patterns of bird migration as well as breeding behaviors. Gardeners like me who rely on birds as part of their pest management strategy might one day find ourselves wondering, "Where are all the birds?" I count on chickadees to capture the cabbageworms that compete for my broccoli and cauliflower plants. A single chickadee feeds her brood up to 500 worms a day. Many birds are adapting to climate change by doing three things: moving north, moving up in elevation, and advancing their reproductive schedules. Still, that may not be enough.

There will be temporary benefits to climate change, including longer growing seasons and the ability to grow new crops in areas unhospitable to them before. And plants do grow better with higher levels of carbon dioxide, which is an effect of climate change. However, these advantages will be short-term, as harmful insects, weeds, water shortages, and heat stress increase.

Ten years ago, I wrote in *Pollinator Friendly Gardening* that a single garden acting to support pollinators doesn't move the needle, but when millions of gardeners do this it is possible to make meaningful change. Ten years later, the idea of pollinator friendly gardening is common practice.

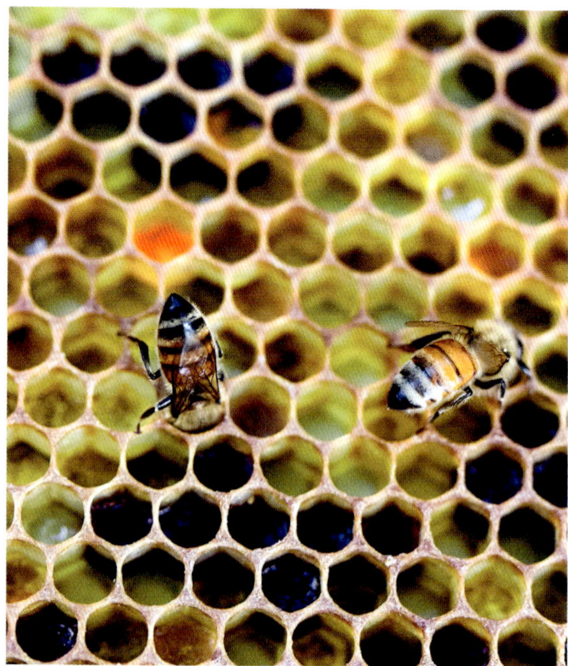

Honeybees collecting different shades of pollen.

HOW WE CAN HELP

As we adapt and enhance our gardens to suit our changing

lives and a changing climate, there are plenty of things we can do—both big and small—to practice sustainability and help to mitigate the effects of climate change to collectively combat this crisis:

- Plant trees to support wildlife habitat; provide shade for other plants, our homes, and ourselves; and combat excess urban heat.
- Create wildlife habitat in our gardens: food, shelter, and nesting sites to help make up for habitat loss caused by development and other land use.
- Build healthy soil in your garden to enhance plant growth, reduce pest and disease problems, and manage rainfall.
- Seek out resilient plant varieties that can survive erratic weather and withstand pest and disease problems; they'll save you time, energy, and money in the long run.
- Wean yourself from peat-based products. Peat extraction damages critical ecosystems and exacerbates climate change; peat-free products can improve soil structure, provide a better environment for beneficial microorganisms, increase available nutrients, and retain moisture.
- Use permeable paving to minimize runoff, letting the water percolate into the ground.
- Grow your own fruits and vegetables or buy them from farmers markets to help local growers.

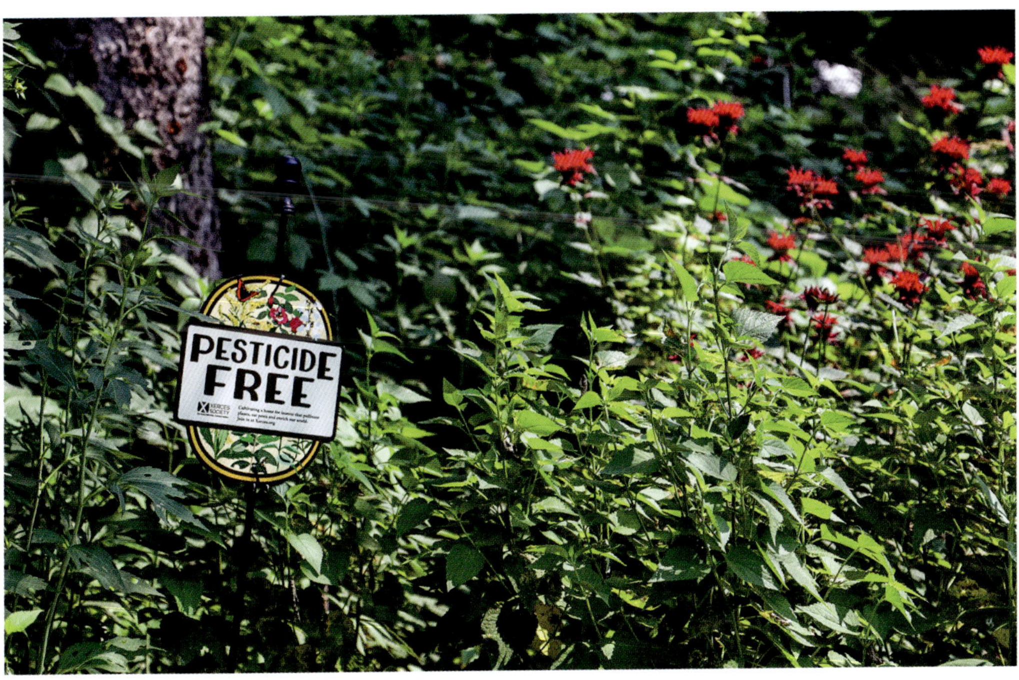

A pesticide-free garden.

GARDENER SPOTLIGHT

Meleah Maynard

It's always a joy to visit Meleah Maynard's garden, which she and her husband, Mike Hoium, have fashioned on their corner lot, a shady retreat in the middle of the city. Passersby always stop and ask gardening questions, and that inspired Meleah, a freelance writer, to write *Decoding Gardening Advice: The Science Behind the 100 Most Common Recommendations.*

Meleah and Mike moved into their house and began the garden twenty years ago, when Meleah first became a Master Gardener. They did away with the lawn and put in a path, and then started with bigger changes, like understory trees, native pagoda dogwoods, and nannyberries, all of which thrived in the shade of two huge bur oaks. Next, they built a rustic picket fence around it. Then they went looking for free plants. They were gifted, and dug up, all sorts of plants, including all of the hostas that she loves. They started filling in with plants here and there. In hindsight, Meleah considers this, "an ill-advised garden design strategy."

In my mind, the garden is a perfect success. It's such a great example of layered landscaping, a style that mimics natural ecosystems by creating multiple tiers of plants to support a wide variety of wildlife. Beneath the oak canopy the understory trees help create a lush, textured garden. For structure, they have extra-large perennials, like black snakeroot, goldenrod, and goatsbeard, throughout the garden. Wild ginger, geranium, lady's mantle, astilbe, hostas, and periwinkle cover the ground below, eliminating the need for mulch and effectively choking out most weeds. The garden shines in spring with Virginia bluebells, trillium, and uncommon plants like mayapple. All the birds and other wildlife that have made a home here seem to think it's pretty nice, too.

Walking by recently, however, something seemed off. As I got closer, I saw that one of the bur oaks was missing, and only a tall stump remained. Meleah explained the pair of oaks "sort of hugged the house," and one had developed some cracks, so they had been trying to figure out what to do. Then an August storm ripped off a huge limb and destroyed the tree.

- Switch from gas-powered tools to electric and manual to reduce noise and pollution; these lightweight tools offer ease-of-use and help older gardeners maintain independence for longer.
- Remove invasive species to give native plants and crop plants a better chance to re-establish themselves.
- Reduce water consumption to reduce stress on community resources; water more effectively—deep and infrequent watering makes plants more drought tolerant and resilient.

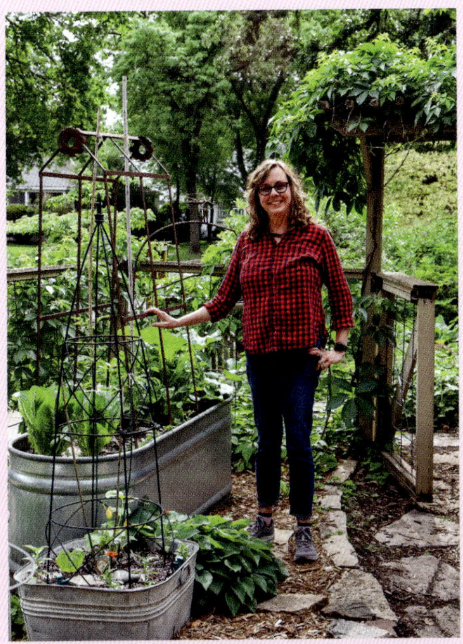

Putting a positive spin on this tragic turn, Meleah and Mike decided to leave the stump and do more to make it into habitat. They love how the squirrels and raccoons sit on it. They plan to bore more holes to make the stump even more welcoming for wildlife. The oak's absence has added more sun to the side yard, so they moved metal troughs there to make a "little, tiny farm" where they are growing veggies and herbs high enough to hopefully foil the rabbits. And the troughs make it easy to tend the plants without bending or stooping.

Many of Meleah's shade-loving plants aren't happy with the new exposure, and she plans to move some and give away others. They miss the shade, too: "That's been part of aging; we used to like the sun but now that we are older—we like shade."

The bur oak's demise isn't the only change they are going through. She and Mike have both retired so they have more time to garden; however, they have to travel frequently out of state to care for her aging parents. This has left her mindful about how she manages her garden for the future.

MELEAH'S TIPS

- Buying smaller plants is better because you'll save money and it's easier for the plants' young root systems to get established quickly. They don't have as much growth to support.
- Think carefully about whether or not plants need to be moved, and be strategic about it by knowing where to move plants before digging up an area.
- Protect your skin from the harmful effects of the sun when working in your garden.

- Use LED bulbs, solar-powered fixtures, and timers for outdoor lighting to conserve energy and protect wildlife from nighttime light pollution.
- Compost kitchen and garden waste to feed your soil and reduce waste sent to landfills.

GARDENERS, UNITE!

The pace at which nations and governments have moved to tackle what is called the greatest existential crisis of our lifetime is infuriatingly slow. As lawmakers and administrations seesaw back and forth over policy, it is exasperating, leading many to feel powerless and hopeless.

But as citizens we can help to bring change by working toward a more sustainable food system, helping people reconnect with nature, and building community. Meaningful action can be as simple as growing herbs in a planter, using a few more native plants, removing some lawn, or volunteering at a school garden:

- Create beauty and biodiversity in your garden to boost your mental health while fostering an environment that helps plants and animals thrive.
- Reclaim land for community garden use to improve residents' physical and mental health by increasing food security and creating social connection.
- Share gardening knowledge to ensure that people have successful gardening experiences and positive results.
- Show respect for gardening traditions and practices while providing science-based knowledge for an all-around better outcome.
- Share seeds, plants, and produce so that everyone benefits from the garden's bounty.

You don't have to wave a protest sign; your gardening efforts toward a more sustainable future will speak for themselves.

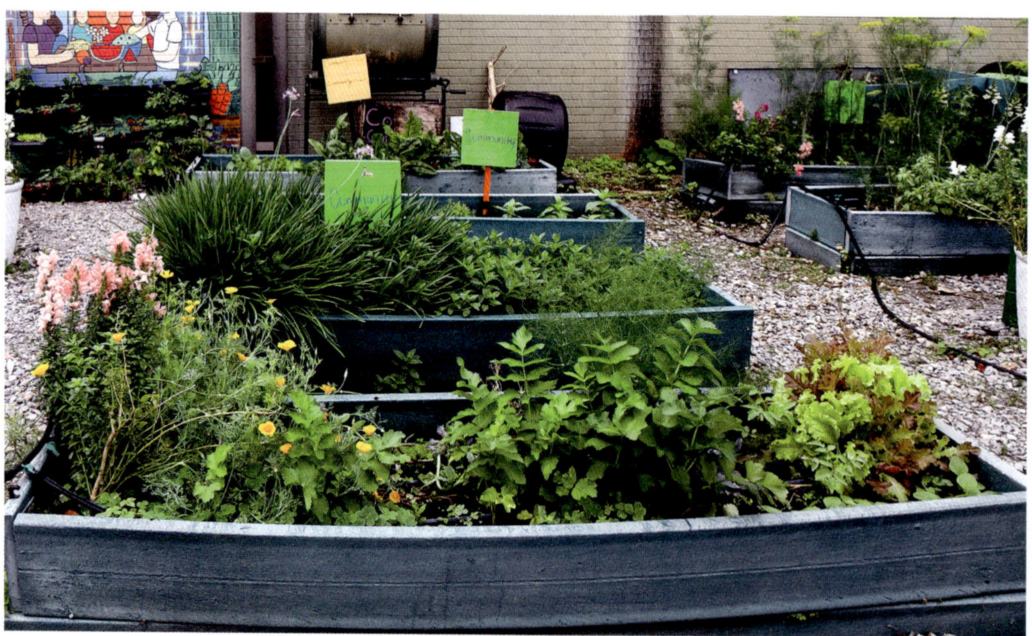

Community garden, SPROUT NOLA, New Orleans.

CHAPTER 2

Evaluating Your Garden

A favorite saying in our family lexicon comes from my mother-in-law. Driving her around the city or countryside she'll watch the houses pass by and exclaim, "There's a whole lotta ways to live." I would add, "There's a whole lotta ways to garden."

Evaluating your garden when considering whether to remain in your present home or move is not a one-size-fits-all proposition. There are countless gardens out there, and each is unique in its own way. Isn't that the beauty of it? The people tending those gardens are all different, too, and have varying backgrounds and situations regarding time, health, energy, budget, and more. Despite these differences, many gardens share common features. Most have a lawn, planting beds, paths and walkways, a patio or deck, maybe some steps. There will also be a variety of vegetation, of course: trees, shrubs, vines, flowers, and often a vegetable patch.

Examining and assessing your garden is a process of thoughtfully scrutinizing all of its elements—from the living things to the hardscape to the overall design and layout—to identify what works and what doesn't, as well as what might become an issue some years down the road. You'll spend most of this time pointing out faults and problems, but don't fear: the next step is to consider new ideas and alternatives. Meanwhile, you might be reminded of what you love so much about your garden now.

Time for Your Garden Gut Check

Start your assessment by doing a thorough walk-through of your entire garden. Circle around the house, crisscross the yard, really give it the once-over. Inspect it with a critical eye to look for current and potential hazards. Ask yourself, "What are possible impediments to my future enjoyment of this space?" If you have time, do this during different seasons as weather conditions and plants change. Take pictures and make notes (see chapter 9

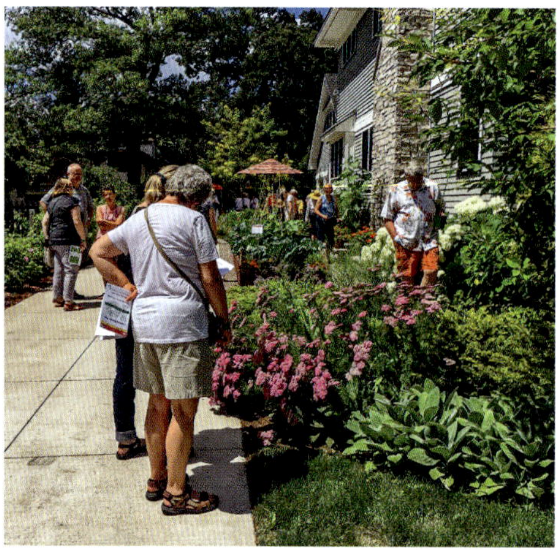

Like garden tour visitors, additional eyes are helpful in evaluating your garden.

for tips on recordkeeping for your garden). You'll have to use your imagination, too. What might not be a problem right now—steep stairs, sharp inclines, uneven or slick surfaces, unruly plants—could become one five or ten years down the road.

This process might sound like a downer. It's not meant to be! In fact, while touring your garden, please notice the things that bring you joy. It might be a plant gifted by a loved one, or perhaps a tree that you've coaxed into its own over the years. For me, it's lots of things, but there are some standouts. When it blooms in spring, my fringe tree (*Chionanthus virginicus*) is a cloud of frothy white blossoms that look and smell divine. It literally stops people in their tracks. Along our well-trod sidewalk people will pause, smile, and then look up to the porch (my outdoor office in summer) where I'm working on my laptop. They'll shout, "What is this?" I'll stop what I'm doing and walk down to tell them about this great native specimen. Some return to tell me they got one for their garden. It reminds me of the many reasons I keep gardening.

For a more thorough assessment, consider taking a second look, this time with a friend or fellow gardener. It's easy to miss a problem or hazard that they readily see. When my garden has been included in tours, I'm often surprised at what people notice or like (or don't like) that slips my radar. In the end it's your garden, but gaining other perspectives never hurts.

While evaluating your garden it is helpful to keep in mind the five core principles for a sustainable landscape:

1. Functionality: supporting your needs, such as entertaining, pets, growing food, composting, etc.
2. Maintainability: reducing maintenance and supporting best practices for mowing, pruning, mulching, watering, and other tasks.
3. Environmental soundness: minimizing or eliminating negative effects on the surrounding environment and wildlife through wise plant selection and establishing favorable growing conditions.
4. Cost-effective: designing within budget (cost, labor, time, etc.), choosing and siting trees for their long-term health and your enjoyment,

planting the right plants for the right places, installing hardscape to minimize extra costs in the future.

5. Visually appealing: designing the garden for what you want to see in your landscape, including plant and hardscape choices and optimizing views both inside and out.

Evaluating Hardscape

Hardscape includes any of the human-made structures around your garden. These elements play a big part in how your garden functions for you. Here are some examples:

- Porches, patios, and decks
- Sidewalks and walkways
- Stepping stones
- Paths
- Driveways
- Walls or retaining walls
- Fencing
- Lighting
- Edging
- Firepits
- Water features
- Swimming pools

Hardscape done right enhances your garden experience: It draws people together outdoors, it guides you through your landscape, it protects you from the elements, and it defines boundaries. However, it can fall into disrepair over time and become unsafe, and some hardscape materials aren't appropriate for aging owners.

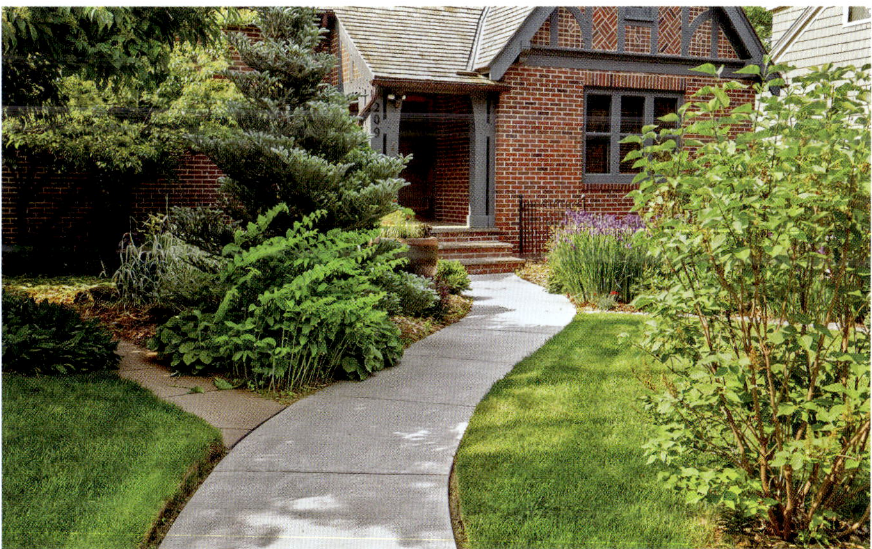

Concrete walkways are some of the safest hardscape solutions.

WATCH YOUR STEP

In the US, falls are the leading cause of injury and injury-related death among adults 65 and older, according to the CDC.[1] This underscores the importance of identifying and eliminating hazards in your garden that might cause you to trip and fall. Not all falls are garden-related by any means, although some happen while in the garden; health conditions, medications, foot issues, vision problems, and loss of balance are some of the frequent causes of falls. But often it's a loose paver that precipitates a fall—one with potentially significant health repercussions. And that's an easily prevented fall.

Even the best-planned gardens can contain dangerous elements. As a cautionary tale, consider my first time visiting the High Line park in New York City. The planting beds, designed by Dutch garden designer Piet Oudolf, have a series of parallel grooves meant to mimic the lines of the old, elevated railway the park now occupies, and these extend to the walkways in places. My shoe caught in one and, before I knew what had happened, I fell backward. Luckily, a paramedic was strolling by and he assessed me and my bloodied head on the spot. It is so easy to get distracted by a beautiful garden, especially your own. Since that incident I've made sure to move more deliberately in gardens.

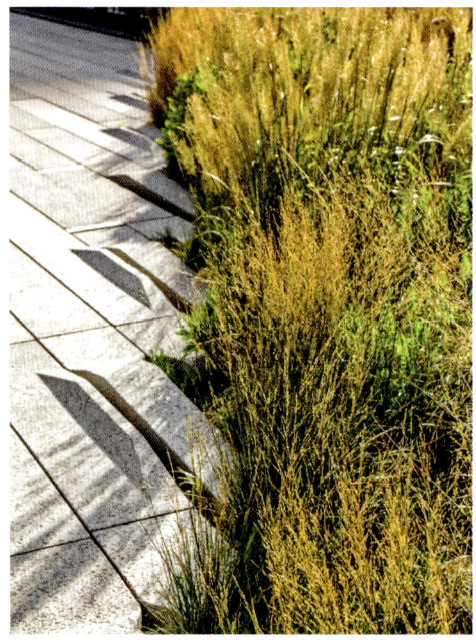

Even the well-designed High Line park has hazards that can cause someone to trip and fall.

STEPS AND WALKWAYS

To assess the safety and condition of pathways, start at the house door you typically use to access your garden. Pay close attention to how you exit your home and follow your usual traffic patterns. First, note the material of the steps and whether there is a handrail. The handrail should be stable and a shape that is easy to grip; this is especially important given the diminished hand strength that occurs with age. Next, note the materials and surface treatment of these steps (the same applies if you step straight onto a deck or patio). The following are some common conditions associated with popular step, deck, and patio materials.

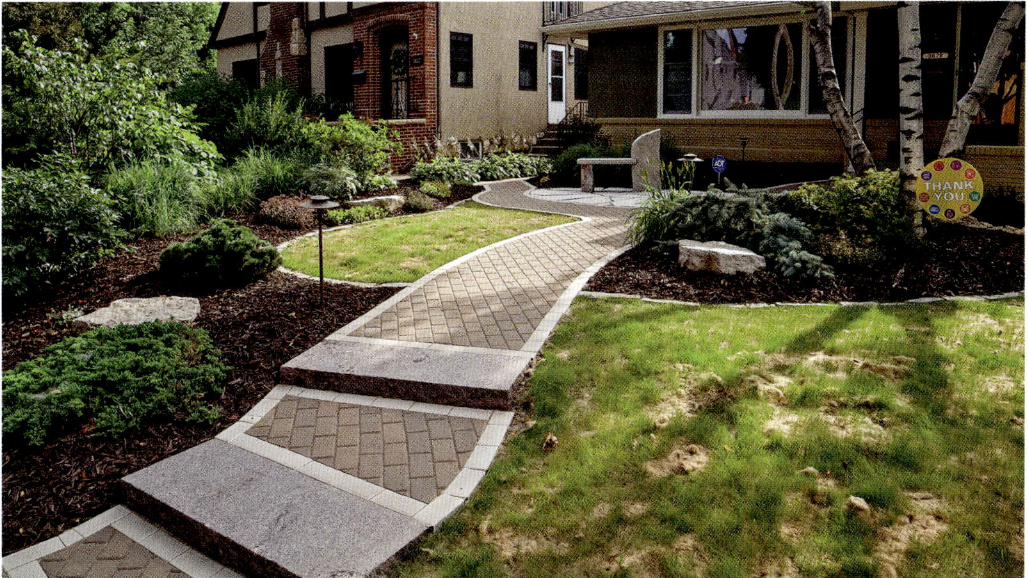

The paver walkway in this newly installed landscape looks great now, but it might shift or develop other problems over time.

Poured concrete (concrete slab) typically has texture and it is one of the safest surfaces when it's flat and in good condition. Painted or highly finished concrete can be slippery when wet, and badly cracked or shifted concrete contains trip hazards.

Wood decking and steps can warp and twist with time, become loose, or splinter. In wet climates or seasons, algae can grow on wood, making it slippery. Wood needs regular upkeep to maintain good condition.

Composite wood materials have a variety of different textures and properties. Some have a smooth, plastic-like finish that can be slippery when wet. Unlike real wood, composite wood does not need stain or paint and is not prone to cracking and splintering, but it holds heat and can be very hot for bare feet. Heat and sunlight can also damage the material and cause it to warp or crack, and mold or mildew can make it slippery.

Pavers, including traditional clay bricks and modern concrete pavers, come with a number of potential problems. Clay bricks can be slippery when wet and are relatively prone to cracking and chipping. Concrete pavers typically are nonslip and stronger than clay brick. Both can grow moss and algae on their surfaces or grass and weeds in the joints between pavers. Most notably, all pavers are susceptible to shifting and sinking with ground movement, creating uneven surfaces, grooves, or raised edges between pavers that can catch a shoe heel. Correcting widespread shifting is an expensive proposition.

A Nonslip Solution

One inexpensive fix for many surfaces that are slippery when wet is a nonskid coating. These products are heavy-duty, paint-like coatings that stick to their host material to give it texture that reduces the risk of slips and falls. They are used to increase traction on floors, stairs, and decks, both indoors and outdoors. Nonskid coatings are designed for specific surfaces, and their effectiveness can vary depending upon the condition and porosity of the host material. It's important to choose the right product for the surface you want to cover; you can learn more through coating manufacturers or knowledgeable staff at a good hardware or paint store.

Flagstone is a generic term for various types of natural sedimentary stones that are split into flat, irregular shapes and are commonly used for walkways and patios. Most flagstones have a gritty surface texture that adds slip-resistance and a natural look. Granite, bluestone, and marble are other popular paving stone materials. They are often slip-resistant in natural form but can be very slippery if polished. Stone is undeniably beautiful and durable, but it comes with a few significant drawbacks. It can be very expensive, especially large pieces of cut stone. It is quite heavy and can be tricky to install properly, and irregular shapes can make for a challenging puzzle. Split stone can have a bumpy, ridged, or contoured surface that creates trip hazards. As with pavers (and bricks), stones can shift or sink over time, and cracks or gaps between stones can harbor weeds and grass, creating additional maintenance and potential trip hazards.

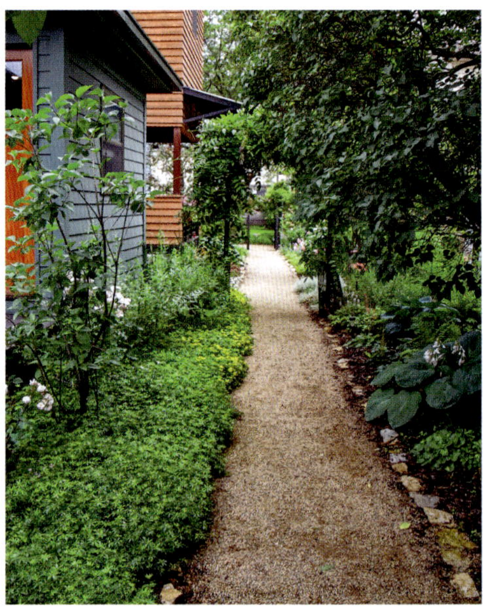

Smooth, stable pathways without clutter or debris make for safe, easy walking.

Walkways close to the house are usually made of more permanent materials like concrete, pavers, or stepping stones. Here the risk is more for tripping rather than slipping. On concrete, look for large cracks and for

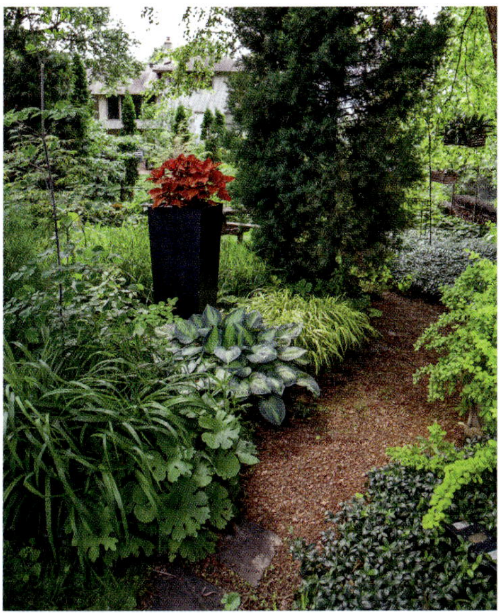

Landscape designer Cory Barton uses Class 5 gravel for her paths.

places that have heaved, leaving gaps or one side higher than the other—a toe-stubber at least, or worse.

With pavers and steppingstones, they should be stable and flush with the ground or their surrounding surface. In addition, look for areas with poor drainage, such as where the ground or lawn meets with the walkway or where there are changes in elevation, noting whether mud, leaves, or other debris collect there on a regular basis, making it slippery. If seed pods or acorns accumulate underfoot, they can cause you to lose balance or roll an ankle. Of course, it all gets trickier if your property is hilly or on an incline.

LOOSE AND NATURAL WALKWAY MATERIALS

As you move farther from the house, walkways or paths usually consist of loose or less fixed materials, such as crushed stone, gravel, mulch, grass, or packed dirt. These materials tend to be highly permeable, which promotes sustainability by reducing runoff and allowing water to percolate back into the soil (pavers and stones also can create a permeable surface with the right design). Check out your paths to see what they are made of; each comes with pros and cons.

Decomposed granite, known as DG in the landscaping world, is granite that has naturally broken down to the size of small gritty gravel and smaller. It's natural, permeable, and inexpensive, and it can be graded and compacted to create a stable, good-looking path. It requires proper installation so that it is level, and a stabilizer might be added to keep the fine particles locked together. Over time, it can erode or settle where drainage is a problem. Some particles might stick to shoes and can damage indoor floors. It needs to be replenished with use.

Gravel is an inexpensive and attractive material. Lots of people love that crunch beneath their feet. It drains well so it is slip resistant. Often called pea gravel, the preferred size is .55″ (10–14 mm), just like a pea. Edging is needed to keep it contained and out of the lawn or planting beds. A depth of 2″ (5 cm) is recommended; any more can make it difficult for walking, especially for older adults. Class 5 gravel is a mixture of rock, sand, and clay that is prized for its stability and good drainage properties, making it a good choice for pathways.

Mulch made of chipped or shredded wood looks natural in the garden but eventually decomposes into the soil and adds substrate for weed growth. Without edging, it can wash away with heavy rains and paths become muddy. It needs regular freshening up.

Grass paths are elegant looking in formal gardens and lend order to native plantings; however, they need regular mowing. They can be soggy and slippery with dew in the morning and after a rain.

Packed dirt paths are practical on large properties with natural or wooded areas. They are muddy after a rain and can be especially slippery when sloped. Erosion can lead to surface damage that is potentially treacherous to walk over.

MAKING PATHWAYS SAFE

Keeping paths in good condition and free of mud, overgrown vegetation, moss, and other natural debris will go a long way toward making them safe. Tree roots that cannot be removed should be clearly marked. It's also important to keep walkways clear of items like garden tools, toys (kid and dog), and hoses.

Another important consideration is the width of your walkways. Are they wide enough to allow two people to walk side by side or to accommodate a wheelchair? Are the walkways connected with steps, and how much of an elevation change is involved? You should determine if those are problems for far off into the future or if they might soon deny you access to the garden, or at least parts of it.

On sloped or hilly lots, retaining walls make more usable space up top, whether for landscaping or gathering places. However, the drop-off they create can be dangerous, especially if a gardener needs to walk, weed, or mow along the top of a wall. Handrails or fencing is a must to make this situation safe. Weather, structural defects, gravity, and time also affect retaining walls. They should be checked regularly for cracks, bulges, tilting, or buckling, which can indicate developing or serious problems.

If you like to visit your garden at night, or even just pass through on your way in or out of the house, it's essential that you do another walk-through after dark to assess the lighting situation. Lighting is one of the best investments you can make for your garden, both for its safety and its aesthetic benefits. Be forewarned, excessive lighting can harm the natural cycles of wildlife as well as your own sleep cycle; you don't want a spectacle. Here are some general rules of thumb for effective and safe outdoor lighting.

- Low-voltage lighting, like LED or solar, pointed downward should light up shadowed areas along the ground at entry and exit points, along paths, at all elevation changes, and up and down driveways. Low-voltage lighting systems operate on 12 volts, while standard outdoor lighting uses 120 volts. This makes it safer for DIY installation and repairs.
- An automatic timer will save you the trouble of remembering to turn them on and off.
- Motion-detector lights for security purposes should not shine upward or sideways so as to avoid glare or deep shadows.
- Well-designed lighting will make your outdoor area a more inviting place to spend time after dark—a safe and comfortable spot for observing the stars, night-blooming plants, and, perhaps, fireflies.

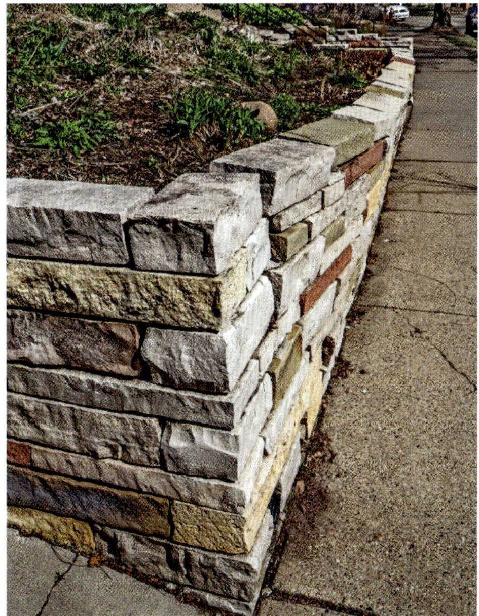

This stone wall is beginning to buckle, a common problem with aging retaining walls.

Firepits, water features, and swimming pools are a bonus to any garden, but they can be dangerous, and even deadly, for older adults, particularly for people with memory issues. Adequate lighting here is critical. Fencing off these areas for children and vulnerable adults can be expensive and complicated; sometimes this can be a deal-breaker when considering whether or not to stay in the house.

Problematic Plantings

While building our forever house in Minneapolis, we took special pains to blend in with the historic neighborhood. A foundation planting of old-fashioned 'Annabelle' hydrangeas along our front porch mirrored the beautiful old homes along the block. Each spring, the fresh green foliage and billowy white blooms were gorgeous—until the first rains fell onto them from our slanted roof. Then, those mop-headed flowers flopped and assumed a forlorn appearance.

It was a common sight to see me shaking the hydrangeas, looking to lighten their sopping wet load, hoping they would bounce back to their original glory. I tried staking them but that looked worse. My Master Gardener training told me I needed the right plant for the right place, and I made the tough decision to replace them with 'Bobo' hydrangeas, a cultivar with sturdier stems and pretty enough blooms that better tolerate a downpour.

It is difficult to pass judgment on a seasoned landscape, nurtured with loving care and settled into itself. But it's important to consider maintainability. Robust, mature plants are the backbone and blessing of any garden. However, some trees, evergreens, and shrubs outgrow their welcome, overwhelming the house, blocking the windows and pathways, and, if they're in poor condition, dragging down the entire landscape.

There's no need to get out the chainsaw yet. In fact, this book encourages older gardeners to put down the power tools and opt for different strategies. For now, though, take note of which trees, shrubs, hedges, and ornamental grasses require the use of power tools to maintain their shape and health. You cannot always prune your way out of a problem. Now is the time to decide if they're high value, high maintenance, or high risk.

Next up for consideration are perennial borders, a delightful feature of many gardens, providing color, texture, and interest. Every perennial comes with its own set of needs to keep it looking its best, and some are more needy than others. Instead of a once-a-year pruning, like some trees and shrubs, perennials might require continuous care throughout the growing season. Some people like the instant satisfaction that comes with deadheading, while others dislike the never-ending job; it greatly depends upon the size of your perennial garden, and your temperament.

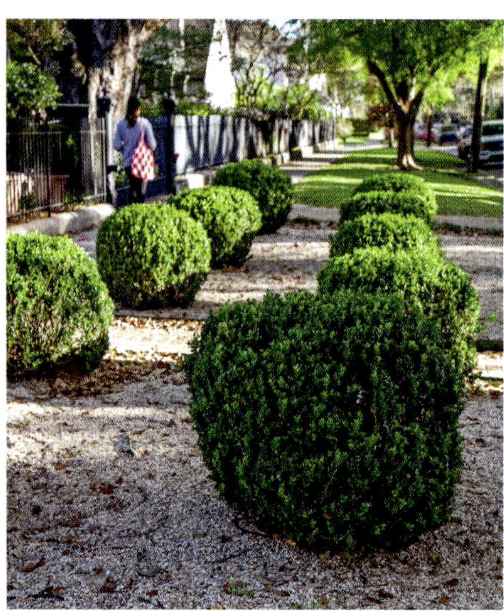

High-maintenance landscapes that require lots of trimming and shaping are too much trouble late in life.

Survey your plants to identify the high-upkeep types. For example, a long border of daylilies along the driveway looks great, but true to their name, the "mush mummies" need picking daily, and the dead stems must be removed later. A stand of bearded iris asks for a

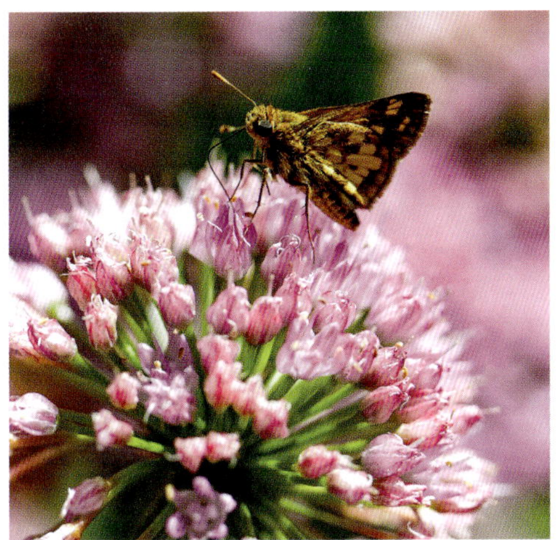
Leave tall grasses for overwintering skipper butterflies.

similar treatment but only once a year. For me it's the coreopsis flowers, so lovely swaying in the breeze, until I have to snip all the leftover blooms on hundreds of those tiny threadlike stems. In addition to these types of tasks, the average perennial needs dividing every three to five years to maintain its health and appearance.

As for the big job of winter cleanup in the perennial garden, the current thinking is: Don't! It is recommended to leave perennial stems at least 12″–15″ (30–38 cm) tall for wildlife habitat over winter. Many native bee species use the hollow stems of spent perennials for nesting purposes. The same advice goes for ornamental grasses, unless they are flopping across walkways, as bumblebee queens frequently nest and hibernate below the tufted crowns. Above ground, skipper butterflies use the grass foliage for overwintering, curling silk around the blades and snuggling in from the cold. Of course, you will still have to cut them back in late spring.

As you continue your walk-through, you should think about which plants provide you the most enjoyment for the time and energy they demand. You might decide that providing crucial habitat is worth the effort. If not, consider reducing your workload with a plant sale or giveaway. Younger, nimble new gardeners might be willing to dig for free plants. They might appreciate some mentoring, too.

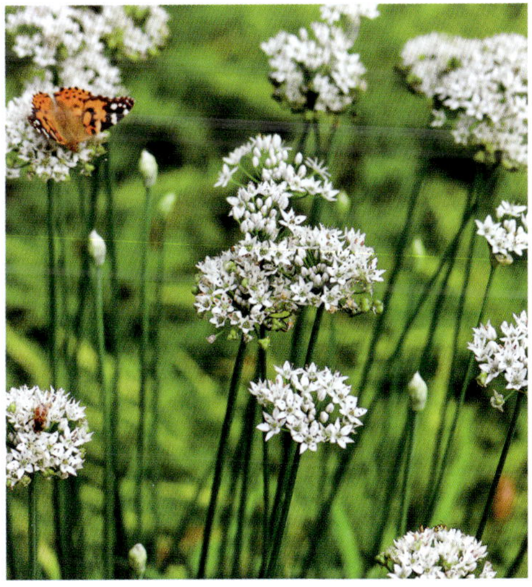
Garlic chives are prolific re-seeders, but they are not invasive.

Invasive Plants

As you inspect the garden, scan the grounds for invaders and thugs, those uninvited plants and others that have worn out their welcome. Invasive plants can ruin your garden, not to mention your time spent in the garden. It is important to define what *invasive* really means, as the term is commonly misused to describe vigorous plants. An invasive plant is non-native and causes, or likely causes, harm to the economy, environment, or human health. Invasive plants disrupt ecosystems, outcompeting native plants and animals for resources, spreading diseases, and altering habitat. In your garden, they are unwanted guests that make themselves comfortable and never leave. They spread rapidly via rhizomes and seeds, hogging light, nutrients, water, and space.

It's common for certain plants to be designated as invasive in some geographical regions and not others. English ivy (*Hedera helix*) is a good example. Native to Europe, it's invasive on the West Coast and around the eastern half of the US, where it crowds out native plants and can spread into tree canopies (check with your local extension office to learn about invasives in your area).

Here are some other well-known invasives:

Barberry (*Berberis thunbergia*) (Some new cultivars are sterile or semi-sterile but are still restricted in some places.)
Buckthorn (*Rhamnus cathartica*)
Burning bush (*Euonymus alatus*)
Chinese privet (*Ligustrum sinense*)
Garlic mustard (*Alliaria petiolata*)
Japanese honeysuckle (*Lonicera japonica*)
Leafy spurge (*Euphorbia esula*)
Lily of the valley (*Convallaria majalis*)
Multiflora rose (*Rosa multiflora*)
Scotch broom (*Cytisus scoparius*)
Tree of heaven (*Ailanthus altissima*)
Yellow toadflax (*Linaria vulgaris*)

Many invasives are pretty plants, but like my mother always said, "Pretty is as pretty does." You may even find garden centers selling invasive plants—I fell for Chameleon plant (*Houttuynia cordata*), with its colorful heart-shaped leaves and perky flowers, before I knew better. Sometimes invasives show up in plant swaps. You might have brought one home without knowing it, and now it's a scourge. Always do your homework before you buy or plant. Take a picture of the tag—get the Latin, or scientific, name for accuracy—and look it up first.

As noted, not every prolific, spreading plant is necessarily invasive. Some non-native plants, like bishop's weed (*Aegopodium podagraria*) and periwinkle (*Vinca minor*), are just extraordinarily successful at what they

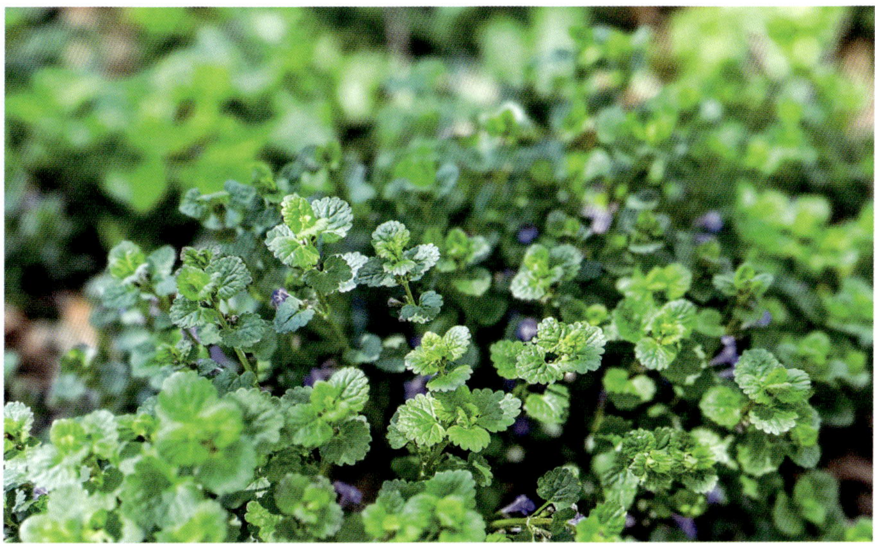

Creeping Charlie is a vigorous spreader that can be tolerated in certain areas.

do, thriving beyond the bounds you have set for them. Whether invasive or simply aggressive, battling these bullies gets old, no matter your age. You will need to decide whether you want to contain it or eradicate it, or if any of these plants might someday make you throw in the trowel.

Other times it helps to reframe the problem. Creeping Charlie, or ground ivy (*Glechoma hederacea*), is a problem in lots of places. It's a delicate low-spreading plant that takes over lawns and gardens with stealthy speed. However, it has a small blue flower that attracts bees and other insects. So, many of my fellow gardeners and I have made peace with it. I pull it out by hand where it detracts, but in other areas, like the narrow, north side of our house, I let it assume the role of a groundcover. As seasoned gardeners already know, you must pick your battles.

Recurrent Pests and Diseases

In early summer, my driveway hedge of pink rugosa roses literally buzzes with bees—bumblebees, honeybees, gorgeous green sweat bees—their high-pitched whine mingling with the wonderful fragrance of the blooms. Unfortunately, a few weeks later the blooms are sullied by hordes of Japanese beetles. You know the drill. I head out with a bucket of soapy water to dispatch them. It's gross and time-consuming. Every year I ponder replacing the rugosas with some other shrub, but I can't because: the bees.

For some folks, the Japanese beetles prove to be too much, and they replace their roses with other blooms. Some gardeners dig up their beloved

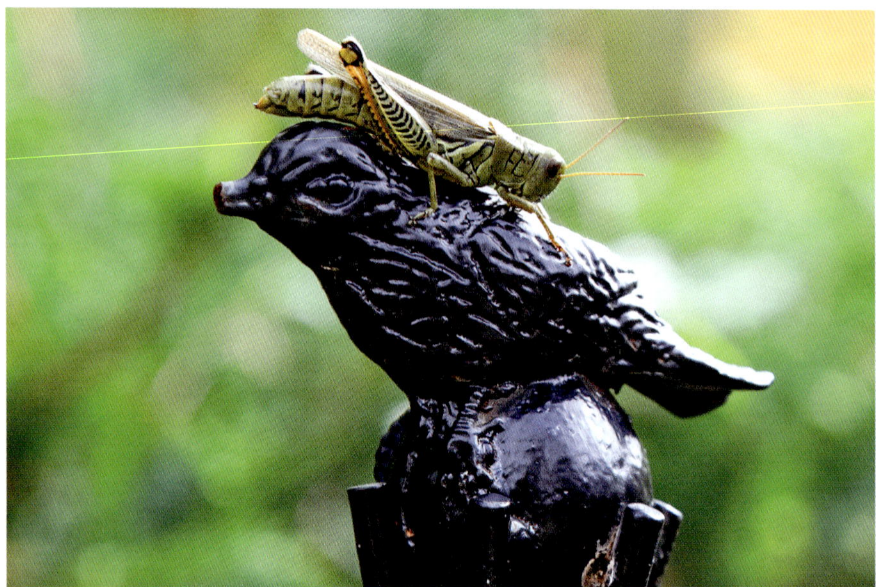

Think of grasshoppers as bird food.

hostas after battling slugs for too long. Vegetable gardeners might give up growing squash because of squash bugs and borers.

I like to encourage people to think of bugs first as bird food that brings in our feathered friends that in turn provide natural pest control. I ask them to consider whether the plant damage is temporary and cosmetic or truly fatal before they give up on their gardens. Most insect populations wax and wane through the years. The trick is to have a balance of good bugs and bad bugs. However, some, like the Japanese beetle, have no natural predators, while other pests reproduce several times per season with no relief. I like to remind frustrated gardeners to do their homework. Identify the culprit and then start with a nontoxic solution. A good spray with the garden hose often disrupts or dislodges pests.

Then there are the larger kind of pests: rabbits, voles, woodchucks, and deer, to name the usual suspects. These hungry critters can test us to our limits, especially in rural or suburban areas. Don't get me started on rabbits. They are frequently the culprits that drive the decision to hand off the house and garden to someone else. While animal repellents claim to work, they need to be reapplied after every rain, making them unsuitable for most gardeners with busy lives or limitations. I find the only effective way to control large pests is by installing some type of barrier. There are entire books devoted to deer- and rabbit-resistant gardening (see Resources, page 213).

Plant diseases that show up every year like clockwork are frustrating, too. Think through your growing season and list the plants that come on bright and strong, then succumb to fungal diseases, like powdery mildew, rust, blight, blackspot, and more. These diseases leave beautiful flowers such as phlox, monarda, hollyhocks, and zinnias disfigured and with unsightly foliage. Vegetable crops like tomatoes and cucumbers can suffer a similar fate. Here the fix is easier. There are plenty of disease-resistant varieties of these same plants that you can swap in. Look for disease-resistant symbols in catalogs and on seed tags, or ask at your garden center. If the disease is in your soil, raised beds and containers are an alternative growing method.

At other times, the plant itself is the pest. Plants with thorns or foliage that triggers allergic reactions should be on the short list for removal. As people age, their skin thins and tears more easily, leaving it susceptible to infection and other complications. As an example, sap from spurge and other members of the Euphorbia family can cause skin and eye irritation that ranges from moderate to severe.

Toxic and Poisonous Plants

Let's be specific. A toxic plant can be harmful through skin contact or inhalation, whereas a poisonous plant is harmful if ingested or eaten. The popular but toxic succulent firestick (or pencil cactus; *Euphorbia tirucalli*) is aptly named; one of these sent my daughter, a budding gardener, to the ER after she broke off a piece and then touched her eyes. Another plant,

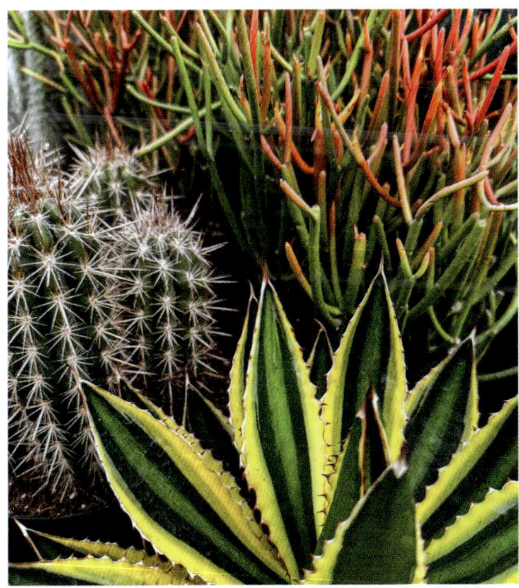

Spiny cacti or toxic succulents should be avoided or removed.

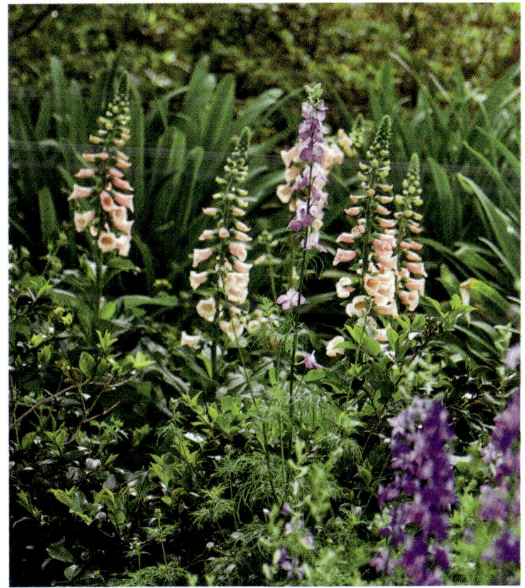

Foxglove and larkspur should be handled with care if they remain in your garden.

oleander (*Nerium oleander*), which is common in southern landscapes, causes rashes and other allergic reactions. If accidentally ingested, the effects are much worse, especially for older individuals.

Wearing protective clothing and gloves can help protect you from irritating and toxic plants, but aging gardeners should think twice before keeping potentially dangerous plants around. It pays to know what you grow in your garden, whether it only causes skin irritation or worse. Ironically, some toxic or poisonous plants might sound familiar since they are also components of life-saving drugs in the right application.

Identify all plants and cross-check them with the USDA website on poisonous plants. Here are some common offenders:

Cape leadwort (*Plumbago auriculata*)
Castor bean (*Ricinus communis*)
European yew (*Taxus baccata*)
Foxglove (*Digitalis purpurea*)
Jimsonweed (*Datura stramonium*)
Larkspur (*Delphinium* spp.)
Lily of the valley (*Convallaria majalis*)
Monkshood (*Aconitum napellus*)
Pride of Madeira (*Echium candicans*)

Lawn: Love It or Leave It?

For some, cutting the grass is the most gratifying part of maintaining the yard for others, it is a Sisyphean task. Even if you land somewhere in between, it's still worth discussing how the lawn fits into your gardening future.

Lawns do have benefits. They produce oxygen, reduce carbon dioxide, cool the surrounding area, and filter rainfall. They provide the eye with a place to rest. Your decision might hinge upon the size of your lawn and how it is configured. Depending on who does the mowing, a lawn might be a deal-breaker, eventually becoming an arduous task for an aging gardener or an expensive job to hire out. Granted, for those with bigger properties, using turf is an uncomplicated way to cover a large piece of land, and mowing does not require a special skill set. On the downside, if an acre of sod isn't used as a gathering place, play space, or for other beneficial activities, it's not much more than a thirsty, hungry, polluting monoculture that is not earning its keep. By contrast, an environmentally sound landscape benefits everyone by reducing inputs like fertilizers and pesticides, conserving water and improving water quality, and providing food and habitat for wildlife.

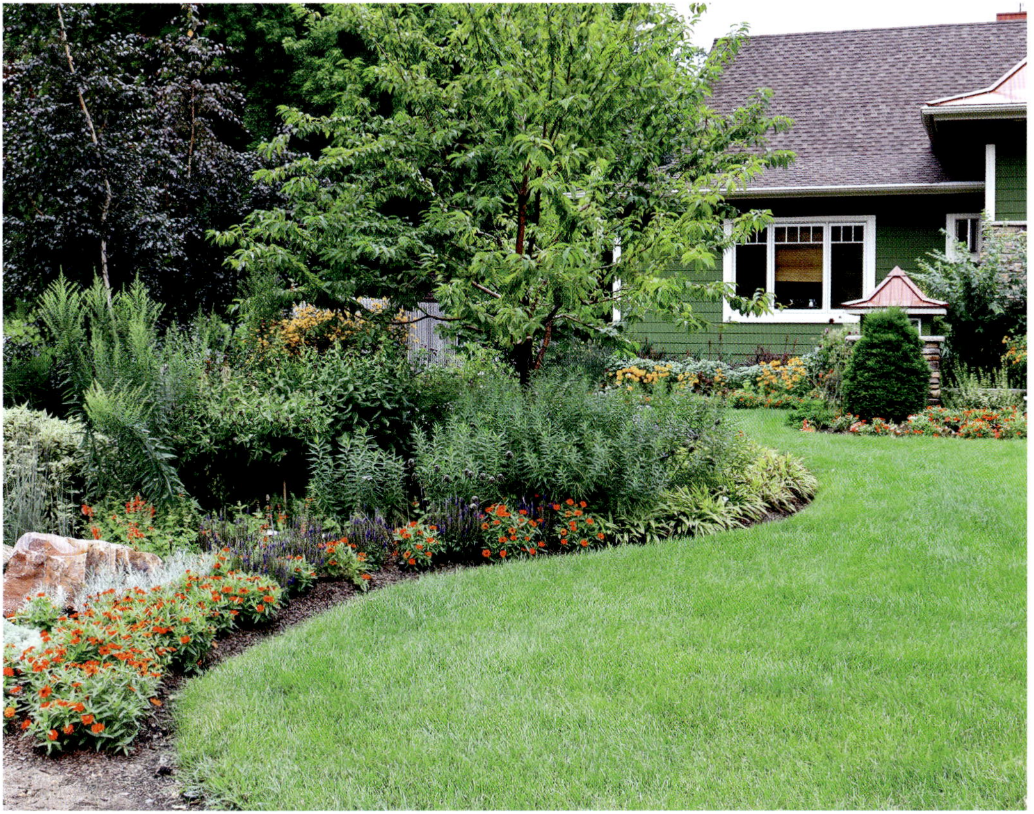

A gently curving lawn makes for more efficient mowing.

Mowing is made more difficult when there are structures, fences, and trees situated within the lawn, making it necessary to use a string trimmer to tidy and finish the edges. Narrow strips of turf and sharp angles are time-consuming to mow and look awkward. You can end up with compacted soil and ruts in those places as well. Areas of turf should be ideally three times the mower width for easier turns. A lawn with gentle curves takes less fuel and effort to mow than a straightedged or angular lawn. Mulched or edged mowing strips along houses, sheds, and fences eliminate the need to string trim those places, once again reducing inputs by using less fuel, not to mention reducing unnecessary noise while saving you time. Generous 6′ (2 m) mulch rings around trees protect the trees from wounds made by string trimmers; such wounds can make trees more susceptible to pests and diseases. Stressed trees need more interventions, such as pesticides or expensive removal. Healthy trees are one of the hallmarks of a sustainable landscape.

For a long time, it has been a given that a stand-alone house has a lawn, even if it is very small, but that is not as true anymore. Looking to make their

GARDENER SPOTLIGHT

Kylee Baumle

Kylee Baumle is a lifelong gardener and photographer with an endless curiosity about nature. She is also a writer, penning columns for her local newspaper and *Ohio Gardener* magazine, along with other publications. I think it's safe to say that Kylee and I both found our passion for pollinators through gardening. Her love for the monarch butterfly inspired her to write *The Monarch: Saving our Most-Loved Butterfly*. In an effort to share the miracle of their migration, she has led tours to the monarch's overwintering grounds in Mexico. As a citizen scientist, Kylee participates in several programs that provide data to researchers studying monarchs.

Kylee started her garden in 2005, after she attended the Cleveland Flower Show. She wanted to grow everything she saw! She and her husband, Romie, went big, tearing out lawn over 10 percent of their one-acre property, the acre that inspired her blog, ourlittleacre.com. Each year they tore out more grass, her theme being "buy the plants and find somewhere to put them." Touring other gardens, she gleaned ideas and adapted them to her own situation.

Kylee's acre is part of the former Great Black Swamp in northwest Ohio. In the early 1800s, this densely forested region with tannin-stained water produced thick, dark mud and clouds of mosquitoes. The area was eventually drained to make rich farmland, and efforts are now being made to restore its role in the region's ecology. Kylee's challenge was to learn more about what would grow in the heavy clay soil in hardiness Zone 5b/6a. She began to focus on plant choices and incorporating more native plants into her landscape. They use no chemicals, and they fertilize only with compost. They mulch with triple-ground hardwood and fallen leaves.

The garden has been a source of peace and joy, and although she enjoys weeding and deadheading, it's overwhelming in spring. That spring work drove the decision to downsize. Now nearing seventy, Kylee says, "It's more difficult to keep up with the gardens as we grow older and don't move as well, or have the stamina

landscapes more sustainable, many homeowners now opt to reduce or eliminate lawns. If your lawn struggles to grow in shadier areas of the yard, that is a perfect excuse to try something else, like a native groundcover that provides habitat and visual interest.

Finally, think of your lawn like this: every curb is a lakeshore or riverbank. Organic matter like leaves and grass clippings end up in the gutter. Runoff carries that along with fertilizer, nutrients, and pesticides into our waterways. Beyond the environmental implications are cost factors. If your

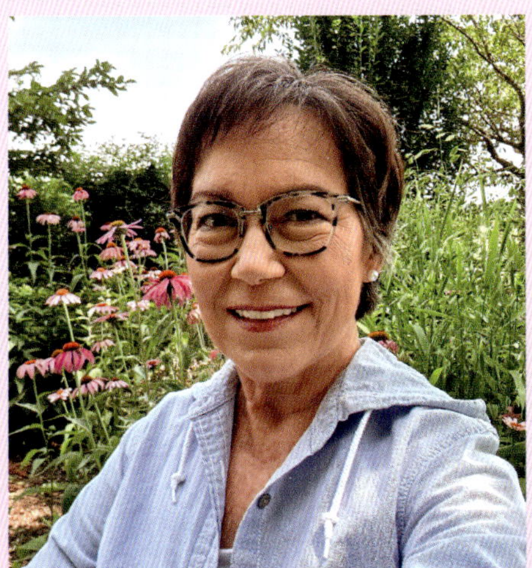

Photo courtesy of Kylee Bauml

we once had. We don't enjoy marathon gardening days like we used to."

The idea to downsize the gardens began a couple of years ago, when they had a horrific hot, dry summer. She called it, "The Year I Didn't Garden." Changes in the climate in their area made it clear that hot and dry was going to be more the norm for a big part of the summer, making it hard to find plants that grow well and thrive—not just survive.

Kylee looked at the garden and took note of what did really well and what was challenging to maintain. No longer up to the task of maintaining the garden to the quality she wanted, she and her husband discussed paring down things to a more manageable level. They evaluated the overall landscape situation—trees, wet spots, shade, sun—and decided which areas to keep and which areas to eliminate, marking plants she wanted to move that fall. They decided to wait until spring to move plants to reduce stress and assure their survival.

As for her gardening future, Kylee says, "I can't imagine myself not gardening. I enjoy the actual work of it, when it's a manageable level, and I certainly enjoy the results. I'm trying to look at it in the same way I look at our home—simplifying where we reasonably can."

KYLEE'S TIPS FOR DOWNSIZING THE GARDEN

- Evaluate the whole landscape to decide what to keep or move.
- Mark the plants you want to move beforehand. Keep your favorites; share the extras with others.
- No more plant heroics! Stop growing things that need too much extra attention.
- Slow but steady wins the race.

lawn care and water bills are sky high, or your city imposes watering restrictions, those are great reasons to lose your lawn. Some townships even offer incentives to do so.

During your garden evaluation, calculate how much of your gardening efforts and costs are involved in managing this stretch of turf. Are there other garden activities or projects you would rather be doing?

In the end, size is a key factor, maybe the biggest when it comes to aging along with your landscape. If you live in a rural or suburban area with an acre, maybe more, that's a lot of garden. Even an average city lot can be a challenge. However, it pays to think about how any landscape is laid out, how much is allotted to lawn, how much is cultivated, and, in some cases, how much can be left to its own devices.

This is the time to think about how much cultivated area and lawn you really need or want, and if there is a portion of your property that can do with minimal upkeep, or left a little wild around the edges.

In the next chapter there are suggestions for concentrating the cultivated areas of your garden closer to the house for easier maintenance. However, if the garden still looms too large, a move might be the best move. Or, a smaller garden could be just the ticket, but small does not have to diminish enjoyment.

Tastes Evolve, Needs Change

As you conclude the tour of your garden, make a formal approach to the front of your house to see how it feels to "arrive" home. If your walk-through netted only a few mentions of room for improvement, you might feel relief, and keen to keep on gardening in place. At this point you'll need to make realistic decisions about what you can do within your limitations and how much you are willing to, or can afford to, hire out. If you returned with a long laundry list of changes and repairs, you might feel overwhelmed and ready to let go.

Pollinator
Habitat
This space is planted with
native wildflowers and grasses
to provide habitat for
pollinators, birds and wildlife

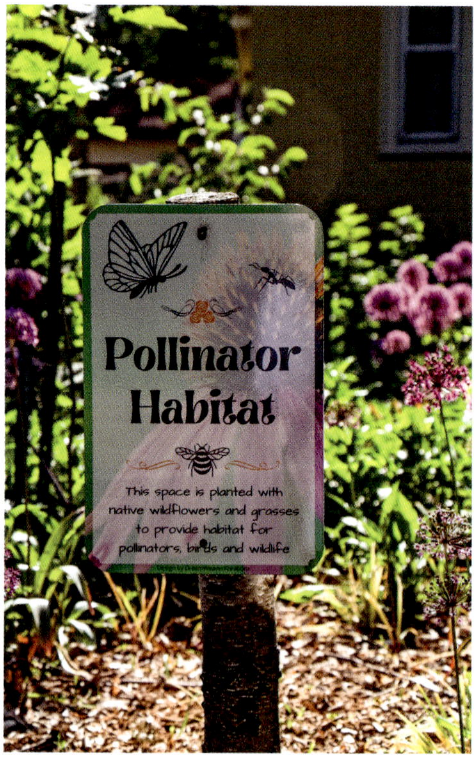

Planting for pollinators and wildlife makes for a more vibrant and biodiverse garden.

There are other factors besides maintenance that merit a change. The garden must be visually appealing to you. Tastes evolve, manicured gardens can seem stiff, sterile, and time-consuming as you learn more about pollinators and creating wildlife habitat. You might want a more naturalistic landscape with fewer demands and a different kind of pleasure. There are strategies for using more native plants and informal designs without offending the neighbors. Finding new ways to garden fits in with a healthy mindset and staying active and curious and open to change.

Twenty-five years ago, I certified my garden in Kansas as a Backyard Habitat through the National Wildlife Federation. This changed my whole thinking about how and why, and for whom, I was gardening. It was the impetus for my burgeoning interest in pollinators. Since then, I have certified my subsequent gardens as Monarch Waystations and Bee-Safe Yards, too. Pollinator Pathways is another opportunity. These programs offer additional ways to evaluate your garden for sustainability, by determining if there is food, water, shelter, and nesting sites for pollinators and backyard wildlife. You can certify a habitat without regard to size, whether a one-acre plot or a patio.

If you are still not sure about your gardening future, consulting a landscape architect can be very informative. Unlike landscape designers, landscape architects are trained in more than just hardscape and vegetation; they are experts who focus on how people utilize their landscapes and how they move through the various parts of their gardens. They can also identify site and structural problems as well as hidden assets. A quick one-hour visit could generate novel ideas for a whole new outdoor environment. Landscape architects (and designers) are discussed in detail in chapter 8.

There are just as many reasons to garden in place as there are to move on to a more manageable garden. Needs change—you might be empty nesters who no longer need a big lawn for playing kids, but you've decided to foster rescue dogs and need an even bigger one! Or maybe you no longer need a large vegetable garden and would be content growing herbs in containers on the patio. You might want to devote more backyard space to entertaining. Or maybe you've decided to plant more trees on your property to develop a personal arboretum. Not everyone is ready to downsize their ambitions as they age. In fact, some people choose to go big with a new gardening dream.

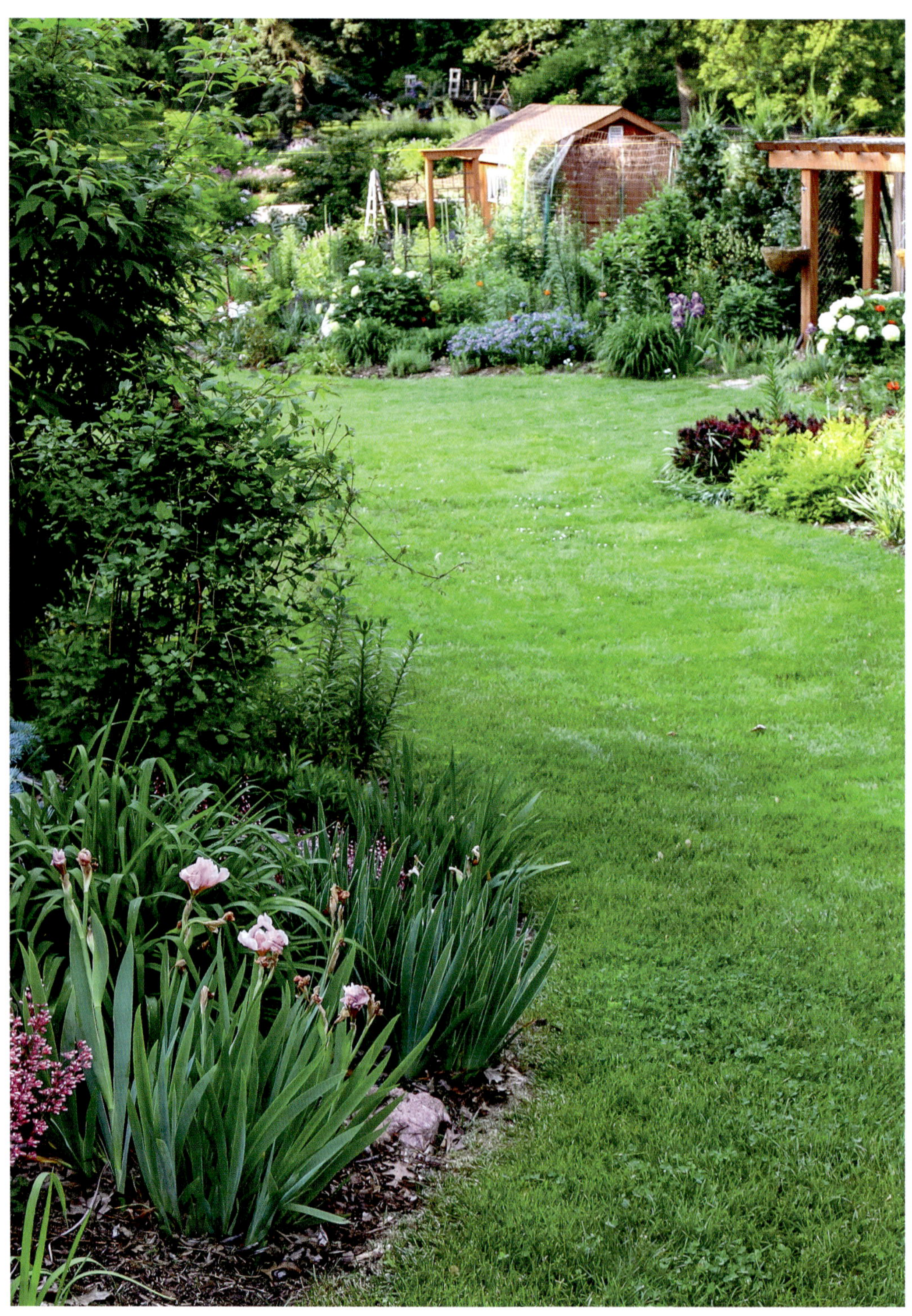

Maintaining a big, beautiful garden like this might become less doable—or desirable—over time.

CHAPTER 3

Deciding to Simplify, Downsize, or Move

Our homes and gardens are so closely connected that it's difficult to make a decision about one and not the other when thinking about the future. One scenario might satisfy the needs of aging in place while the other is all wrong, or vice versa. It seems straightforward to adapt and outfit a house for aging: eliminating trip and fall hazards, fixing rickety stairs, installing grab bars in the shower, enhancing lighting, reducing clutter, etc. By contrast, a home landscape is in constant flux at the whims of the weather and the changing seasons. Plants keep growing!

Talking with so many gardeners, I found each of their gardens was unique, but I heard common themes regarding their desire to continue gardening while making accommodations for a new reality. Folks told me they wanted to keep gardening, but not so intensely. They often felt overwhelmed by the garden and suffered anxiety when maintaining it became too much. A guilt-free garden was one of their goals. They wanted to focus on just the plants they loved. Many wanted freedom to travel without worrying about who would mow the lawn or shovel the snow. They all wanted to return to gardening as a joyful pastime rather than another line on the to-do list.

Just as no two homes or gardens are exactly alike, everyone has a different situation with health, family, income, and outlook. With that in mind, this chapter doesn't offer black-and-white solutions but rather suggestions for simplifying and rightsizing your existing garden, or, when it makes sense, making the move to a more perfect garden (and home) for you.

The Upside of Downsizing the Garden

Although many of us came by our interest in gardening at an early age, there probably was a time, perhaps around the time you hit forty, when your

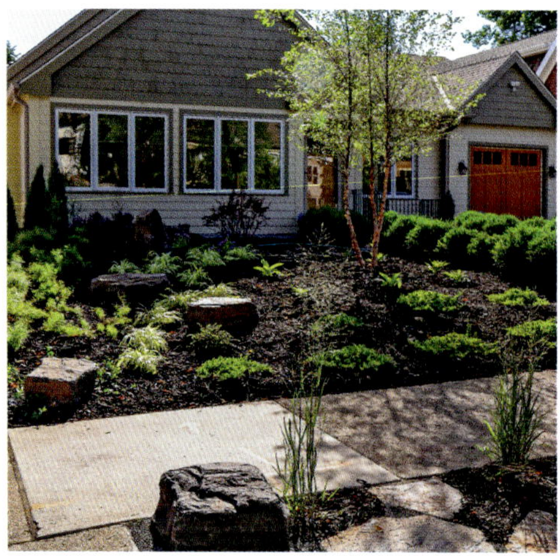

This new front garden is designed to be both beautiful and manageable—and there's no lawn to mow.

gardening passion began in earnest. It might have happened suddenly, as in one moment you were "down at the club" and the next thing you know you're swapping compost tips at parties. For twenty or more years you went hard, never missed a plant sale, sowed seeds like crazy, sought out unusual cultivars, dug hundreds of holes, and created your own personal Eden. Some might have described your gardening as overzealous, but what a muddy, exhilarating ride. Yet, somewhere in that journey, the garden became more a chore than a hobby. Now that it's time to downsize the garden, where do you begin?

Downsizing the garden can be emotional; you might even feel you've let down your plants. I compare it to the philosophy of Marie Kondo, who wrote *The Life-Changing Magic of Tidying Up*, a timely book that encourages a decluttering and organizing method that focuses on simplifying your home and life. Per her philosophy, your home should "spark joy." You can apply similar principles to the garden: paring down so that you can focus on the important stuff, ridding yourself of stress and feeling overwhelmed, and aiming for a more restorative environment.

There's a practical aspect, too, in making the garden more manageable: saving the best of it for the next generation. Grown children might live across the country or simply not be in a place to inherit such a project when they are busy with careers or raising children of their own. Younger homebuyers could be put off by an elaborate garden, although some are thrilled by the prospect. With this you are doing a favor to those who survive you while making the garden more enjoyable for you in the here and now. As I talked with people who rightsized their gardens, they all reported a sense of relief and renewed energy, as well as a fresh outlook for their gardening future.

Break It Down and Prioritize

According to psychologists, the longer you put off formidable tasks like this, the more likely you won't do them, ever. Whether you are doing it by yourself or enlisting help, it helps to make a plan by breaking down jobs like this into doable portions. Define your garden in zones by where you want to allocate time, money, and energy. Areas that are nearby and are seen every day should get the most attention. You should prioritize views from inside, too. As you go further out, the less care those zones should need.

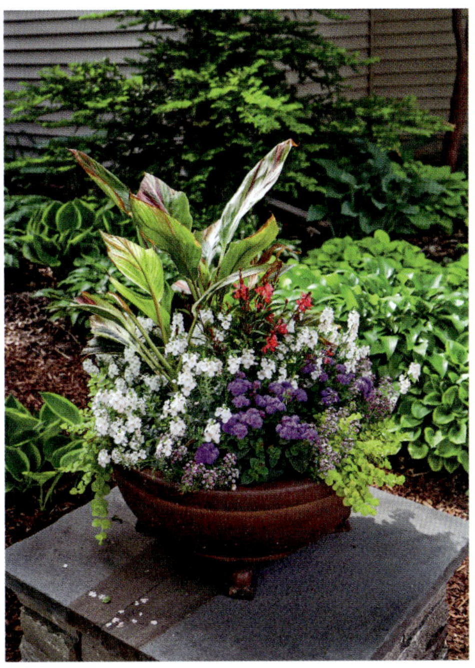

Place containers so they can be viewed from both inside and outside.

Focus on those closest areas first. Consolidate the "keepers" whenever possible, and try to showcase favorite plants in new ways in containers or prime viewing spots. Some people will tell you to cut down on containers, while others will say double down and do more than ever. You'll have to search your heart for the answer that is right for you. Keep the most demanding plants close to the house and near a water source, or perhaps ditch the divas altogether. Pay attention to microclimates, such as extra-warm or sheltered spots (or whatever conditions are favorable in your area), around the house and use them to your advantage.

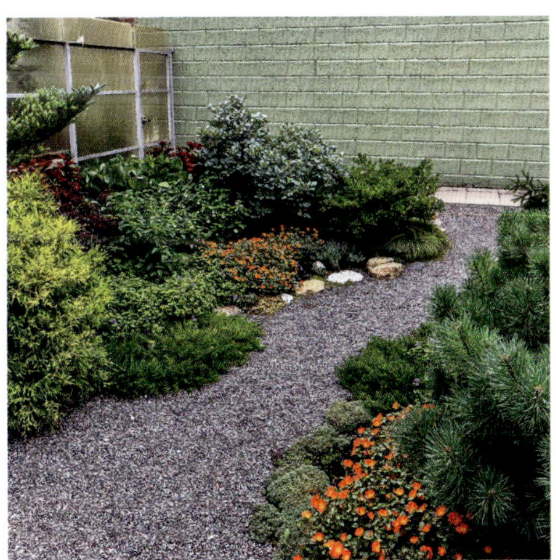

This stylish urban courtyard benefits from its warm, sheltered microclimate.

Depending upon how your property is arranged, determine if you can let the back forty get by on its own or with minimal care, letting it go a little wild around the edges. This might hinge on how your neighbors, if any, feel about it. Perhaps they've been waiting and wanting to do it themselves? An over-the-fence neighborly chat will smooth the way.

For those areas and large borders and beds farther from the house, replace perennials with shrubs, evergreens, ornamental grasses, and smaller trees. The idea is to fill up space with low-maintenance plants

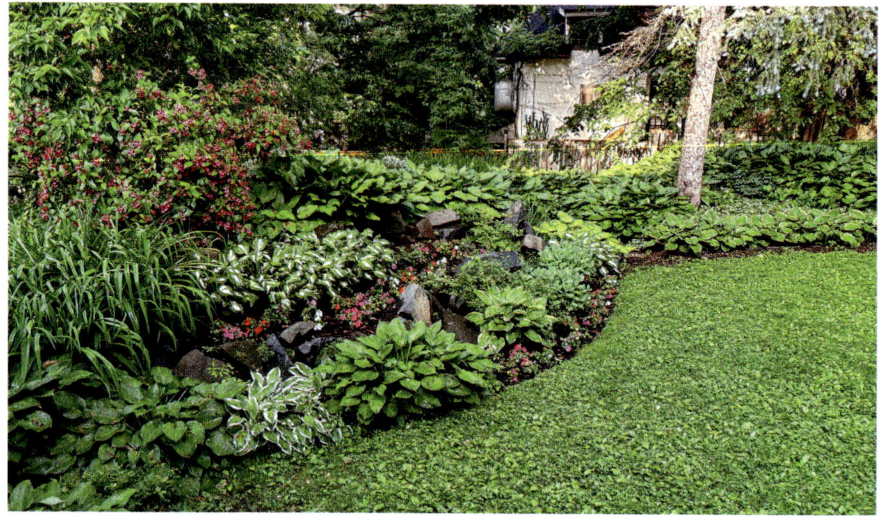

This large back garden is tidier up front and left wilder in the back. *Photo courtesy of Donna Hamilton*

without leaving it barren. In fact, you might find the opposite, that birds find it a welcoming habitat. While clearing out planted areas, it's a great time to apply compost and other nutrients to refresh the soil.

So, what does this look like in real life? Follow along here and in the next chapters as real gardeners find workable solutions to the next phase of their gardening lives.

Rightsizing a New Garden

Rightsizing a new garden at a new home, whether you are starting from scratch or working with an existing garden, can be both exciting and daunting. I've moved enough to know that you should give the home and garden a grace period before you dive in with new ideas. Let the garden speak to you. Observe it at different times of day or, if you can stand it, through a few seasons. But as time marches on, who wants to wait to create your new and improved patch of paradise?

Here is your chance to design a safe, comfortable, and accessible garden. Begin with a plan. Think about how you will use the new landscape. Will it be a sanctuary, a party place, a vegetable garden, or a little of all three? Decide how it will connect to the house, where the landing zones are, and what the pathways lead to. Balance the plantings with the scale of the home and in keeping with its architectural style. And what about the work: Can you do it in phases or hire a crew to do it all at once? Top of mind, how does it all fit with an ambitious but aging gardener?

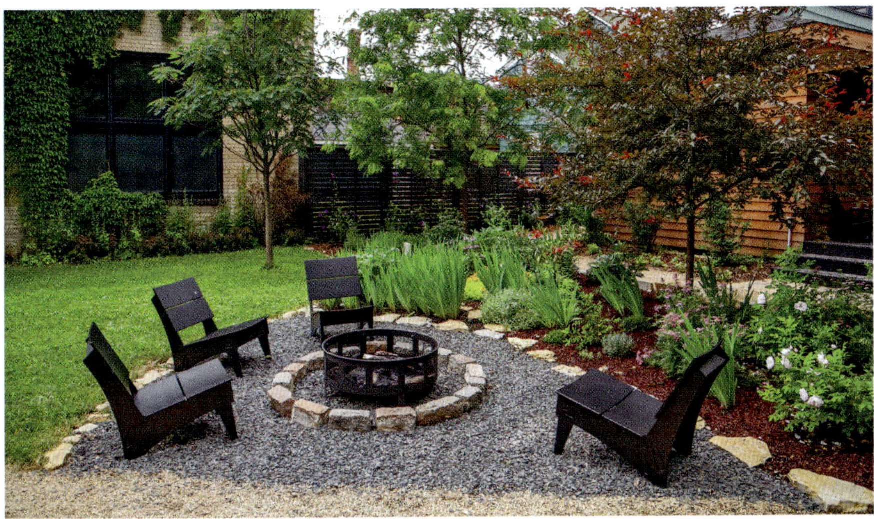

Concentrate cultivated parts of the garden closer to the house.

Look at neighboring gardens and note which ones you find attractive and what plants are thriving, what elements you might use in your new design, or what you might overhaul. Evaluate existing trees and shrubs for health and how they benefit the overall landscape to know what to keep and what to remove or replace. Begin the design with tree placement to get a sense of how light and shade fall. Ask yourself how much lawn you need, if any. These will be big determining factors going forward. Until you have a cohesive plan, quell your plant cravings with container plantings; they are much easier to undo than digging up a tree.

Downsizing Your Home

Moving to a townhouse, condo, or apartment doesn't have to mean giving up gardening for good. Do your homework and you could find yourself with a Goldilocks garden—just right for this time of life. However, it might be an adjustment living in a community setting where certain rules and regulations apply, such as what color you can paint your front door and what you can plant. Read those rules carefully before you sign on the dotted line.

HOA rules can be subject to the whims of those in charge, and board members change as the years go by. You might also be at the mercy of neighbors' varying tastes and ideas. You can often win people over if you explain the motivation behind your gardening efforts, such as supporting pollinators and attracting songbirds.

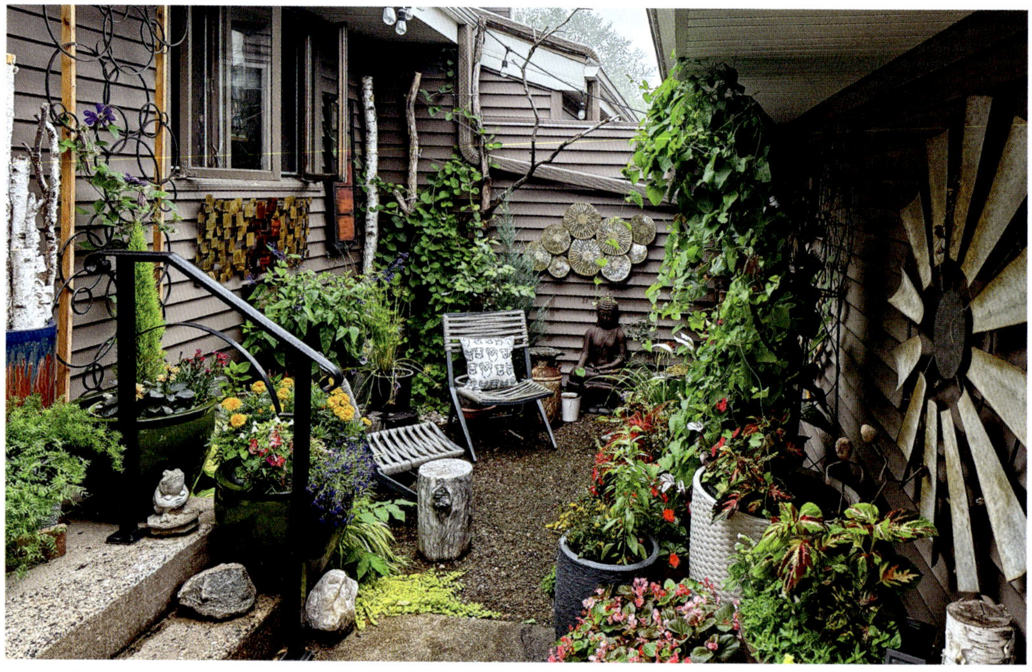

Eric Johnson makes the most of his town house's courtyard. *Photo courtesy of Eric Johnson*

When looking for a townhouse, condo, or apartment, it pays to do more than one drive-through. Get a sense of the vibe during different times of the day. Look for traffic patterns, noise levels, parking, and the general condition of any amenities. Take a walk and see whether people are out and about. Is it a collection of buttoned-up buildings, or does it feel warm and welcoming? And, most important for green thumbs, look on the balconies, decks, porches, patios, and front steps to see if there are signs that people are growing things.

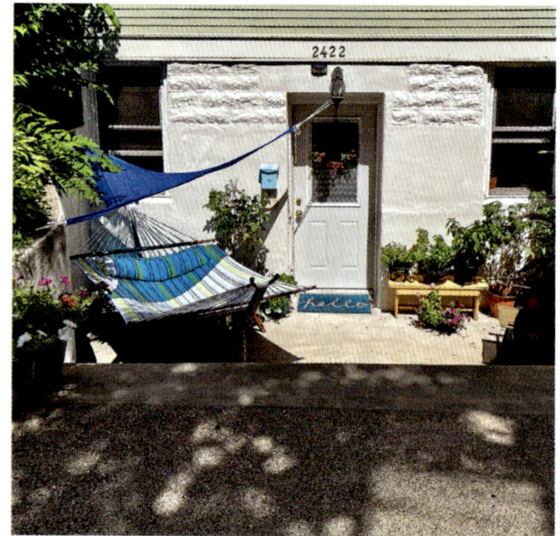

A garden grows at the front door of this garden level apartment.

GARDENING ON HIGH (FLOORS)

I always like to scan apartment balconies when I pass by to see what's growing up there. Some people have a few pots while others go full-tilt and tend a lush jungle in a small space. I applaud their efforts and always send a good thought upward, wishing them happy gardening adventures.

When choosing an apartment with the hope of balcony gardening, there are a few things to consider before moving in. First of all, think about how high you will go; wind can be a challenge, and the higher you go the stronger the wind. On the ground, friction from obstacles like buildings and trees slows down wind, but as you ascend, the influence of these ground-level obstacles decreases, leading to faster wind speed and, at times, a wind tunnel effect. It will quickly dry out plants and possibly knock them over. It might also determine how much you will enjoy sitting out there with your plants.

Think about what type of plants you want to grow, keeping in mind the exposure; a sunny south side will be extra hot if additional heat is reflected off the windows or radiated from the building. Add strong wind and you better choose tough plants. An exposure with afternoon shade might be more ideal.

Also consider how you will move and water the plants. Wet soil is heavy, so plan to use lightweight containers and soil (you can always add nutrients to a soilless mix). Is there an elevator to facilitate hauling soil and plants? Containers need frequent watering; is there a spigot, or will you have to use a watering can? If there's a water source, a drip system will help out. But make sure the plants don't drip on neighbors below.

With all that said, there's a plethora of no-weed, no-bend plant options using containers and vertical methods: houseplants in summer, an herb and salad garden, tomatoes, annual flowers, foliage plants, and more. Depending upon your climate, you might even be able to grow small shrubs or trees in containers.

Community Garden Plots

Dowling Community Garden sits close to West River Parkway in Minneapolis, the scenic road along the Mississippi River where my husband and I walked our dog for miles during the pandemic. It is one of the last two original Victory Gardens in the US; the other one is in Boston. Started in 1943 to help the war effort, the Minneapolis garden continues to offer almost 200 residents the opportunity to grow their own bounty in a safe and beautiful space while building community. According to the Trust for Public Land neighborhood gardening statistics, there are over 29,000 community garden plots in city parks in the 100 largest US cities.

A community garden plot can replace or supplement a home garden, helping gardeners with different living situations keep their fingers in the dirt and healthy food on their table. These plots are popular; if you are considering one, don't procrastinate, as lots of them have waiting lists.

Every garden is different, but you'll find they all encourage you to respect your neighbor, maintain your plot, avoid pesticides, keep paths clear, and obey water rules. When looking for a community garden that fits your needs, be sure to get the scoop on watering and where the spigots are located. I once inquired about a garden plot that didn't have a piped water source, but they cheerfully assured me there was a creek nearby. At Dowling, longtime gardener Jeffrey Loesch designed and helped implement a system where no gardener is more than 100′ (30 m) from a faucet.

Other requirements might include minimum service hours to common areas, background checks, planting and cleanup deadlines, and restrictions on subletting or transferring plots without approval. Some community gardens serve people with special needs or disabilities. Excess produce might be donated to food banks and other programs.

Learning from other gardeners is one of the advantages of community gardening. Experienced folks will tell you to start small and plant crops that don't need lots of attention, since you might not always visit as frequently as you would like. While things like beans and peas need picking every day once they start producing, it's better to stick with crops that can "sit"—cabbage, eggplant, kale, onions, garlic, leeks, peppers, potatoes, beets, and chard. Tomatoes need more tending, as do cutting flowers.

Community gardens grow more than produce; they create all-important social connection, provide exposure to diverse cultures and foods, promote

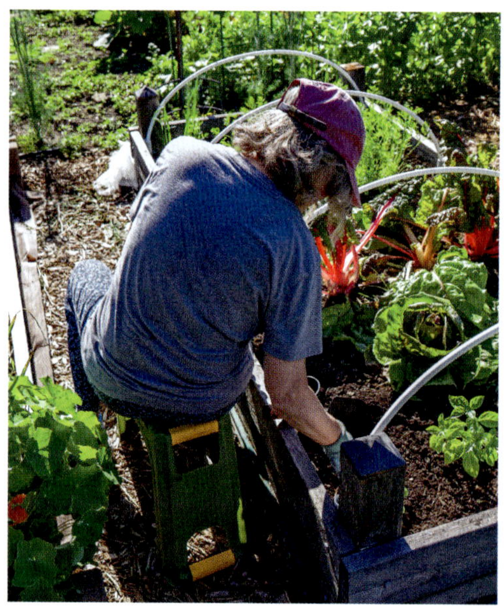

Biology professor Mary Montgomery secured a plot at Dowling just as COVID-19 struck. The garden served as a safe social outlet for her through that time.

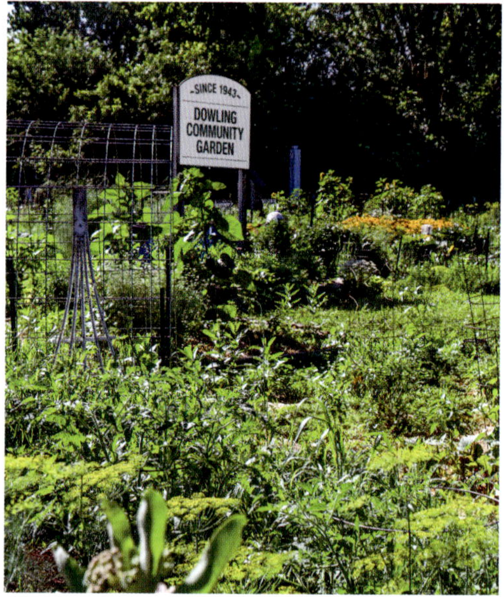

Dowling Community Garden in Minneapolis.

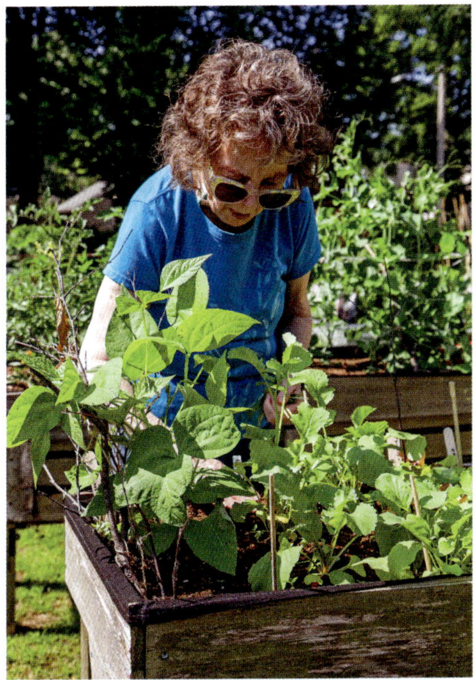

Hennepin County Master Gardener Flo Golod tending her tabletop garden.

sustainable practices, and extend outreach and education. In a booklet my neighbor brought back from Sweden (where the government encourages community gardening for exactly those reasons), one gardener exclaims, "*Här har man sommar vänner*"—Here you have summer friends!

What are you waiting for? Apply for a plot right now!

Senior Living, Still Gardening

As my fellow Master Gardener Flo Golod describes it, there are 200 apartments in the Nokomis Square Cooperative Senior Living Community, housing around "300 souls," and three gardening committees. She and

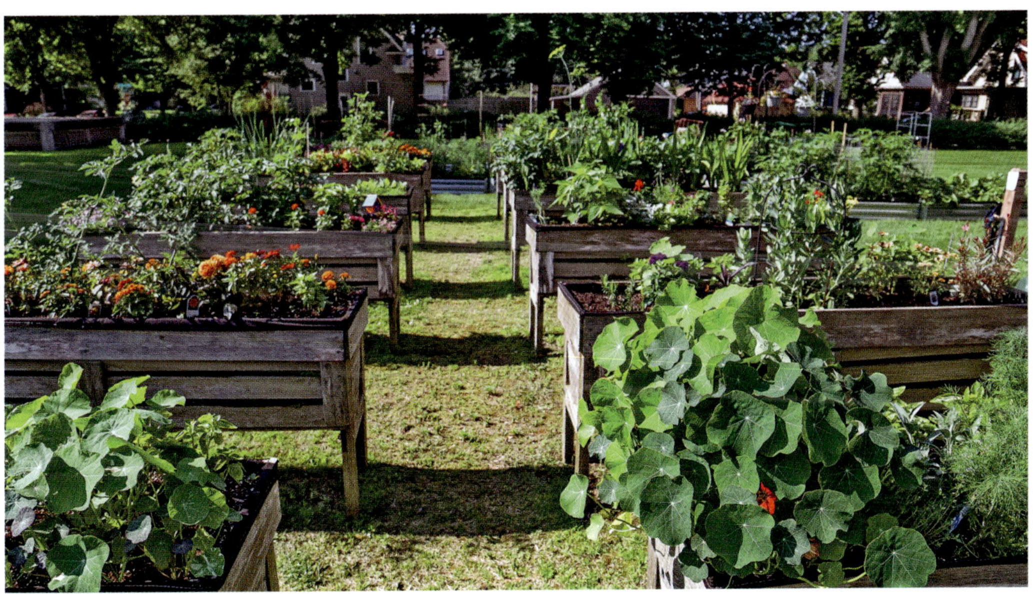

Elevated gardens are a popular amenity at Nokomis Square Cooperative Senior Living Community.

GARDENER SPOTLIGHT
Mary Yee

My fellow Master Gardener Mary Yee and her husband, Paul, are still in the process of creating the new garden at the house they recently built, designing it with sustainability as well as aging in mind. They took a long time searching for a flat lot, as they were keen to avoid slopes and icy steps, although this was hard to find in the hilly St. Paul neighborhood where they landed.

Mary left behind a lush landscape she had tended for years, including 80 peonies. Wisely, she made sure to include a line in the sales contract stating that she could remove any plants she wanted, and she ended up taking some of the peonies with her. She was still sad to leave her pawpaw trees and heavenly scented Korean viburnum, which were too established to transplant.

Known for growing a wide range of plants, including some not recommended for the far north, Mary impresses people with her diverse plant collection. I am always in awe of her vast plant knowledge. However, not everyone is so admiring; she once had a neighbor tell her she had too many plants. Thankfully, her new neighborhood is more environmentally conscious and tolerant of different garden styles.

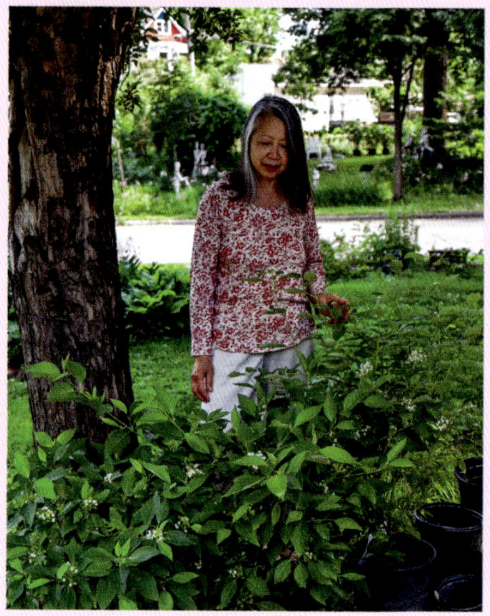

another Master Gardener, Doris Wickstrom, both moved in at the same time four years ago. Flo came from a bigger house and garden, with a smaller one in between, while Doris came from a townhouse where she was allowed to garden on three sides of the property. They both feel that it all became too much, and that it was sad to leave. As Doris said, "You build up all these tools and plants, your plant inventory that's so dear to you." It was hard to give up, but they knew they could garden at their new home.

Their community has extensive flower gardens tended by the seniors at the front and back entries of the high-rise residence. Out back are a series of elevated garden beds they refer to as "tabletops" filled with flowers, herbs,

Even though Minnesota is the Land of 10,000 Lakes, several years of drought have motivated Mary to think about water usage at this new address. There is little lawn, and what is there is pollinator friendly: a bee lawn that borders perennials, shrubs, and trees, along with groundcovers. Eschewing an irrigation system, she is trying to match new plants to the site according to their water requirements. Mary and Paul are still evaluating sun and shade patterns as they make plant selections and decisions about existing trees to minimize heating and AC needs.

Mary is substituting shrubs for many perennials to create more structure, citing her lower level of energy as she grows older. She's okay with this because there are so many great shrubs, including native species. As she tells it, "Despite advancing age—I just turned 67—I am still planting for the future . . . new trees, including sure things like many pagoda dogwoods and red buds, and iffy things like Metasequoia and Japanese maples." You can tell she still likes to gamble with the planting zones!

She has about 30 pawpaw seedlings from the fruits off her old trees that will enable her to plant a little grove in the new garden. She will donate the rest of the seedlings to other Master Gardeners who are interested in this native American fruit, and to the city forester who is nurturing and planting saplings grown from Mary's offerings.

Rest assured this new, smaller garden will be low-maintenance but still high-interest. After all, during Mary's extensive international travels, her favorite souvenirs to buy are seeds.

MARY'S TIPS FOR CREATING AND ENJOYING A NEW GARDEN

- Pay attention; take a second and take in your natural surroundings. Something as simple as a pollinating bee on a flower could spark a shift in mindset.
- Try to plant a garden that's friendly to nature—for bees and other pollinators.
- Avoid pesticides.

and vegetables. Beyond that are in-ground beds, the result of Flo and Doris' lobbying efforts. With more potential gardeners than beds, there are hopes to make even more beds. However, people trade beds and switch from raised to elevated beds according to their circumstances. Everyone here is considered independent. One woman still tends another garden at her cabin. Another uses a walker but doesn't let that stop her from caring for her tabletop garden.

Although Doris, 79, would like a bit more space for growing fresh vegetables, she and Flo agree that this arrangement satisfies their gardening needs. Doris has packed her beds full; besides tomatoes and eggplant, she

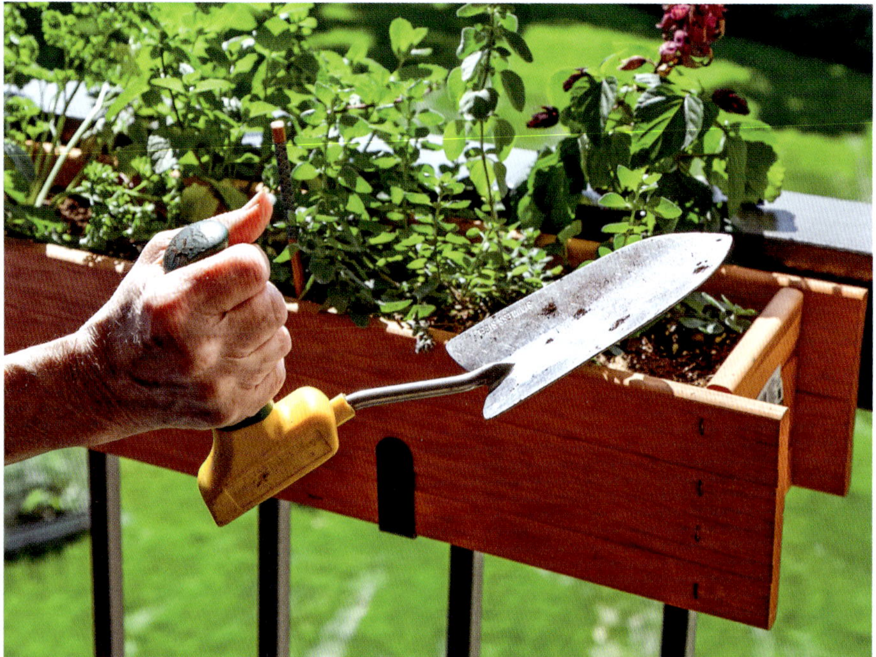

Flo uses an ergonomic Easi-Grip trowel for her balcony garden where she grows herbs in small troughs and pots.

likes to grow Asian long beans and is trying Albanian cucumbers. Flo switched apartments to gain a balcony for more plants. She can grow herbs in her tabletop bed below as well as on the balcony above and has found that the basil is happier with the hot, sunny exposure of the balcony. Doris explains that the balcony next to Flo's is surprisingly shady, and the neighbor there grows begonias. This is a good example of how balcony conditions can vary, so you should think about what you want to grow.

Moving to a senior living facility doesn't have to be the end of the road for gardening but rather an opportunity to do it differently. In fact, Flo, 77, still teaches two online gardening classes. As she tells it, "Everyone here brings their own gardening experience, and we all learn from each other."

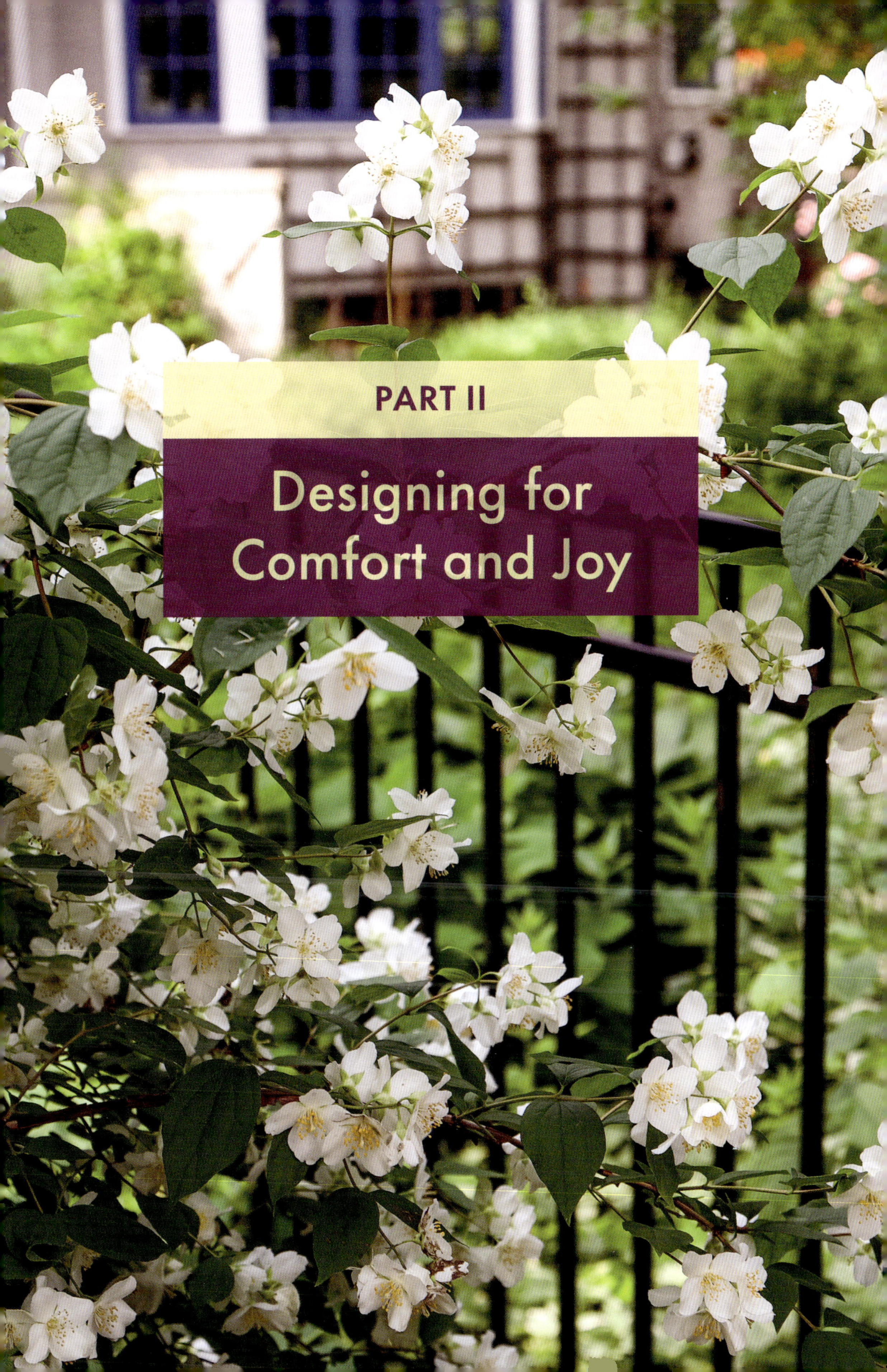

PART II

Designing for Comfort and Joy

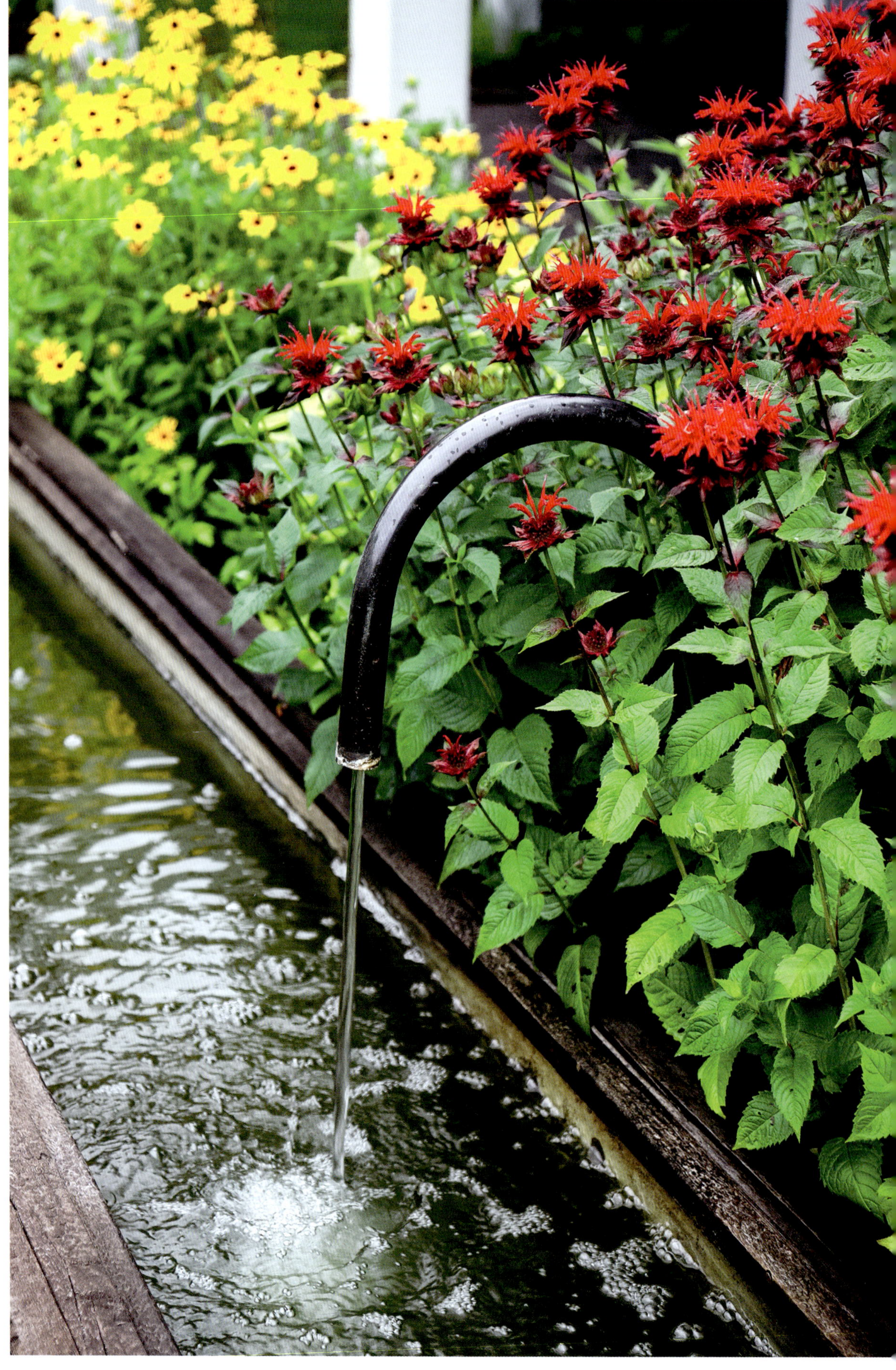

CHAPTER 4

Garden Diversions (Beyond Plants)

Every day in the garden is different. There are moments that come and go—sunlight shining through paper-thin petals of a certain bloom, a migrating bird passing through, new shade patterns as a tree stretches outward, an uncommon bee species spied on a blossom. When I experience one of these small events, I remind myself: You won't see these things if you aren't out here. You can't live in the garden 24-7 but you can make it more inviting, so you don't miss those life-affirming moments that contribute to greater longevity.

If you called a carpenter, plumber, and electrician to renovate a fixer-upper, each would approach it through their own eyes and expertise. The carpenter might move a wall, the plumber transform the bath into a spa, and the electrician install dramatic lighting. When rethinking a garden, gardeners will gravitate first to plants as a solution. It might seem counterintuitive, but making the garden more welcoming could require more hardscape elements and fewer plants. You're not paving over paradise; you're making it easier to get out there and more enjoyable once you do.

Create an Oasis with a Water Feature

Water is life. A spiritual and symbolic component of many cultures, it adds a new dimension to a garden, providing beauty and tranquility along with practical benefits. Even the smallest offering brings life to the garden. Add water and a simple patio becomes a sanctuary; the relaxing sounds of water can mask outside noise, and its movement releases negative ions. Negative ions are odorless, tasteless, and invisible molecules that we inhale in abundance in certain environments. Think mountains, waterfalls, and beaches. They are believed to produce biochemical reactions that increase levels of the mood chemical serotonin, helping to alleviate depression, relieve stress, and boost our daytime energy.

Important to seniors who are heat-sensitive, water has a cooling effect that happens through evaporation. As water evaporates, it absorbs heat from the surrounding air, which can create a microclimate that is slightly cooler than the general environment. At the same time, it increases humidity in the air, which can help to make the air feel cooler, especially in dry climates.

But not all is peaceful and relaxed; expect wildlife to appear once water is in the mix. Birds, frogs, and dragonflies are among the visitors you can count upon to show up, boosting biodiversity in your garden and taking the vibrancy level up a few notches. You'll find yourself heading outside more to enjoy their company.

There are many ways to incorporate water into your garden, from simple fountains to traditional inground garden ponds. Ponds are wonderful but can be lots of work, and possibly dangerous for older people to maintain. Pondless features that recirculate water without a visible pond are a better solution. They are designed for smaller gardens and are perfect for courtyards and patios. Water contained in an inground or hidden reservoir is pumped out as a fountain or waterfall, then flows back down into the reservoir. They require less cleaning and maintenance than traditional ponds, as they don't accumulate algae or debris as quickly, and the absence of a pond makes them safer for older gardeners, children, and pets. And birds love them.

Pondless water features come in different configurations. The most common are tall ceramic urns, with water spilling onto a bed of polished pebbles below. Stone basalt columns of varying sizes offer a natural look. Water walls are another form. You'll want to match the style to your home and garden. Another aspect to consider is its "water song." Determine what water sound is most pleasant to your ears. Depending upon the feature, water will bubble, gurgle, spill, or spray. The distance between the feature and where you'll spend the most time outside will affect the sound volume.

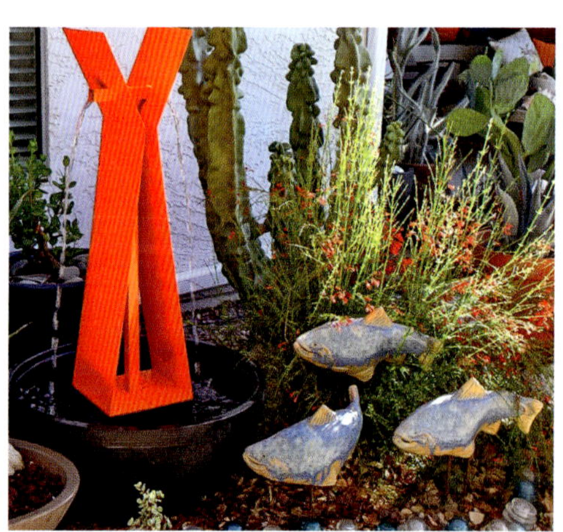

This sculptural fountain cools off a desert patio. *Photo courtesy of Shawna Coronado*

Be aware that some pondless features require a hole for an

inground reservoir, and anything with a pump needs an electrical source, so you might need a professional installation, but after that cost is minimal. Energy consumption for this type of electric pump is low compared to other household appliances.

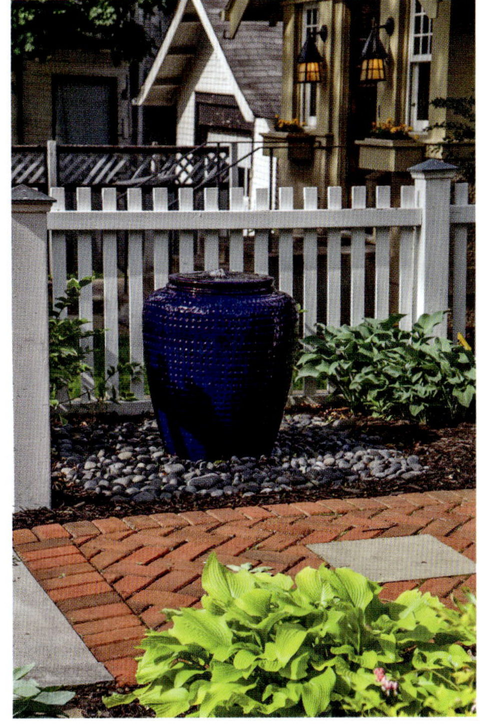

Pondless water features offer gentle splashing sounds and attract birds to your garden.

If you want to have water plants and a few fish, you'll want to go the no-dig route. Small aboveground water features, or patio ponds, made of fiberglass or metal offer almost instant gratification. Once it's set up (exactly where you want it, since you can't move it once it's filled), you can add plants of different heights and growth habits—some have shelves for easy placement of plants that require different water depths. Place rocks and gravel at the bottom to naturalize the look and provide habitat if you plan to have fish. You can add a spitter for interest, and motion to keep mosquitos at bay; the fish will help with this, too.

If you live in a cold climate, you'll need to accommodate for the fish and bring them inside when the temperature drops. My metal pond is built into the patio and is not deep enough for fish to hibernate in freezing temps. And since we go away in the winter, I found a nice lady on Nextdoor.com—she's in my phone as "Trish for Fish"—who takes the goldfish or small koi for her aquariums at the end of the season. I get to enjoy them for the summer, and she acquires new fish for her growing aquatic menagerie.

Make Waystations for Respite

Traveling backroads around the country you still come across basic rest stops called waystations, an old-fashioned word for a stopping point in a journey. These are usually nothing more than a few picnic tables on the side of the road, but sometimes that's all you need. A place to refresh and gather your wits before carrying on. Why not a waystation, or two, for your garden?

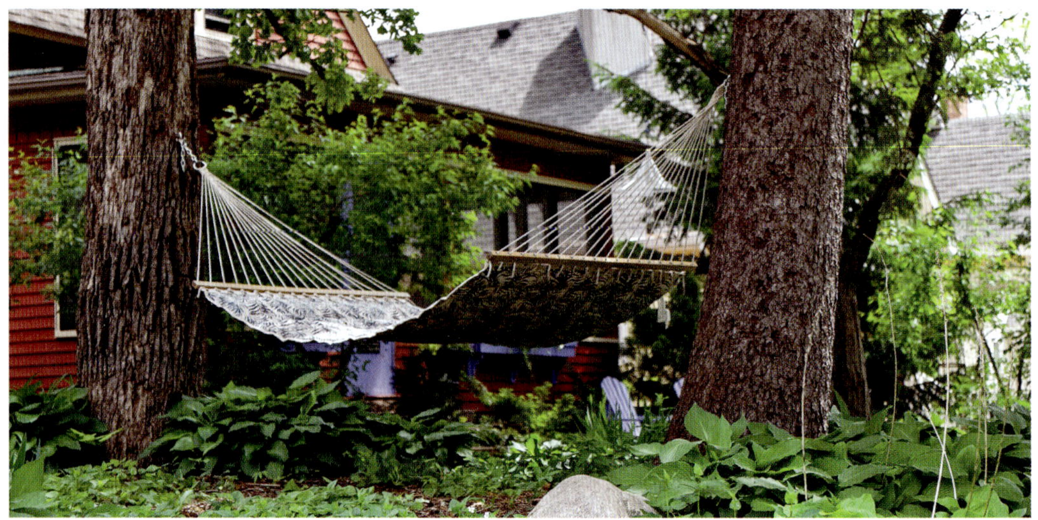

Hammocks promise a moment of rest and relaxation, but make sure they are hung low and above soft ground. You might need a spotter or helper to get in and out.

You can also have resting spots for when you're staying on your feet. A decorative garden totem, art pole, newel post from an old staircase, or any other sturdy vertical structure can function as an accent piece as well as a place to lean on. You can make your own or find them at craft fairs and flea markets. Occasionally you just need to grab on to, or rest against, a solid object while you center yourself, like when you get lightheaded rising up from a kneeling or seated position (a side effect of some medications). Other times, you need a bit of support to steady yourself while thinking about your next garden task.

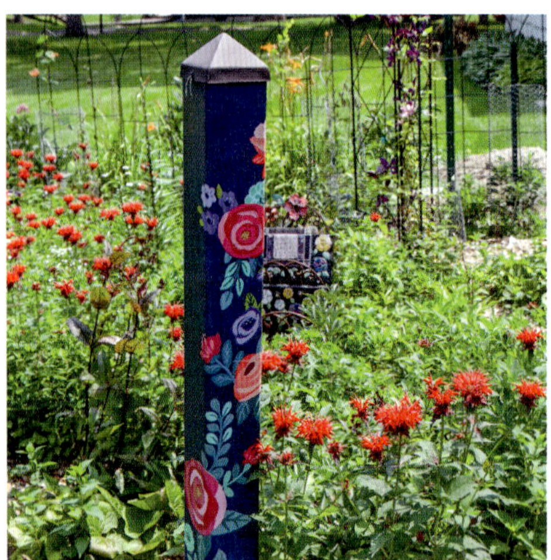

Decorative posts or poles make great garden accents as well as a "shoulder" to lean on.

A leaning post can be embedded or anchored into concrete for permanence, or it can be supported with rebar (metal reinforcing rod used in concrete work), a tree-stand base, or other type of anchor. If a suitable material, a post can also be partially buried in the ground like a fence post. When you aren't using your stand-up waystation, birds will use it as a perch. Birds like perches for various reasons, including observation, resting, and as a natural part of their behavior.

Make Way for Monarchs!

Speaking of waystations and wildlife, is your garden a certified monarch waystation? Everyone knows that monarch butterflies are in serious need of assistance as they make their miraculous migration. Here is a summary of the guidelines for setting up your own monarch waystation.

- A recommended minimum of 100 square feet (30 m) of area, which can be divided among multiple sites; ideally areas that receive at least six hours of sun daily.
- Ten or more milkweed plants of at least two different species to provide season-long habitat.
- Nearby nectar plants that bloom all summer; can be annual, biennial, or perennial.
- A plan for maintaining and sustaining the waystation and its plants, such as weeding and thinning like in any garden.
- A saucer of mud or wet sand for puddling, from which butterflies siphon salt and minerals.

By registering your monarch waystation you join the over 50,000 other backyard conservationists and citizen scientists in doing your part. You can also purchase a metal sign that identifies your monarch habitat as an official waystation. This display helps convey the importance of monarch conservation to all those who visit your habitat and might encourage them to create their own. More information is available online through the program website (see Resources, page 213).

Design a Dedicated Destination

Destinations in your garden differ from waystations in that you are visiting these places for a purpose, rather than a quick rest. Sure, having an outdoor eating area, a grill, or even an outdoor kitchen for dining al fresco is a no-brainer, but there are other activities that merit a special nook or corner—away from the main gathering spot—to help you make full use of your garden space.

As discussed in chapter 3, one solution for rightsizing a garden is to concentrate cultivated areas closer to the house, leaving the farthest reaches to get by with less maintenance or perhaps to rewild. Another option is to utilize more of this area and create secondary sites for whatever you like: relaxation, hobbies, exercise, reading, meditation, yoga, or just sitting and enjoying a cup of coffee or tea. Set it up with an easel for plein air painting or a daybed for napping, or create a quiet place to use your Merlin bird app and listen for birdsong. Build a place to picnic with your grandkids—all the ingredients for a backyard staycation. Maybe you want to sink into the latest garden trend with an outdoor bathtub!

Add a public-facing destination to the front yard for more opportunities for that social connection so important for a long life. It can be as simple as placing a pair of Adirondack chairs out front—you might meet neighbors you didn't know you had.

Even a smaller garden can provide opportunities to make what one Master Gardener called "nodes of interest." Our friends Christine Scotillo and Doug Peine have created such a garden, a combination of craft and choreography. She designs and he builds. Within the bounds of their backyard, there's a circular deck cantilevered over a large pond for daydreaming, another smaller deck to the side for drinks, a pebble mosaic "rug" denoting another zone for reading or quiet time, a shaded table for dining, and then a firepit with a cozy "inglenook" fashioned from wooden pallets. Lush greenery separates each node. When you visit for a

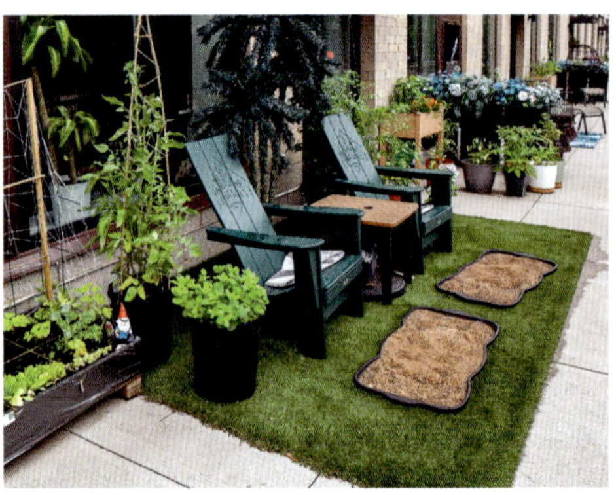

Apartment living doesn't stop these folks from "going to the lake" while also growing container veggies on their charming patio.

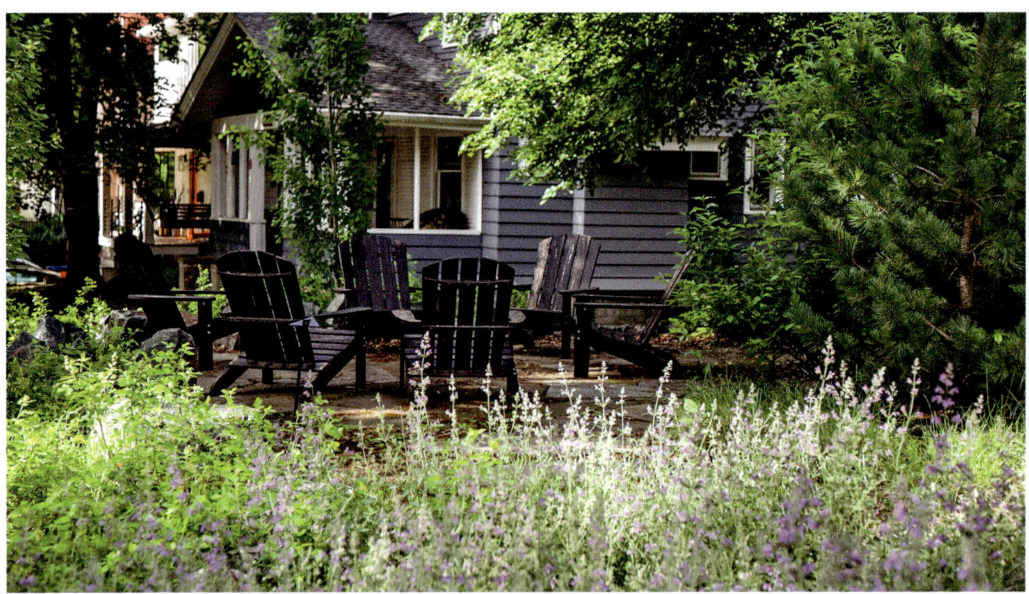

A front yard gathering place to meet with neighbors and greet passersby.

meal, it's like a progressive dinner in different settings, yet you never leave the property.

So many of us like to make the rounds every day to check on our garden, no matter our abilities. A series of small destinations on a patio or courtyard—container plantings, vignettes of garden collectibles, a grotto or altar, even a simple labyrinth—can establish a daily ritual or comforting routine for older gardeners with limited mobility or cognitive issues.

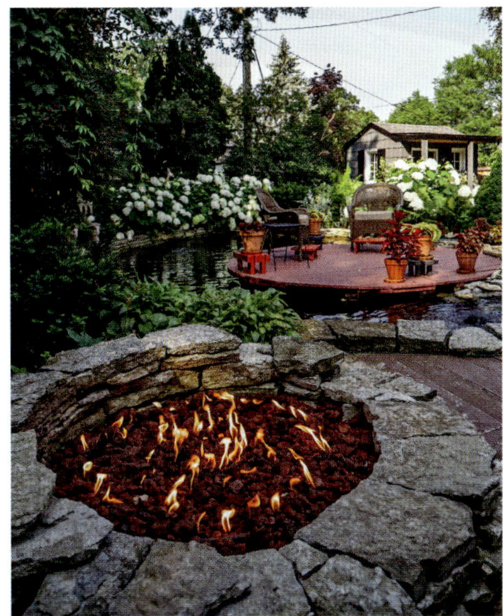

The waterfront deck in Doug Peine and Christine Scotillo's backyard is perfect for unwinding and daydreaming.

Circular paths offer a sense of accomplishment, as walkers or wheelchair users return to their starting point feeling they've completed a loop. While some prefer the feeling of accomplishment and predictability of circular paths, others prefer the sense of achievement from linear paths. Knowing the route's length and having a sense of the remaining distance can be reassuring.

Let the Games Begin

Make better use of your lawn (or do away with an uninspired planting area) and make a "playground," a place where you set up simple backyard games like ring toss, cornhole (they call it "bags" here Up North), horseshoes, croquet, ladder golf, or giant versions of Connect Four or Jenga. Set up one game or make a circuit of several. These low-impact games can be adapted for individuals with varying mobility levels and don't require intense physical exertion. An added benefit: Strategic thinking and problem-solving within the games help keep the mind sharp.

Grandkids aren't mandatory, but having a dedicated play zone is a great way to lure kids off screens and into a garden setting. Sure, the games might seem old-fashioned, but that's the beauty of it; the rules are straightforward and can be grasped quickly by everyone, regardless of their athletic ability or prior experience with similar games. These simple diversions encourage gentle competition and camaraderie that can reduce stress and improve mood in the best of times; they also offer a great alternative to tense

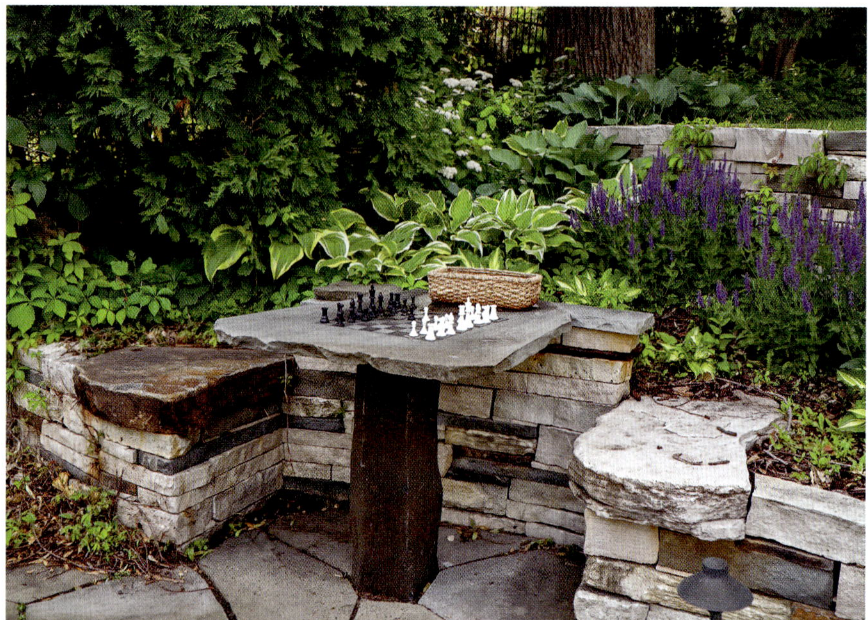

Chess in the garden.

dynamics that can occur at some gatherings of family or friends. Just being in the garden takes down the temperature.

Make sure the playing surface is stable and level and there are no lumps in the grass—caused by critters like gophers, moles, and voles—that create a trip hazard. Some people are serious about their backyard games and use rubber matting or synthetic turf (forgivable in this situation) or even go as far as poured-in-place (PIP) rubber surfacing for dedicated areas devoted to fun.

On the quiet side, outdoor chess offers fresh air in combination with a brain challenge, as well as the potential for social connection. Oversize sets give an Alice in Wonderland vibe to the landscape.

Admire Art in Your Garden

Not all garden solutions involve plants. Artwork can be a low-maintenance element with big impact. Using art in your garden does more than add beauty. It can heighten visual interest, provide a unique focal point, and enhance a garden's overall aesthetic—all without the need for deadheading. Garden art can add a touch of whimsy or invite deeper contemplation. It can be silly or serious or somewhere in between, a vehicle for self-expression or perhaps a home for a piece by your favorite local artist.

Garden art can take many forms, such as a statue or sculpture, or functional art like a birdbath, bench, or sundial. It can be DIY, maybe a scarecrow

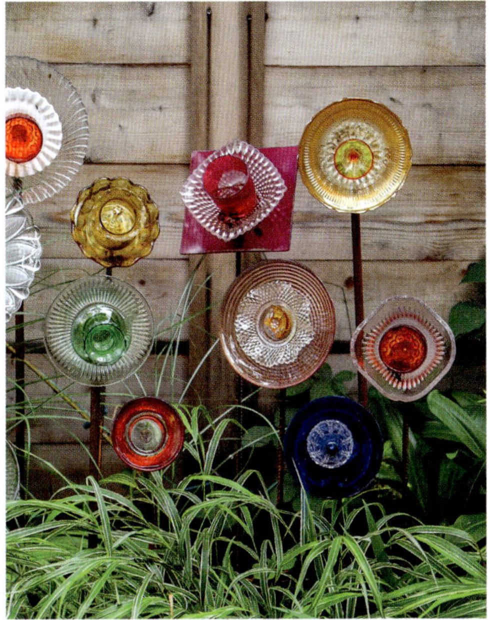

Garden art: flowers that don't need deadheading.

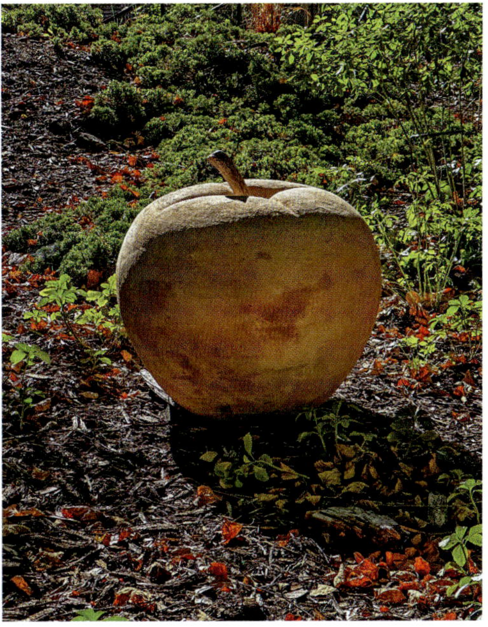

This apple sculpture draws the eye when the garden is resting.

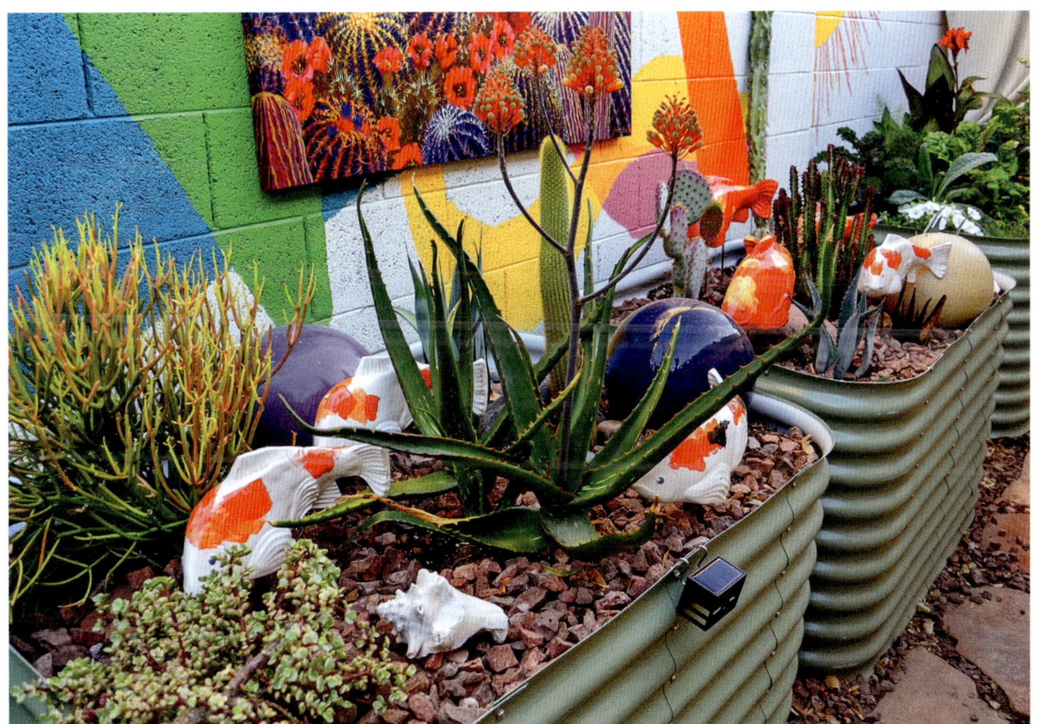

Outdoor paintings and decorative fish in Shawna Coronado's side yard art gallery. *Photo courtesy of Shawna Coronado*

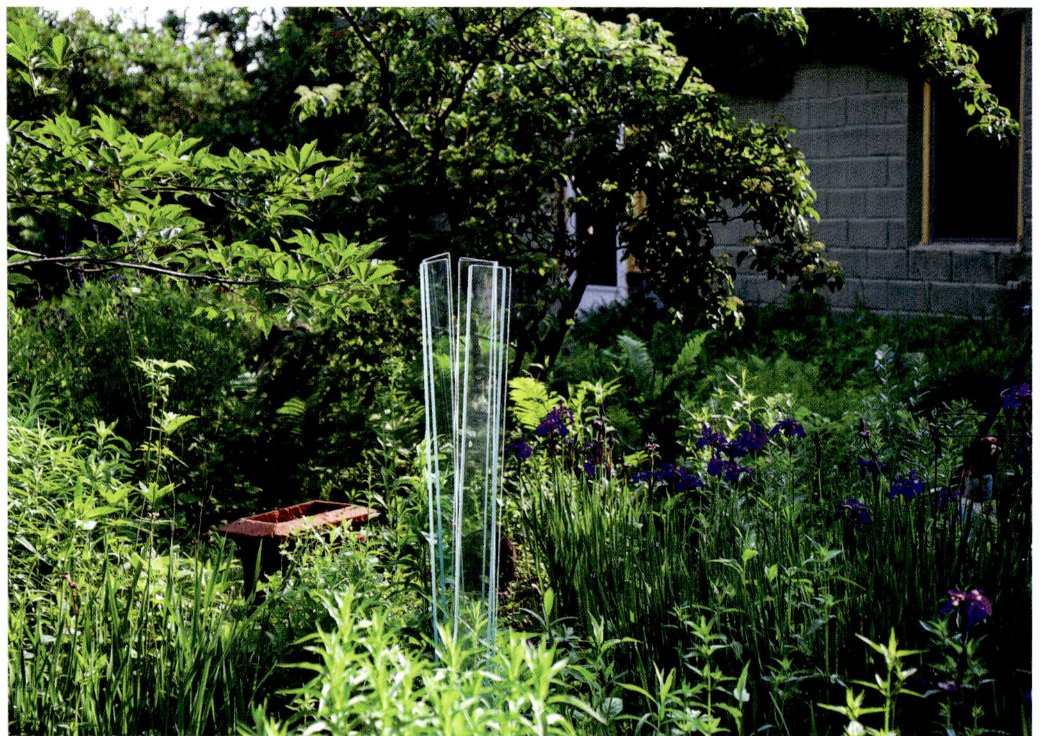

This glass sculpture captures the changing light that moves through a native planting.

or salvaged thrift find, mirrors, upcycled objects, or unusual containers. Mine is a bottle tree, a nod to my Southern roots: a collection of blue, green, aqua, and lavender vessels that mark my travels and memories. It catches my eye when the light slants just so through the trees.

Garden art should have a reciprocal relationship with the landscape, adding value to the entire design. Think about how an artwork contrasts with the color and shape of flowers and foliage around it. Keep it in proportion and style to the garden, so that it doesn't detract or overwhelm the space. In a small garden, art might be the main focal point or an accent off to one side; it can be the primary attraction or complement other landscape features. In larger gardens, you can use one art piece or several to draw the eye and lure visitors through the garden, guiding their way as the path turns or changes elevation, lending an element of mystery.

You can utilize that sense of discovery to create a visual scavenger hunt for small but delightful surprises by placing art of varying sizes at different levels—a petite turtle sculpture at their feet or an abstract object suspended in tree branches.

When placing a piece of art, consider the views from inside and outside. It will change during the day as the sun travels overhead, and with the

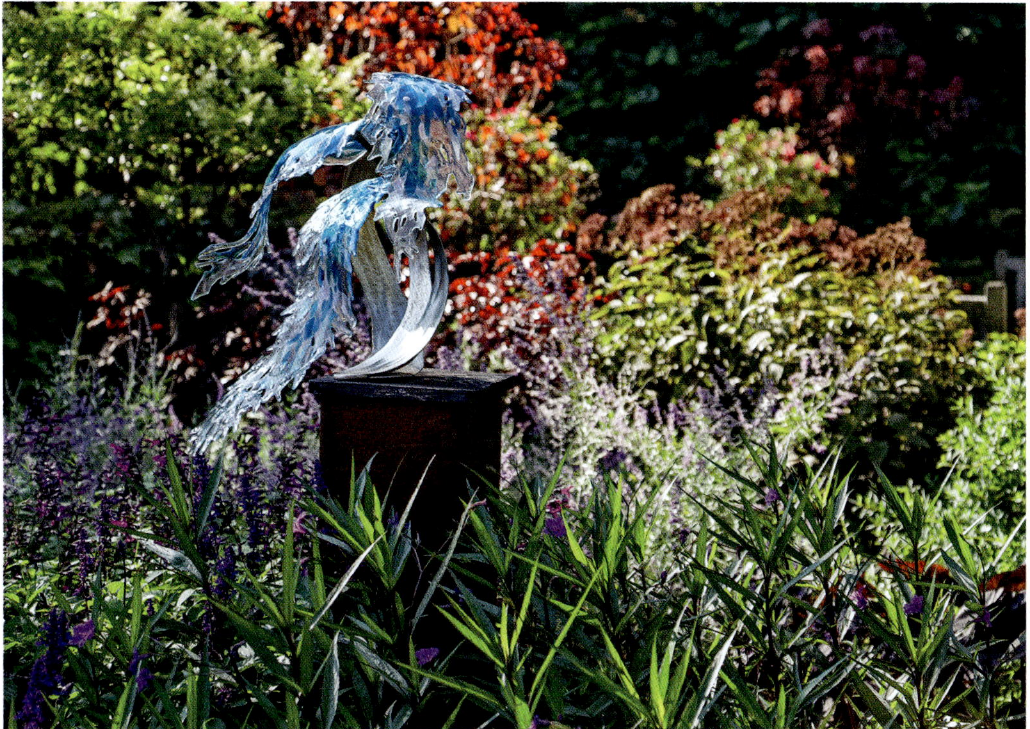

A dynamic glass sculpture among lush plantings.

seasons, but in the monochromatic landscape of winter it might truly carry the whole scene.

Art signals a human presence and, in a garden, conveys purpose. This "cue to care" is especially helpful when employed among native plantings, where a looser plant composition might appear haphazard; a simple bench or a birdbath tells people that this is intentional. Suddenly, a residential plot of goldenrod, aster, and prairie grasses makes sense to the casual onlooker.

Natural objects, such as driftwood, a fallen limb, or a weathered stump, can be just as powerful as human-made art. In my front yard a granite boulder takes pride of place. I call it my "rescue rock." A glacial remnant of Minnesota's prehistoric past, this huge rock lived several houses down from mine, and I admired it every time I passed by walking our dog. When the neighbors had new landscaping done, the rock wasn't included. Right before it was loaded on a truck, I ran down and asked the guy driving the skip loader if he could dump it in my yard. I made a snap decision as to where it was placed. It sits firmly by the front porch and anchors the landscape, glowing in the morning's warm sunlight. The backside is a mosaic of lichens. Birds, chipmunks, and squirrels often survey the garden from its gentle hump. I treasure it like a priceless sculpture.

GARDENER SPOTLIGHT

Mary Schier

Mary Schier and I go way back. She's the former editor of *Northern Gardener* magazine, where I found my footing as a budding garden writer newly moved to Minnesota. She is a writer, speaker, author, and editor who offers information and encouragement to gardeners tending small spaces and growing in cold climates. I've followed her gardening evolution as she has downsized not once but twice.

When I first met her, Mary gardened on a third of an acre in Northfield, Minnesota, which was situated on a steep hill and backed up to a nature area. As she cultivated the garden for over seventeen years, she grew native plants and traditional Minnesota plants, like peonies, viburnum, and dogwood, as well as raspberries and a vegetable garden. However, she admitted the nature area was more weeds than nature and her attempt at making a meadow was less than successful. In addition, the hill made mowing difficult, so she wasn't all that sad when they left it behind.

Moving up to the Twin Cities after her husband retired from college teaching, Mary wanted a smaller, flatter garden, a blank slate. She found exactly that, and after three years she had shaped a garden that was, "the perfect size garden for me at age 60." It included an insectary, vegetable beds, trees, and perennials. It turned out to be the most enjoyable gardening she had ever done.

Although she dearly loved that garden, she also supported their next move. No one blames older Minnesotans for escaping the cold winters and wanting to spend more time in Florida. She and her husband made the decision to buy a townhouse so that shoveling snow no

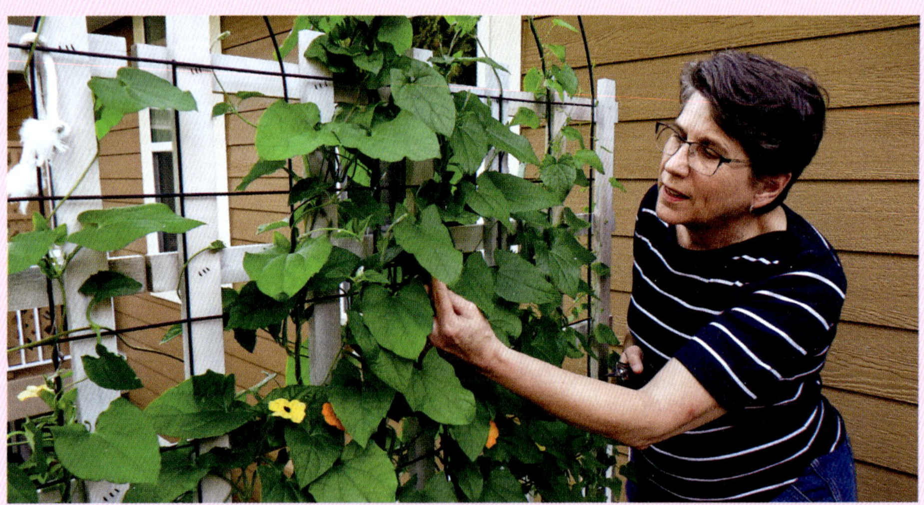

Photo courtesy of Mary Schier

longer weighed on their minds or bodies. Now it's easier to shut the door and leave town for the winter.

Buying the townhouse during summer, she was able to see "evidence of gardening," and they found an end unit with extra space for planting. Still, she read the HOA documents closely. In this case, they sounded stricter than they are in practice. Her husband became president of the HOA, and now they are working to get a greater variety of tree species planted around the development.

Mary has found that the front plantings are what concern people and the HOA most—that and mowing. She's made sure that all personal gardening done at the back and side of the house do not interfere with mowing accessibility, and she hasn't encountered problems. When she wanted to change out barberry bushes in front, she had to get permission, but it was granted, and that encouraged others also wanting to rid their landscape of the invasive shrub.

Her favorite place by far is the deck. A 6′ × 2′ (2 × .75 m) elevated planter box with a trellis affords privacy from the neighboring deck. She has been surprised at how many tomatoes she has been able to grow in pots. She puts out lots of other container plantings and finds it a relaxing spot for her morning coffee. Next, she is planning to grow some herbs, a salad garden, and plants to attract hummingbirds.

One of Mary's solutions to decreased gardening space has been to secure a spot at a community garden. Just an eight-minute drive away, she visits her plot every other day during the growing season. She also maintains the garden beds at a nearby retreat center. She says that volunteering to tend gardens is a good idea for people without gardening space of their own: "It scratches the itch, and you meet nice people."

As for the downside of downsizing, Mary misses having a more personal, cohesive space. Her garden beds are disjointed, and she wishes she could view more of the garden areas from inside. If she had it to do again, she would like a courtyard. She acknowledges it's hard to leave a garden you've loved and cautions that you might suffer transplant shock; you should give yourself time to think about how you will live and garden in the new home.

MARY'S TIPS FOR MOVING TO A TOWNHOUSE

- Do your due diligence before you purchase, read through the HOA documents thoroughly to see what they specifically allow or disallow in the development, and look for signs of others gardening in the neighborhood.
- Figure out the watering—townhouses don't have as many faucets outside as houses do!
- Lean into container gardening; you can grow perennials in containers or even shrubs if you figure out how to store them in the winter and you can create a very lush deck or patio with a lot of containers.
- Even if it's small, create a garden space that feels like you; many developments tend to be cookie-cutter, so planting a deck or a patio that reflects your personal style will make your space more comfortable.

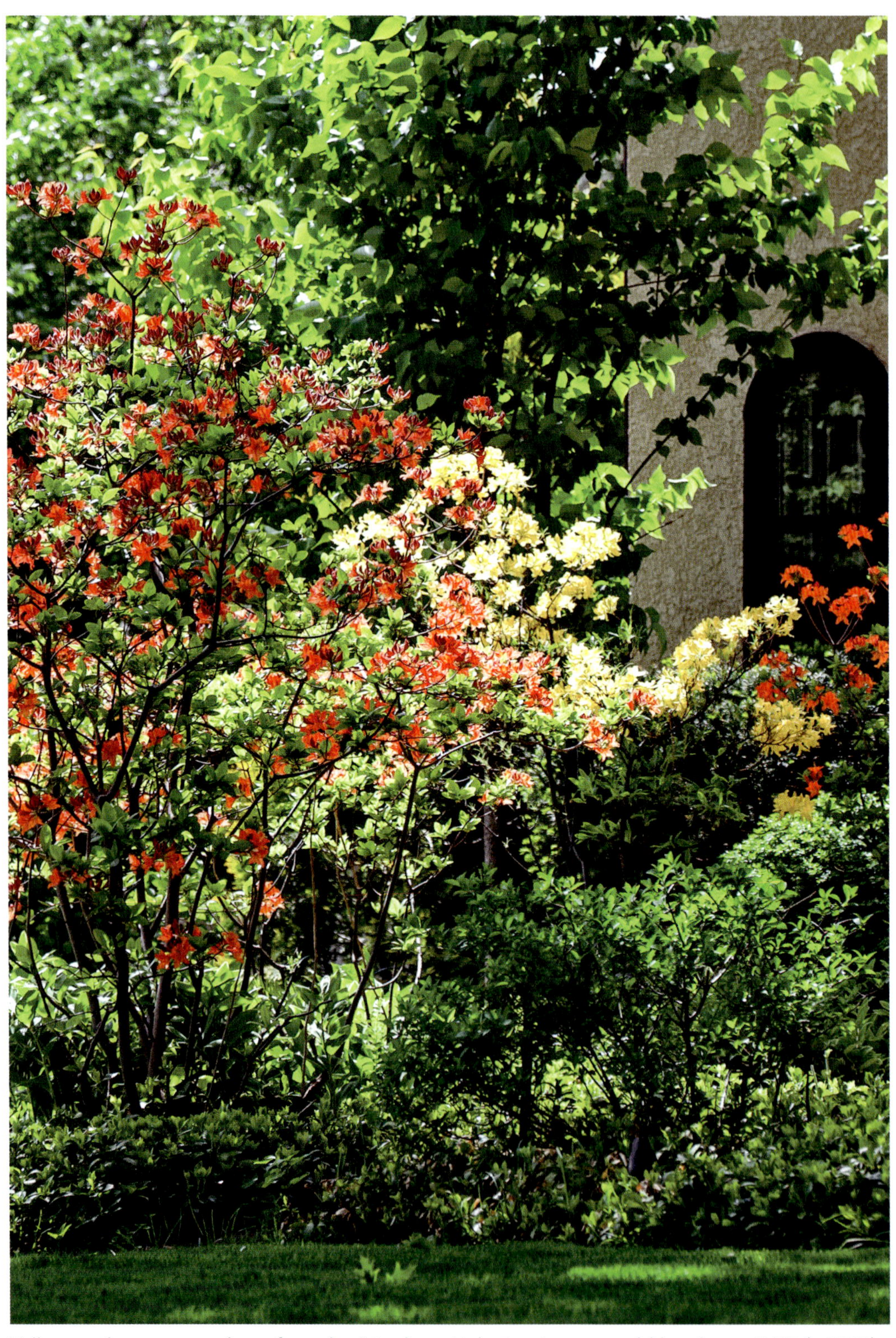

Yellow and orange azaleas, from the 'Northern Lights' series, are cold hardy to −35°F (−37°C).

CHAPTER 5

Reimagining Your Garden

I love to imagine you, my readers, living and gardening all across the United States and beyond. I picture you in a chair on a sunny patio or shady porch, perusing the pages and dreaming of next year's garden—it's always the best one; it doesn't have any weeds yet. You might be in Arizona or Vermont, Mississippi or Michigan—the United States has the most diverse landscape of any country, with mountains, plains, coasts, swamps, deserts, and rainforests. It's difficult to always give the right gardening advice for so many ecosystems, but there is common ground that binds us as gardeners.

Now that you've looked at your garden from several different perspectives—big picture, the good and the bad, hardscape and structures, ideas for enhancements—it's time to turn to the discussion to new plants. As you adapt and optimize your garden for the near and distant future, an important goal is to identify the plant species that will serve your needs best, plants that will thrive not only with less care and maintenance but also will endure increasingly unpredictable and record-setting weather conditions.

In the second part of this chapter, we seek out plants that actually give back, thinking in terms of function beyond aesthetics. Lots of trees do this: They boost curb appeal and increase property value while providing shade, wildlife habitat, and more. But the same can be said for humble groundcovers. A conventional turf lawn looks great, sure, but a bee-friendly lawn looks great, is low-maintenance, and provides food and habitat for some of the most important pollinators in the global ecosystem. Now, that's a hard-working plant!

Needed: Resilient Plants

No matter where they live, older gardeners want to keep going, but their gardens might start to look different. In reimagining future gardens, resilience will be a key factor. With less energy and patience to give, older gardeners should look to tough, trouble-free plants that can withstand erratic weather; plants with grit, plants that can bounce back, much like they themselves have been doing as they go through life.

In many cases these will be native plants, species that have historically occurred in a particular region or habitat, without human introduction or influence. These plants have coevolved with wildlife over millennia and adapted to the local climate, soil, and ecological conditions of their region. They are crucial for supporting local ecosystems, providing food and habitat for native wildlife, insects, and pollinators.

At other times they might be selected cultivars bred for more than visual appeal, including exceptional cold-hardiness, heat-tolerance, disease- and pest-resistance, strong growth habit, and adaptability to other environmental stresses. Nativars—cultivars of native species bred for specific traits like larger flowers and more compact growth habits—will become more attractive to home gardeners. Stalwart plants typically considered ordinary might deserve another look. As one of my favorite garden columnists, Ann Treneman, an American but longtime UK resident, suggests in *The Times*, "Instead of trying to grow the impossible, it pays to love those that thrive."

A Word About Plant Lists

Every gardener loves a good plant list. I know I do. It's like a treasure hunt where you might find the perfect new plant, or perhaps just confirmation of plant choices you've already made. But as a garden writer, plant lists make me a bit nervous. A basic plant list with common names, Latin names, and USDA Hardiness Zones doesn't begin to tell the whole story.

Hardiness Zones are the first data point you should use when determining if a plant is right for your garden. The USDA Plant Hardiness Zone Map (see Resources, page 213) is the standard by which gardeners and growers can determine which perennial plants are most likely to thrive at a location. The map is based on the average annual extreme minimum winter temperature. Nowadays, gardeners should also check the American Horticultural Society Plant Heat-Zone Map to see how plants respond to high-heat days (see Resources, page 213).

Given all this, USDA Zone 6 in Utah is vastly different from Zone 6 in Pennsylvania, just as Zone 9 in California is different from Zone 9 in Florida. You have to consider differences in soil composition, humidity, rainfall, wind, nighttime temperatures, length of growing season, and more. And then there are the unique differences in your own garden and its microclimates.

'Peggy Martin': A Plant with Grit

I am lucky to garden in two places, albeit both with extreme conditions at times. My main garden in Minneapolis endures frigid temperatures and, as of late, weather that whipsaws between warm and cold in the middle of winter, confusing plants and confounding gardeners. Here, we wish for snow, not just for recreational opportunities but also for its insulating properties that protect plants like a cozy blanket. This garden rests, if sometimes uneasily, from November to April.

My little patch in New Orleans where my husband and I now spend our winters (our daughter lives there) has been a learning experience. We inherited two dwarf Meyer lemon trees that sat tilted, partially uprooted by Hurricane Ida. We managed to re-dig and gradually reposition them, their thank you a bumper crop of luscious fruit.

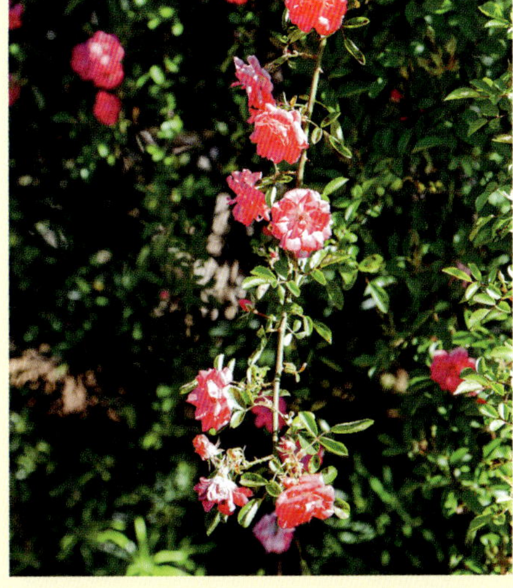

Miraculous Katrina survivor, Rose 'Peggy Martin.'

Spend enough time in this historic city and you'll see a particular pink climbing rose, everywhere. It has a remarkable story. Peggy Martin of Plaquemines Parish grew hundreds of roses until Hurricane Katrina. When she returned home after the storm, her beautiful garden had been under saltwater for two weeks. She found nothing but gray mud and devastation, except for the tiniest bit of green: a rose of uncertain origin gifted to her by an elderly woman. She grew it out and started taking cuttings to local nurseries to help fund the replanting of public spaces along the Gulf Coast, at which time a rose expert named the hardy survivor after Peggy.

For the western states there is even a more detailed model within the Sunset Climate Zones—twenty-four Zones that account for mountain altitudes, coastal moisture, desert conditions, and more (see Resources, page 213).

As native plants become more mainstream, some advocates are telling gardeners to ignore hardiness Zones and to instead go by ecoregions. An ecoregion is a major ecosystem defined by distinctive geography that receives uniform solar radiation and moisture. The US EPA Ecoregion Map divides North America into 15 broad levels (Level I), all the way from tundra to tropical wet forest and all places in between. Two more levels (Level II and Level III) drill down deeper into the intricacies of our continent's wildly varied landscape (see Resources, page 213).

Don't let this scare you! Start at the plant's hardiness zone, and then look at light, soil, and moisture requirements. If you still aren't sure, consult a reputable garden center or check with your state's Extension office. Extension websites offer a wealth of information about your local growing conditions.

Finally, pay close attention to the full names of specific plants, including the Latin name and any cultivar name. Different cultivars of the same plant species can have dramatically different characteristics. For example, there's a world of difference between the straight species of giant goldenrod (*Solidago gigantea*) and the adorable, diminutive cultivar 'Little Miss Sunshine' (*Solidago*).

Native Plants for Smaller Gardens

When you see native plants in wild landscapes, they grow together cheek by jowl, vying for any available space. Their survival tactics vary; some play well together while some seek world domination. Others bide their time until the moment comes to bloom, and afterward they seem to disappear, a sort of shrinking violet. This is most apparent to anyone who has planted the "meadow in a can" and after a few seasons found that nothing but black-eyed Susans remain.

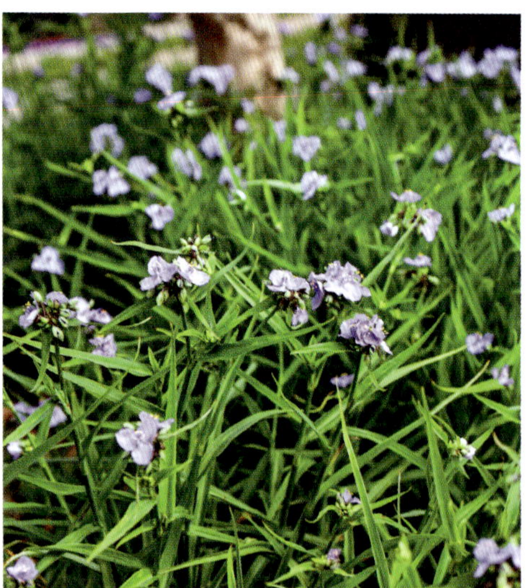

Vigorous native spiderwort (*Tradescantia ohiensis*) fills up this bed but is contained by the sidewalk.

When I wrote the newspaper story on strategies for aging gardeners that inspired this book, one of the comments I received stood out among the others: "Just tell them to use native plants." It stuck with me not for its blunt tone but because it was unhelpful for seniors looking to simplify their gardening lives. No doubt, native plants are great, but there are a few caveats to consider before using them in smaller spaces, lest they colonize your courtyard.

Some native plants are better for filling up prairie acreage or battling invasives on a large property, if that is your goal, but as most older gardeners are seeking to go smaller and easier, these beneficial but bountiful beauties should be appreciated from afar. Attractive but aggressive native species like Canada goldenrod (*Solidago canadensis*), cup plant (*Silphium perfoliatum*), and obedient plant (*Physostegia virginiana*) are simply successful at what they do; you can't blame them, but they're not necessarily the right plant for your place.

NATIVES FOR SMALL GARDENS

The best native plants for small gardens should be well-behaved, ones with a clumping growth habit with fibrous roots, or ones that spread slowly with rhizomes. They shouldn't re-seed willy-nilly or throw out too many suckers. You'll still get the benefits of lower maintenance (ditch the fertilizer and the deadheading) and wildlife support without creating a new problem to solve. Don't worry if you aren't growing 100 percent natives; most gardens are a mix. Pollinators and other wildlife prefer some plants to no plants. Don't let guilt get in the way of your gardening joy.

The following list is for perennial natives; we'll talk about shrubs and small trees in the next section. It's just a sampling to give you some ideas. These are great candidates for small beds, narrow strips, corner pockets, downspout gardens, and mailbox gardens. Use them to design as you would any garden vignette, in graduating tiers, short in front to taller in back, in threes, fives, and sevens, in natural drifts, etc.

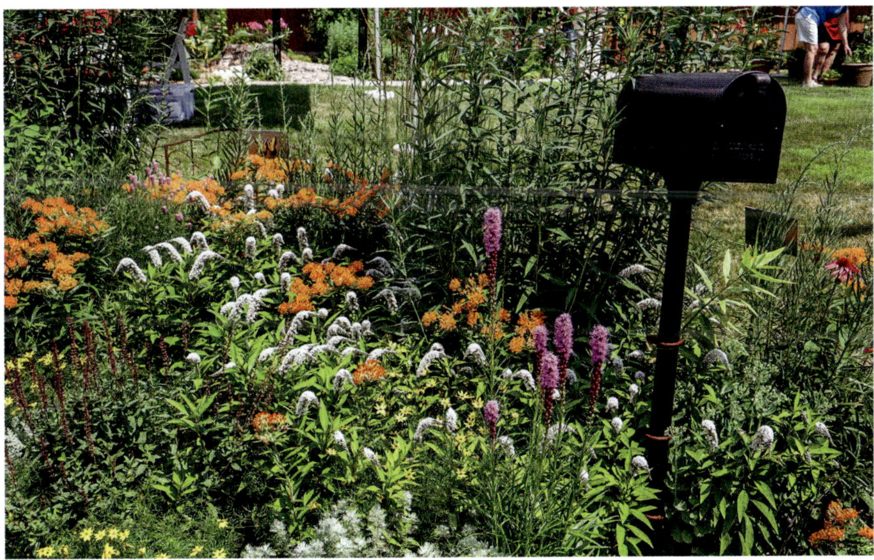

Well-behaved natives grow in this lovely mailbox planting. But watch out for that nonnative gooseneck loosestrife (the plant with the graceful white "goose-neck" bloom); it can be a bully.

For sunnier spots—some will tolerate partial sun; it's important to check for soil and moisture requirements before planting:

Butterfly weed (*Asclepias tuberosa*): Zones 4–9
Prairie alumroot (*Heuchera richardsonii*): Zones 3–9
Aromatic aster (*Symphotrichum oblongifolium*): Zones 3–9
Nodding onion (*Allium cernuum*): Zones 4–8
Blazing star (*Liatris aspera*): Zones 3–8
Blazing star (*Liatris spicata*): Zones 3–9
Threadleaf coreopsis (*Coreopsis verticillata*): Zones 3–9
Purple coneflower (*Echinacea purpurea*): Zones 3–8
Helenium (*Helenium autumnale*): Zones 3–8
Garden phlox (*Phlox paniculata*): Zones 4–8
Rattlesnake master (*Eryngium yuccifolium*): Zones 3–8
Amsonia (*Amsonia tabernaemontana*): Zones 3–9
Virginia bluebells (*Mertensia virginica*): Zones 3–8
Little bluestem (*Schizachyrium scoparium*): Zones 3–9

For partial or dappled sunlight:

White tinged sedge (*Carex albicans*): Zones 4–8
Canadian wild ginger (*Asarum canadense*): Zones 4–6
Jacob's ladder (*Polemonium reptans*): Zones 3–8
Wild columbine (*Aquilegia canadensis*): Zones 3–8
Prairie dropseed (*Sporobolus heterolepis*): Zones 3–9
Maidenhair fern (*Adiantum pedatum*): Zones 3–8
Wild geranium (*Geranium maculatum*): Zones 3–8

PLANTS ARE SOCIAL CREATURES

When considering native plants suitable for smaller gardens, Benjamin Vogt, Nebraska native plant designer and prairie advocate, thinks in terms of plant communities: "A plant community is both mutually supportive and mutually combative. In the wild, plants jockey and tussle for resources—what we see in a meadow, for example, isn't balance so much as it is a blood-thirsty fight for water, sunlight, and soil nutrients." Because of that, many native plants aren't meant for the confines of your typical flower bed.

He recommends "low sociability" plants for small gardens. These are plants that tend to grow individually or in small clusters in their natural environment and therefore are less likely to spread beyond the bounds of the garden. His favorites for shade: White tinged sedge (*Carex albicans*) and

Early meadow-rue (*Thalictrum dioicum*); for sun: Prairie alumroot (*Heuchera richardsonii*), Blue grama grass (*Bouteloua gracilis*), Dotted blazing star (*Liatris punctata*).

His design tip: "Small gardens follow the less-is-more rule. Less diversity means more aesthetic punch and more ability to manage the space sanely without any one species taking over. In 100 square feet (9 m^2) I wouldn't use more than ten species."

A Case for Flowering Shrubs

In my discussions with gardeners aiming to rightsize their gardens, front and center is the plan to replace perennials with more shrubs or with small trees with shrub-like qualities. Many shrubs and shrub-like trees offer multiseason interest with flowers, fruit, and fall color, and they make so much sense for gardeners looking to lighten their load. They're also a boon to birds seeking food, shelter, and nesting sites—and more birds mean more natural pest control.

Shrubs and small trees can provide structure to larger areas, especially if you're adding evergreens to the deciduous mix. If you are hoping to fill up space with low-maintenance plants, a shrub can take up the space of three to five perennials, if not more. Where perennials typically need three years to do their "sleep-creep-leap" thing before they make a real contribution to a garden design, in that same time frame some shrubs will reach maturity,

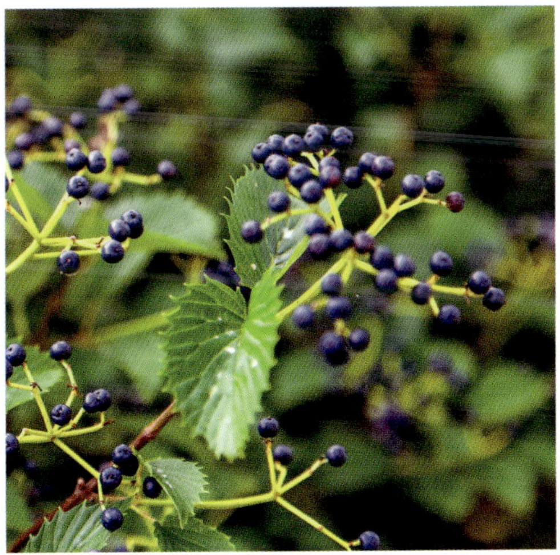

Arrowwood viburnum (*Viburnum dentatum*) is known for its beautiful white blooms in spring and its dark blue berries and vibrant foliage in fall.

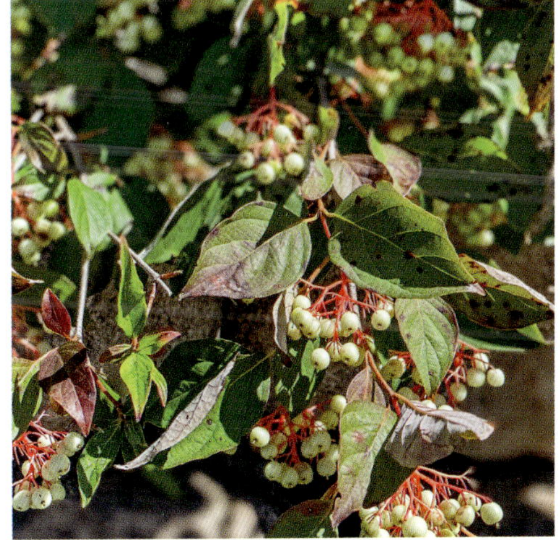

Red osier dogwood (*Cornus sericea*) produces clusters of white berries and has striking red stems that stand out in the winter landscape.

or at least put on substantial growth. That said, there are some supersized shrub-like perennials, such as baptisia, goatsbeard, Joe Pye weed, queen of the prairie, and black snakeroot, that should be considered.

I've heard shrubs called "one-touch" plants. After planting one, you might need to touch it once a year, pruning an errant branch or doing some mild shaping, maybe not even that. But you'll gaze upon it admiringly many more times. They don't need deadheading, staking, or dividing. And they're beautiful.

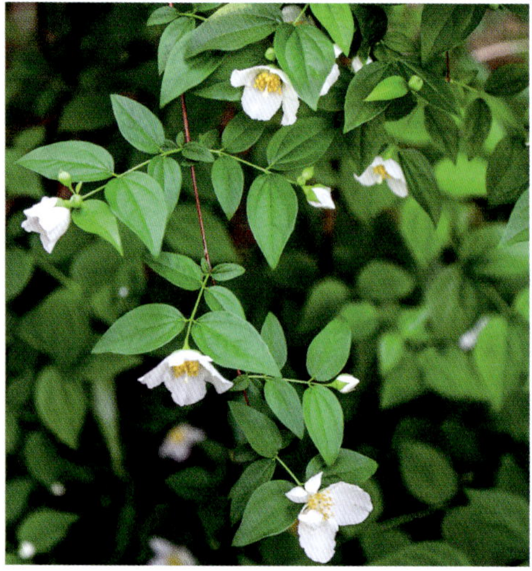

Mock orange (*Philadelphus* spp.) is a tough plant with a delicate orange-blossom scent.

CREATING A BIRD BORDER

Shrubs offer a safe spot for birds to rest and reproduce; they also provide food in the form of fruit, berries, nuts, and seeds over summer and fall, in addition to visiting insects (and larvae) for bird moms to ferry to hungry fledglings needing protein throughout the breeding season. By creating a border with a mixture of different shrubs you'll increase biodiversity while decreasing the risk of a pest or disease wiping out an entire border (as is more likely to happen with a monoculture of a single shrub species). I like to think of it as emulating the hedgerows that lined the roads in the English village where we once lived, a rich tapestry of bloom, leaf, and berry full of birdsong.

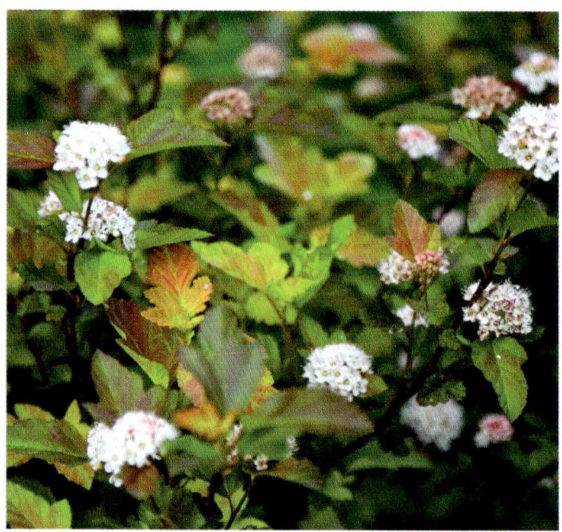

Ninebark (*Physocarpus opulifolius*) has bright yellow foliage in early spring that looks just like forsythia blooming, but this shrub has so much more to give throughout the growing season.

With so many sizes, shapes, textures, and bloom colors it's possible to design a perennial-like border using only shrubs. Plant breeders responding to a general trend toward smaller garden spaces have developed pint-sized versions of our favorite big bushes. In many cases, they have taken native shrubs and selected for size, growth habit, bloom period, and fall color. Some of these nativars might not support wildlife to the same degree as the straight species do, but they can still provide some form of habitat value.

The following lists are a sampling of good habitat shrubs for very general areas of the US. Many of these plant species are also available in cultivars suited for different regions.

For the West

Apache plume (*Fallugia*): Zones 4–8
Desert peach (*Prunus andersonii*): Zones 5–9
Golden currant (*Ribes aureum*): Zones 4–8
Mock orange (*Philadelphus*): Zones 3–8
Red yucca (*Hesperaloe parviflora*): Zones 5–10
Three-leaf sumac (*Rhus trilobata*): Zones 4–8

For the South

American beautyberry (*Callicarpa americana*): Zones 7–10
Black chokeberry (*Aronia melanocarpa*): Zones 3–8
Buttonbush (*Cephalanthus occidentalis*): Zones 5–9
Fragrant sumac (*Rhus aromatica*): Zones 3–9
Oakleaf hydrangea (*Hydrangea quercifolia*): Zones 5–9
Sweet pepperbush (*Clethra alnifolia*): Zones 3–9
Yaupon holly (*Ilex vomitoria*): Zones 7–11

For the North

Common ninebark (*Physocarpus opulifolius*): Zones 2–8
Dwarf bush honeysuckle (*Diervilla lonicera*): Zones 3–7
Highbush cranberry (*Viburnum trilobum*): Zones 3–6
Inkberry holly (*Ilex glabra*): Zones 4–9
Mapleleaf viburnum (*Viburnum acerifolium*): Zones 3–8
Red osier dogwood (*Cornus sericea*): Zones 2–7
White snowberry (*Symphoricarpos albus*): Zones 2–5

For the East

Arrowwood viburnum (*Viburnum dentatum*): Zones 2–8
Fothergilla (*Fothergilla gardenii*): Zones 5–8
Highbush blueberry (*Vaccinium corymbosum*): Zones 3–7
Leatherwood (*Dirca palustris*): Zones 3–9
Mountain laurel (*Kalmia latifolia*): Zones 4–9
New Jersey tea (*Ceanothus americanus*): Zones 4–8
Smooth hydrangea (*Hydrangea arborescens*): Zones 3–9

A Gardening Journey with Rosarian Chris VanCleave

You may know Chris VanCleave as the Redneck Rosarian, one of the country's foremost experts on growing roses. He shares his passion for the beloved blooms as cohost of the popular podcast *Rose Chat*, along with fellow rosarian Teresa Byington.

Chris's love for gardening began when he was around six years old, following his dad around their big vegetable garden. When he was twelve years old, his father died, and he redirected his efforts to helping his mother with her roses, and from there his love of roses was born: "I discovered that she worked through a lot of her grief in that garden—cutting away the dead, damaged, and diseased rose canes; cleaning up beds; and preparing the shrubs for new growth—and in the process found the courage to begin again in her own life. It was those observations and learnings that shaped my lifelong adventure in the garden."

In addition to roses, Chris's Alabama garden is home to favorite perennials, among them iris, daylilies, salvia, Russian sage, 'Walker's Low' catmint, cleome, and others. He loves container plantings of annuals, like calibrachoa, geraniums, lantana, euphorbias, zinnias, and more.

Asked if his garden had a goal or mission, Chris responds, "My garden is a celebration of my love of fragrant roses, heirloom perennials, and vibrant blooms. It is a space where the past is honored and embraces the future and the joy of each new season. It has taken thoughtful cultivation and heartfelt care, but these gardens have also served as a sanctuary to sit and relax and be."

Chris sees his gardening journey in four life phases. Growing up with his par-

SMALL BUT VERSATILE SHRUBS

Often times the cultivar name hints at a smaller version of your favorite shrub, as shown in the following list of compact plants. These are attractive front-of-border candidates and small-space specimens.

'Baby Kim' (*Lilac*): Zones 3–8
Double Play 'Candy Corn' (*Spirea*): Zones 4–8
'Firelight Tidbit' (*Hydrangea*): Zones 3–9
'Fizzy Mizzy' (*Sweetspire*): Zones 5–9
Invincibelle 'Wee White' (*Hydrangea*): Zones 3–8
'Lil Ditty' (*Viburnum*): Zones 3–8
'Midnight Sun' (*Weigela*): Zones 4–8
'Mucho Gusto' (*Abelia*): Zones 6–9
'Strongbox' (*Inkberry*): Zones 5–9
'Tater Tot' (*Arborvitae*): Zones 3–8

ents in the garden, he learned the basics of gardening and developed a love for the soil and growing things. When he was married with kids he focused on easy-grow flowers like zinnias and veggies, hoping to instill that love of gardening into his own children. He also grew a garden of over 250 roses. In middle age, divorced and with his kids grown and on their own, he set out to create a new, larger garden, but with "only" one hundred roses. He calls this fourth phase, "older and wiser." After a cancer diagnosis, he has scaled back and downsized and is building a smaller, compact garden with his favorite varieties and will maintain twenty-five roses.

As Chris has gotten older and faced serious health challenges, he remains resilient, looking for ways to work smarter: using raised beds, gardening more in containers, using kneeling pads, and choosing low-maintenance plants. He likes to work in his garden early in the morning and late in the evening, which reduces stress on his body from heat and humidity. "As blooms emerge," Chris suggests, "focus on the joy of being outdoors and connecting with nature, and less on creating a perfect space."

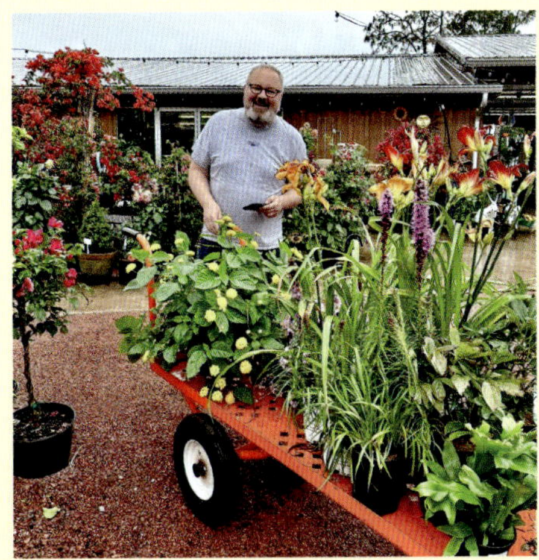

Photo courtesy of Chris VanCleave

The Bright Side of Shade Gardening

I hear so many folks lament, "I don't have any sun." Well, maybe that's a good thing. As temperatures set new records and summers on average are trending warmer and drier, perhaps it's time to seek out the shade. People become more sensitive to heat as they grow older, so shade gardening is a matter of comfort and safety. But there are plenty of pluses beyond that: lower maintenance, fewer weeds, and a wide variety of beautiful flowering and foliage plants from which to choose.

Shade gardens typically retain soil moisture due to cooler temperatures and protection from sunlight. This can benefit plants that prefer cool, consistently moist growing conditions. In shady conditions, there's also less watering and feeding to do, weeds don't grow as prolifically in lower light conditions, and sun-seeking pests often have gone elsewhere. It's still important to grow the right plant in the right place; sun-loving plants will always struggle in shady conditions. But do watch out for slippery moss.

Shade offers opportunities to grow woodland wildflowers, including ephemerals, which are especially treasured for their wildlife value because they are early sources of pollen and nectar for bees when other plants are just getting started. They are the first native plants to pop up and the first to bloom in spring, with a short time to shine, setting seed early in the spring before retreating underground for the rest of the year. They naturalize quickly and provide a lovely welcome mat for spring. They are a less showy but reliable alternative to spring bulb displays that can require intensive work on your knees. They are generally suited for Zones 3–9. You might even grow them only for their whimsical names:

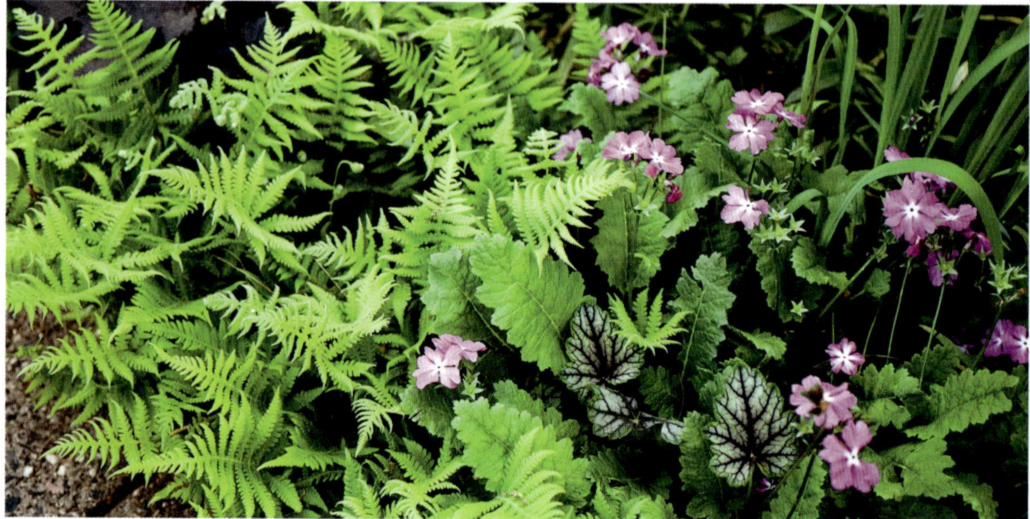

Ferns and primrose thrive in shady gardens.

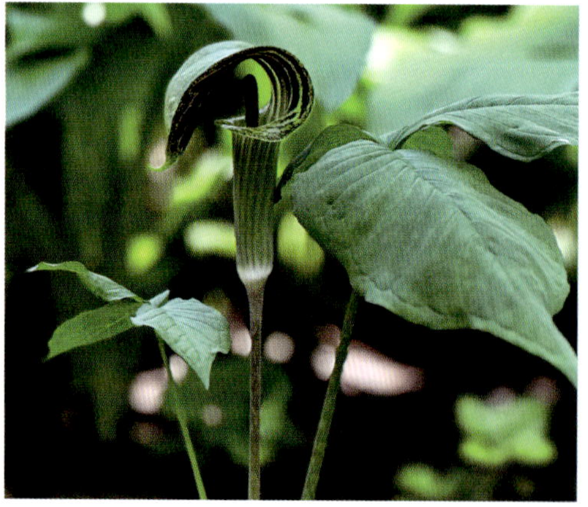

Jack-in-the-pulpit (*Arisaema triphyllum*). *Photo courtesy of Donna Hamilton*

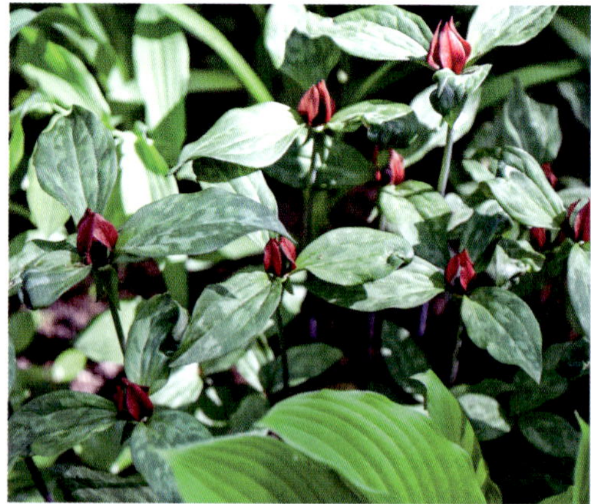

Red trillium, *Trillium erectum*.

Dutchman's breeches (*Dicentra cucullaria*)
Jack-in-the-pulpit (*Arisaema triphyllum*)
Shooting star (*Primula meadia*)
Squirrel corn (*Dicentra canadensis*)
Stinking Benjamin (*Trillium erectum*)
Virginia springbeauty (*Claytonia virginica*)
Yellow trout lily (*Erythronium americanum*)

TIPS FOR SHADE GARDENING

If you want to grow food, fear not. Leafy greens (such as lettuce, beets, spinach, chard, and arugula) and herbs (such as cilantro, chives, chervil, and parsley) can tolerate partial sun to partial shade. Protection from harsh western sun is actually a blessing. Lemon balm and mint also do well in shade, but they can do too well, so be sure to contain them!

While you're at it, take your houseplants outside for a summer vacation in the shade; they'll benefit from the humidity and rain. I always display mine in a grouping on a small table by the front door that gets just a hint of morning sun. Be sure to acclimate them gradually, after danger of frost is gone, and check for pests when you bring them back inside at the end of the season. A good shower with the garden hose will dislodge most stowaways.

Dry shade presents its own challenge but is nothing that can't be worked around, often spurring creative and attractive solutions. You'll find dry shade in areas that are isolated from sun and rainfall, such as under tree canopies, house eaves, awnings, and overhangs; even buildings sometimes block rainfall. Tree roots are also responsible for dry shade, sucking lots of moisture and nutrients from the ground (however, trees that make the dry shade are also a built-in focal point in your garden design).

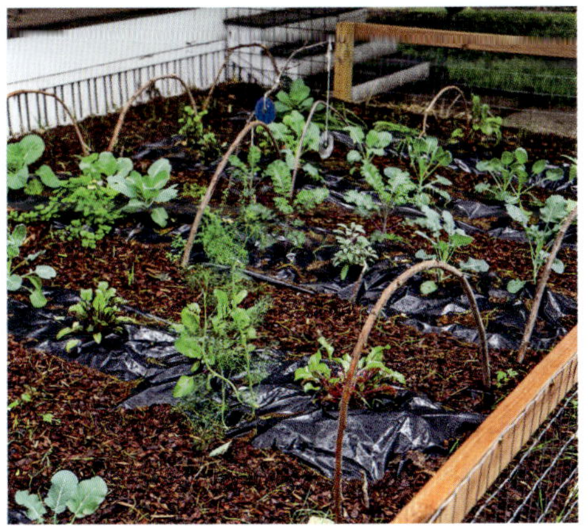

Partially shaded front yard vegetable garden.

You can circumvent competition from tree roots by planting containers of shade-loving annuals and placing them in the beds under your trees. In milder climates, you can even mix hardy perennials into these containers, such as shade-tolerant plants with attractive foliage like heuchera and hosta. Hang baskets from lower tree limbs as long as you have a safe and easy way to water them. If the shade is too dark, consider calling an arborist to thin or limb up the tree to allow for a "better kind" of shade. Dappled shade is a versatile condition suitable for a number of plant varieties. And while you're at it, put a bench out there and sit for a spell.

Container Cottage Garden

Living in a townhouse or condo doesn't necessarily mean you have to give up your herbaceous borders. You can still have an English-style border or bed on a patio, courtyard, or deck, or even along a walkway if it's wide enough. Do this with containers placed, as the Brits say, chockablock, in groupings close together so that they mimic the colorful abundance of a cottage garden. As the plants get bigger the pots will disappear, and the effect is charming.

The plan here is to group many containers tightly together into what you might call a "super container" that is treated as one—and is watered all at once. The result has a concentrated visual impact, as opposed to plants being spotted here and there around the garden.

A container cottage garden can be all annuals, which is best if you live in a cold climate and need the season to be "one and done" at the end. If you live in a milder climate, a mix of annuals, perennials, and even small shrubs or roses can make for a striking combination. Designers recommend using a color theme: monochromatic, as in all shades of pink from cotton candy to wine; or complimentary, as in opposites on the color wheel—purple and orange, yellow, and blue. But a mix of all colors might produce that delightful disarray so characteristic of the classic cottage garden.

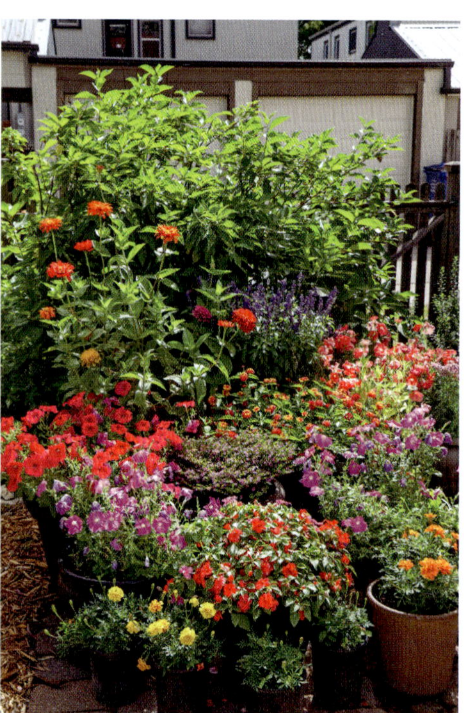

Grouping plants close together creates a beautiful and colorful container cottage garden.

Individual pots with one kind of plant work best, giving you the flexibility to change them around as blooms ebb and fade. Design the "garden" as you would one container, the usual thriller, spiller, filler mantra but think also in terms of climbers, sprawlers, and mounders. You can insert a trellis in the back containers for the climbers. You can also boost individual containers within the group on stands or blocks to vary heights. You might have beautiful containers, like a collection of terra cotta you want to showcase within the grouping. These container groupings can live inside planting beds, too, for a seasonal accent or gap-filler.

Use a slow-release organic fertilizer to keep the blooms coming, maintain watering during hot or dry spells, and tidy up spent flowers when needed. That's a bit of maintenance, but no knees, no weeds, no worries.

Petite Potager—Plants to Feed One Kitchen

There comes a time when you don't have the need or want for bushel baskets of tomatoes and cucumbers but you still want enough for a few salads and side dishes. I remember the great cucumber glut of 2015 when my crop exploded. The cukes kept coming, and a gal can make only so many pickles. That's when I started my free produce box on the front steps with a sign that said: "Take some cucumbers, *please*." It's also when people on our street started calling me the cucumber lady.

A successful harvest shouldn't be a burden, but sometimes life happens, and you don't get around to eating it all. That's another time when guilt and feeling overwhelmed threaten our gardening joy. A *potager* might be the answer for a "just enough" garden. This French word for vegetable garden literally means "for the soup." Nowadays the word brings to mind a scaled-down kitchen garden planted with a bit of flair.

Your potager could be sown in small beds close to your kitchen door or in a courtyard in containers. This garden isn't meant to yield quantities of produce for canning or freezing; it's more for what's ripe right in the moment and might be no more than one tomato plant and some basil and peppers. It could also include a few more herbs and some easy flowers, like zinnias, for your table. Stepping out to your patio or deck and finding a few fresh ingredients is so satisfying. It makes all the difference in cooking and preparing meals.

To plant in containers, look for veggie seeds and transplants labeled as suitable for containers. In some cases, these are regular-sized plants deemed possible to grow in big enough containers—most of these will require a pot of 15–18″ (38–46 cm) in diameter. In other cases, they are plants bred specifically for smaller spaces; for these, look to the name for clues, like *mini, petite, Thumbelina, baby, pixie, patio,* and *personal size.* You'll find carrots, beans, peas, cucumbers, eggplants, squash, and more, but all in miniature. I'm always surprised at the number of cherry tomatoes one patio plant can put out.

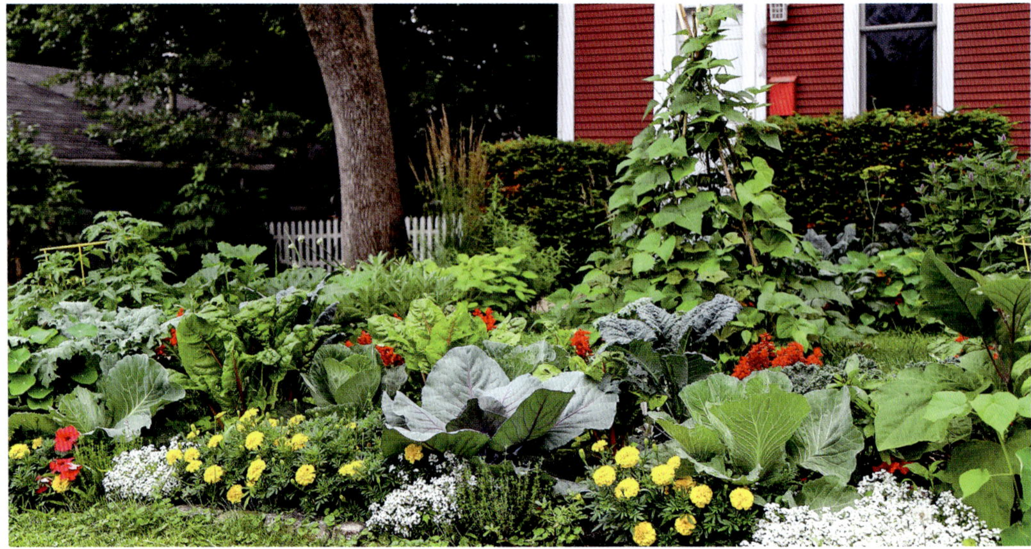

Lara Lau-Schommer's front yard potager combines flowers, herbs, and vegetables.

Determine the veggies you want to grow by what you like to eat, what you want to try, and what will give you the best return in your allotted space. Technically, you can grow anything in a container, but do you truly want to use that real estate for corn, or is it better for strawberries?

Herbs—for Use and Delight

You might be done growing vegetables, but even the smallest space probably has room for an herb garden. Don't underestimate these plants when it comes to providing a sense of gardening fulfillment. You might think of them as little plants with little leaves growing close to the ground, but these sources of use and delight are surprisingly varied in size and stature. The biggest herb in the world is actually a wild banana that grows to 45′ (14 m) tall, while the tiniest is no bigger than a grain of rice, a type of duckweed called watermeal. And then there's parsley, sage, rosemary, and thyme.

You can go down one of those research rabbit holes and find hundreds of herbs to choose from, but you only have to find room for a few to reap the benefits. Herb gardening gives so much bang for so little time and effort. If you don't have the space or the will to grow vegetables anymore, adding flavorful homegrown herbs to meals will give you a sense of creative achievement, a little flourish, and more control over what you eat. Herbs brighten up dishes for people with a dulled sense of taste, a culinary casualty of growing older. Just as Julia Child recommended, a simple sprinkling of chives elevates your eggs.

Herbs lend themselves to containers, planters, elevated gardens, and raised beds. They are low-maintenance once established. Plant them where you can best take in their fragrances: spicy, fruity, lemony, musky, or floral. For an easier harvest, place herb containers on tables, ledges, and other aboveground surfaces. With your herbs raised to eye level you'll also be able to appreciate foraging pollinators attracted to the plants for nectar and larval food. The larvae, those "worms" on your dill and parsley, are black swallowtail butterfly caterpillars, so be prepared to share, and witness the circle of life.

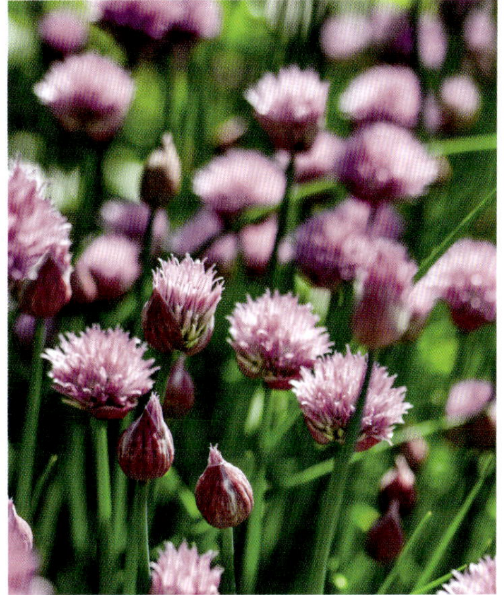

Chive blossoms can be used to garnish salads or to flavor vinegar. They attract butterflies, too.

Savor a Sensory Garden

Having a theme can help you pare down all the plant choices. With an herb garden you're halfway to creating a sensory garden, a garden that appeals to all five senses: sight, hearing, touch, smell, and taste. Something to tickle your brain. Sensory-rich activities promote neuroplasticity, the brain's ability to build new neural connections. The calming, grounding effects of a sensory garden can relieve stress and boost cognitive ability by helping you to engage with your environment. In addition, a sensory garden is the perfect place for strolling with someone who struggles from memory issues, a chance to spark conversation and reminisce with a family member or caregiver.

Herbs play a big role in sensory gardens. Mint, rosemary, lavender, and basil offer distinctive notes, a "scratch and sniff" that can evoke distant memories and pleasant sensations. A single cherry tomato plant covers taste and smell with zingy fruit and pungent foliage. Lamb's ear provides a soft, velvety feel. If your garden has room, and your hardiness zone accommodates it, a fragrant but thornless rose like 'Zephirine Drouhin' can perfume the space. Jasmine, honeysuckle, and citrus are other alluring scents. Flowers in warm, happy hues attract butterflies and hummingbirds.

Bring in the sound of birdsong with a small feeder or, if there's enough space, berry-producing plants or a dwarf crabapple tree. A small fountain or

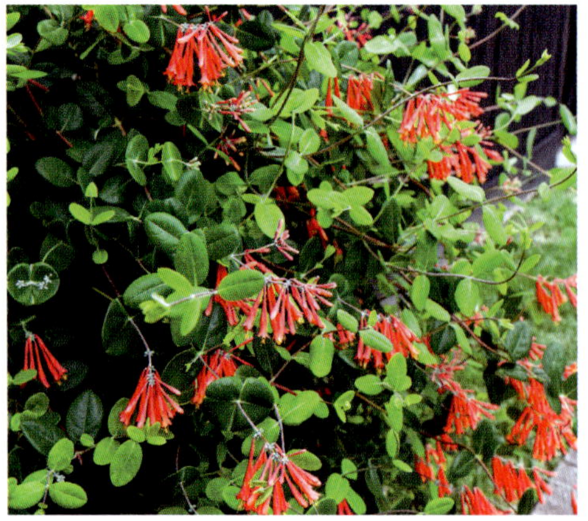

The striking 'Dropmore Scarlet' honeysuckle attracts hummingbirds.

birdbath will draw them in for a place to drink, preen, and splash. Plants like clumping bamboo or ornamental grasses that rustle and sway in the breeze will complete this dynamic and restorative place.

Ask More of Your Plants

Tending plants is much like caring for children: we give them food and water, new pots when they outgrow their old ones, wipe their leaves, trim their scraggly bits, even sing to them. We go out in the dark with a headlamp to see who's pestering them, check on them before we've even showered or dressed in the morning.

Yet as we grow older, we need less needy plants—plants that give back, that go the extra mile. After reducing the size of our garden and the number of plants we grow, we need plants that can multitask. It's not good enough to be just a pretty face anymore. Let's see their resume—what can they do besides bloom?

TREES FOR SHADE AND MORE

As our planet warms, shade becomes a more valuable commodity, especially for heat-sensitive seniors. In addition to shade, trees cool the area around them by releasing moisture in a process called evapotranspiration, and with enough trees to create a sizeable tree canopy, this process can benefit an entire neighborhood—a phenomenon called community cooling.

Count your luck if you already have mature shade trees. If not, you can't conjure up a fully-grown shade tree overnight in your existing landscape, but you can plan for a faster-growing species if there's room. Be advised that fast-growing trees, such as silver maple, may have weak branching that is susceptible to storm damage. It's also important to consider the tree's total height at maturity. Smaller patio trees (page 103–5) might be all you need.

If you're considering a new rightsized home and garden, it's smart to look at existing tree cover and potential tree placement. Planting shade trees might seem overly optimistic for older gardeners, although the saying "The best time to plant a tree was twenty years ago, but the second-best time is now" is so true. It can take five to six years for most trees to provide substantial shade, so they should be a priority when planning your new landscape. These selections from the Arbor Day Foundation list for fast-growing trees are a good starting point; however, consider your specific site and growing conditions:

American sweetgum (*Liquidambar styraciflua*): Zones 5–9
Dawn redwood (*Metasequoia glyptostroboides*): Zones 5–8
Hackberry (*Celtis occidentalis*): Zones 3–9
Northern red oak (*Quercus rubra*): Zones 3–8
Paper birch (*Betula papyrifera*): Zones 2–7
Quaking aspen (*Populus tremuloides*): Zones 1–7
Red maple (*Acer rubrum*): Zones 4–7
Red sunset maple (*Acer rubrum* 'Franksred'): Zones 4–8
Tulip tree (*Liriodendron tulipifera*): Zones 4–9

Get out the compass and orient yourself. A thoughtfully placed tree can not only give you respite from the heat outside; it can also help regulate indoor temperatures and reduce energy consumption and costs. According to the US Department of Energy, "Carefully positioned trees can save up to 25 percent of the energy a typical household uses."[1] Here are some more tips for smart tree placement:

- Planting trees on the west and southwest side of your home can provide shade for the hottest part of the day, blocking intense afternoon sun; this prevents it from directly entering windows and heating up the home.
- Avoid shading south windows, but if you want a tree southeast or southwest of a window, use a "solar friendly" tree, like oak, maple, or birch that has moderately dense foliage during the hottest times of the year, loses its leaves early in the fall as the heating season begins, and has sparse winter branches, which allow for natural warmth from sunlight in winter.
- Trees planted on the east side of your home can provide morning shade to prevent excessive heat buildup during the day.
- Make sure trees shading HVAC units don't shed leaves or debris (such as cottonwood cotton) that can clog the unit and cause a malfunction.

Trees do more than cast shade. They stabilize soil and absorb rainwater runoff. They improve soil structure, provide aeration, and improve water infiltration. They remove pollutants from the air and buffer unwanted sound. Trees offer food, shelter, and nesting sites to birds and small animals. All of that helps to relieve stress: According to the USDA, simply looking at trees can lower anxiety.[2] This, along with increased social

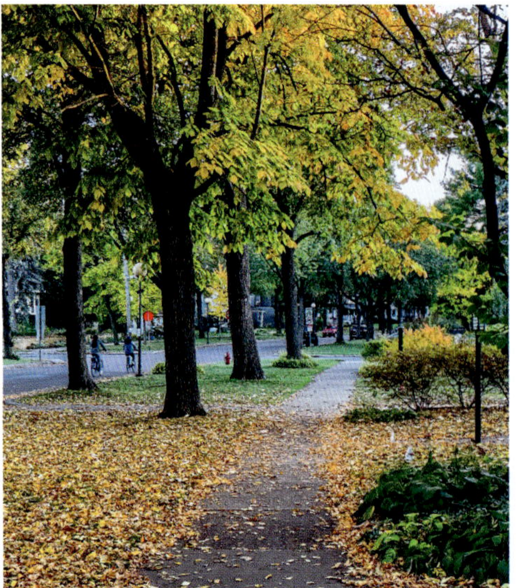

The tree canopy in my neighborhood provides cooling shade in summer and bright color in fall, and it allows warming sunlight to pass through in winter.

interaction in green spaces, bolsters the claim that trees actually reduce property crime.

If that isn't enough, trees are the most important plant in a butterfly garden. Trees like oak, willow, hackberry, and elm are larval hosts to hundreds of species of butterflies and moths.

LIVING MULCH: A BETTER WAY TO COVER GROUND

To talk about living mulch, sometimes called green mulch, first we need to talk about conventional mulch. Should we call it dead mulch or just mulch? Gardening experts tout the benefits of mulch all the time, and they're not wrong. It does a number of things to help our gardens: retains moisture, suppresses weeds, reduces erosion, insulates plants while cooling the soil, and even repels some insects. However, I suspect its most endearing quality is giving gardens a tidy appearance.

Mulch materials vary by region or climate. Pine straw is commonly used in southern states, oyster shells are found in mulch around homes along the Gulf and in New England, and people in the rice-producing state of Arkansas use rice hulls. Gravel and rock are used everywhere, and especially in arid climates. But the most common overall is some form of wood mulch. Each material has its pros and cons, and you should know these if you're planning to use nonliving mulch.

Here's what has convinced me to move away from conventional material (in my case, wood mulch) and toward living mulch: My urban lot isn't large, but it still took a lot of bagged mulch to cover the bare spots. Even as the plants filled in over the years there was still that need to "fluff up" the mulch as it thinned (wood mulch, being organic, slowly but steadily breaks down into soil). Buying, loading, unloading, hauling, and spreading all those bags of mulch is too much time, money, and effort. As we grow older, we've got better things to do.

I began a quest to cover as much of that area as possible with plant life, with the ultimate goal of eventually losing the mulch altogether. I quickly learned that groundcover is the best friend you didn't know you needed.

Something I brushed past at the garden center on my way to attention-seeking perennials suddenly fascinated me. So many colors and textures, like that quiet person at a dinner party you have to draw out only to find they can tell a captivating story. Here is a sampling of options for living mulch.

Low-Growers

Bugleweed (*Ajuga reptans*): Zones 3–10
Canadian wild ginger (*Asarum canadense*): Zones 4–6
Cheddar pink (*Dianthus gratianopolitanus*): Zones 4–8
Creeping phlox (*Phlox subulata*): Zones 3–9
Creeping thyme (*Thymus serpyllum*): Zones 4–8
Maiden pink (*Dianthus deltoides*): Zones 3–8
Sedges (*Carex* spp.): Zones vary by species
Sedum (low-growing varieties)
Spotted dead nettle (*Lamium maculatum*): Zones 3–8
Sweet woodruff (*Galium odoratum*): Zones 4–8
Woodland phlox (*Phlox divaricata*): Zones 3–8

Taller, but Attractive in Mass Plantings

Coral bells (*Heuchera* spp.): Zones 3–9, depending upon variety
Cranesbill (*Geranium* spp.): Zones 3–8, depending upon variety
Dwarf goat's beard (*Aruncus aethusifolius*): Zones 3–9
Lady's mantle (*Alchemilla mollis*): Zones 3–8
Lamb's ear (*Stachys byzantina*): Zones 4–8
Siberian bugloss (*Brunnera macrophylla*): Zones 3–8

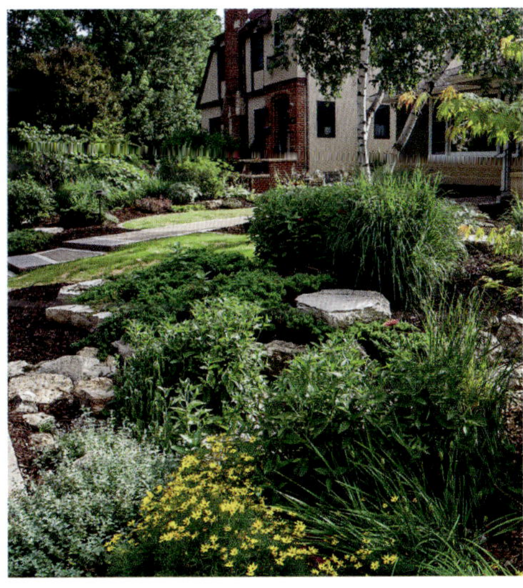

A new landscape benefits from mulch until the plants mature and fill in more area.

In nature you won't find "polka dot" or "meatball" plants growing in isolation like islands among mulch. Yes, you'll see some leaf litter that looks like mulch, but still, plants tend to grow next to one another; they touch and interact. When choosing your groundcovers it helps to mimic that in your design.

Plants have different levels of sociability, as discussed earlier in this chapter. Understanding plant sociability—how they interact with one another according to their

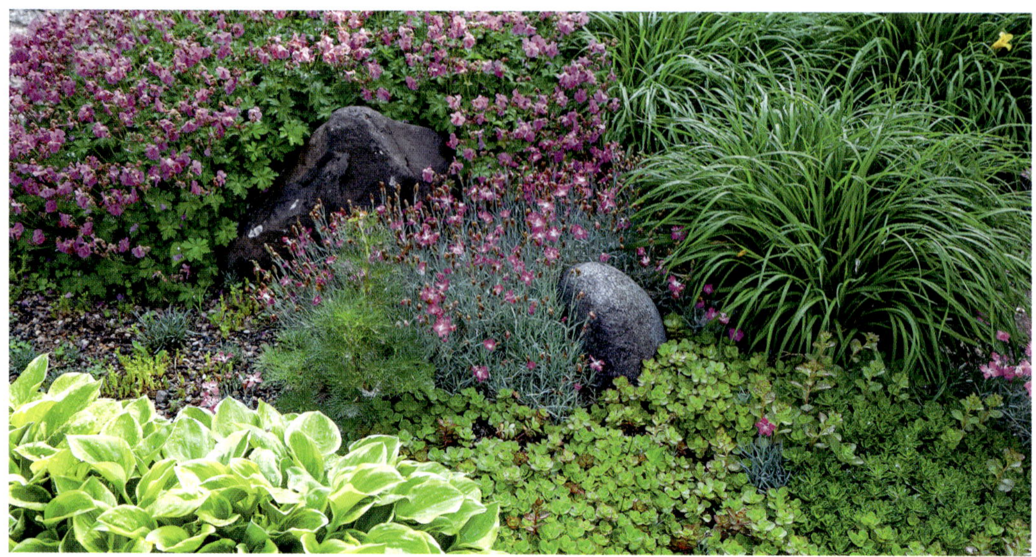

Living mulch with sedum (front), dianthus (center), cranesbill (top left), and sedge (top right).

growth habits—can help gardeners create more natural and sustainable landscapes by imitating the way plants naturally group together in their native habitats. Some grow in colonies, eventually spreading to form a mat, while others grow in individual clumps (but can be spaced closely together to form a a layer of groundcover). That can inform your choice of plants for this first layer of your landscape. Consider bloom time and how they complement the larger plants they grow beneath.

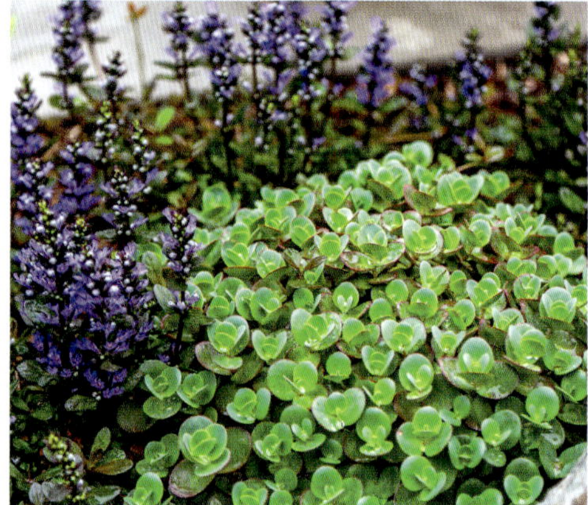

Living mulches 'Lime Zinger' (*Sedum*) and blue-flowering 'Chocolate Chips' (*Ajuga*).

Be aware that some groundcovers can be too aggressive for your needs, so do your homework. Groundcovers sold at informal plant sales (often plants dug from yards) are known to spread quickly—that's why people have a lot to spare. These may be perfect for large areas but maybe not for smaller gardens. The tendency to spread is what makes groundcovers successful at what they do. Once I have a patch established, I don't need to buy more; I just "divide and multiply." I dig up small pieces, poke them in the ground, and water well to keep enlarging the area of living mulch.

Living mulch goes beyond groundcovers. You can select matt-forming plants, or plant shorter plants en masse (mass planting). Low-profile grasses

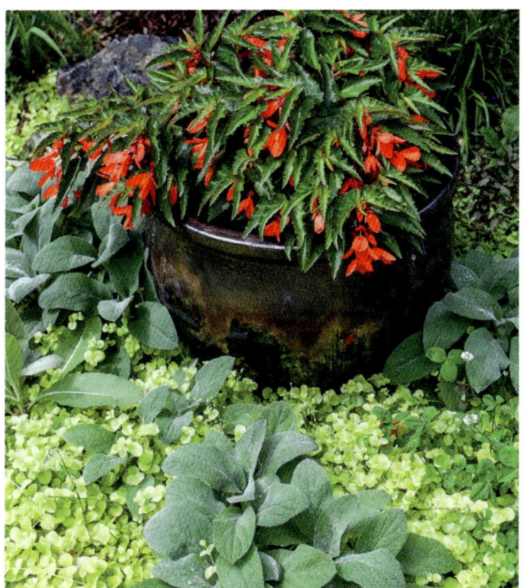

Living mulch of creeping Jenny with its gold-green foliage, and fuzzy, gray lamb's ears.

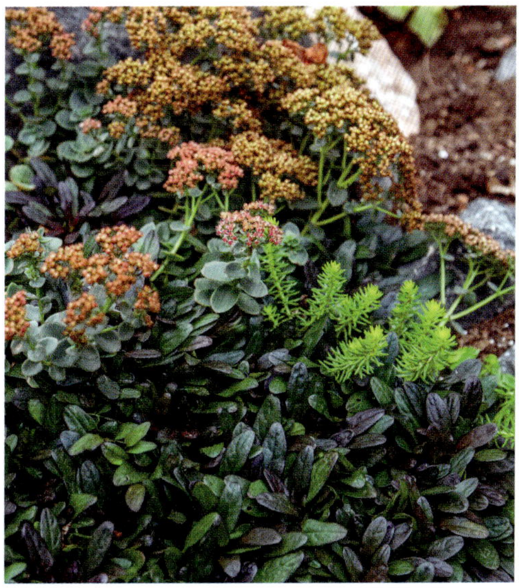

Living mulch helps to prevent erosion on slopes.

and sedges are perfect for creating a cohesive design. I like to think of them as sautéed onions in a savory dish: They act to bind together all the flavors to make something more complex. I love it when the plants that make up my living mulch meet and mingle, forming a living tapestry beneath my feet. I'm not there yet, but I'm well on my way to having living mulch throughout my entire garden.

It turns out that living mulch can do all the good things that dead mulch can do, plus a few more. Like conventional mulch, living mulch suppresses weeds, cools soil, and prevents erosion. Beyond that, it's sustainable and visually interesting, and it saves work. Once established, it's also economical because you don't have to replace it periodically like you do with wood and other organic mulches. In addition, I think it gives landscapes a mature, settled look; I call it "plant patina."

Living mulch also provides an all-important "soft landing" for insects. This term was coined by pollinator conservationist Heather Holm. It refers to diverse native plantings beneath keystone trees, like oak, willow, cherry, poplar, pine, and other natives trees that "provide habitat and shelter for various life stages of insects, especially caterpillars, moths, butterflies, and other beneficial insects like bumblebees and fireflies."

PLANTS FOR GUIDING FOOT TRAFFIC

In your current home, newly downsized garden, or entirely new garden, you'll find yourself taking certain routes back and forth from the house, to the garage or garden shed, and other frequented destinations. They might be newly created paths or shortcuts around the property. In a backyard it will be you and invited guests, and occasionally workers who need to safely follow these paths. It's important that these traffic routes are clearly marked, paved or covered with stable materials, and free of trip hazards like tree roots, clutter, and uneven ground. The way to your front door should be equally accessible, keeping in mind visitors, the folks who deliver packages, and others who might enter your property.

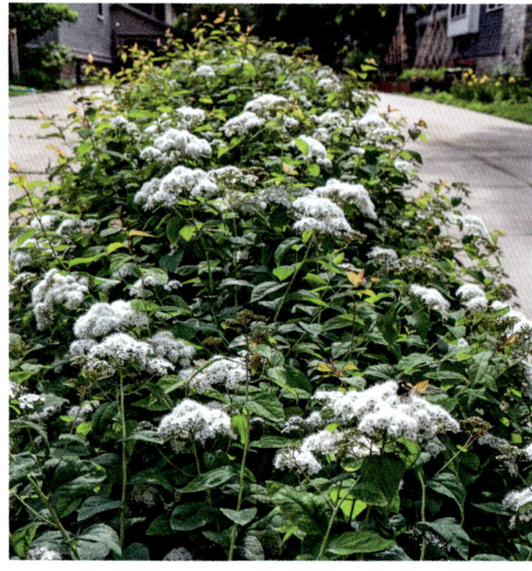

Spirea 'Double Play® Blue Kazoo®' attracts bees while dividing driveways, too.

It's helpful to identify the entry you want people to use, as it's not always obvious to someone unfamiliar. This can be achieved by simply marking an entry with two shrubs or large containers at either side that seem to say, "Enter here." Entrances are symbolic signs of welcome, facilitating that moment when visitors go from public to private space. An entry sets the tone for your interactions and expectations with everyone who passes or stops by.

If you live on a corner, you might find that passersby cut the corner and wear a path through your lawn or trample your plants. Kids, solicitors, utility workers, and landscape crews could cross your front yard with no regard for established pathways. There's a term for that: desire path. It's an informal, unplanned route or path formed by pedestrians who choose to walk along a more direct or preferred path rather than the designated one. Writer Robert Macfarlane, known for his books on landscape, nature, place, people, and language puts it more poetically in *The Old Ways: A Journey on Foot*: "Paths are the habit of a landscape. They are determined and sustained by usage, scored into the land by customary behavior. They are acts of consensual making, and in this sense, quietly democratic."

Considering all that, is it possible to train people to follow another path, one of your choosing? Whether you come from a point of aggravation or simply concern for others' safety, it's possible to use plants to gently guide foot traffic in and around your garden, without saying a word. Plants can work to guide foot traffic and subtly say, "Get off my lawn!"

Our long driveway runs parallel to our neighbor's, with only a narrow planting strip between them. When we built the house, I was worried about the little girl (and then came two more) next door crossing into the driveway before we could see them from the car. I purposely put in thorny plants, a hedge of raspberries, and a row of rugosa roses. It wasn't intended to harm or be inhospitable but rather to do just the opposite—protect those precious girls. It's a sweet deal because we share the raspberries on our respective sides.

There is a single break in the hedge, where we can predictably expect someone crossing, like the mail carrier. This break coincides with the walkway next door, our own front walk, and a flagstone path leading to the next house beyond. Instead of walking up and back to each house on our section of the street, Kelly, our postal carrier, can save lots of steps with our "postman's path." I can't claim credit; it's a brilliant idea I borrowed from a fellow Master Gardener who also happens to be a landscape designer. I often look out to see neighbors using it, too, knowing they are welcome to cross anytime.

Thorny deterrents around ground-floor windows also work to discourage burglars. Even densely planted woody shrubs can make an intruder think twice. You'll want to be careful around thorny plants, wearing gloves to work with them and maybe hiring someone to trim them, since our skin thins as we age and becomes more susceptible to tears and wounds. But you don't always have to employ gnarly species to guide people the right way.

Strategies range from a physical barrier, like a large container, all the way to creating a wildlife-friendly hedge, creating a visual guide to defining the pathway you prefer. You can use plantings to make the shortcut (the desired path) less accessible. Or, if all else fails, make the shortcut safer by lining the path with plantings and using decomposed granite or gravel to create a stable surface and show the way. In other situations, use groundcover that can handle foot traffic instead of turf that wears down quickly and becomes muddy after rain. Making the footpath more attractive and interactive will sway them to your "desired path."

SCREENING FOR PRIVACY, WIND, AND SOUND

Moving from a larger family residence to a smaller home, townhouse, or condo can be a shock in different ways. For one thing, you might not be used to living so close to your neighbors. While this proximity offers great opportunities for socializing and community-building, you don't always want to be on display. As the saying goes, "Good fences make good neighbors."

When we travel, we relish wide-open spaces and broad vistas, but at home we long for a sense of enclosure. It's almost primal to seek a sense of security, cozy but not claustrophobic, before we can relax and let go of the day's worries. But in tight quarters a wooden fence can sometimes seem unfriendly, and the blank panels are not exactly the most attractive sight.

Plants can help soften harsh views and create a private sanctuary, a retreat from the world even when the neighbors are grilling right next door.

Depending upon your situation, you can use hedges, trellises, and strategically placed plants for total privacy, or the illusion of privacy. You'll have to determine the level of visual porosity needed for your sense of comfort. In small developments or townhouse communities there could be rules about fence and tree heights, or even what you can plant yourself. You'll need to assess when you need privacy, seasonal or year-round if you live in a moderate climate. Deciduous shrubs, vines, and ornamental grasses will offer quick "cover" during the growing season but will allow people to see through in late fall to early spring.

For real privacy, plant tall, dense evergreen trees and shrubs, like holly or arborvitae, but keep in mind that this can lead to feeling boxed in, without a view to the outside. Using a single species, you also run the risk of disease or storm damage ruining that perfectly solid green wall. Eliminate some of that claustrophobic feeling by planting a variety of evergreens of differing heights and textures.

On the other hand, you can layer a number of plant species using deciduous and evergreen plants to diminish the lines of an existing fence, or you can start fresh with a livelier mix of colors and textures, possibly including seasonal interest. Choose smaller trees and shrubs that fit better into height

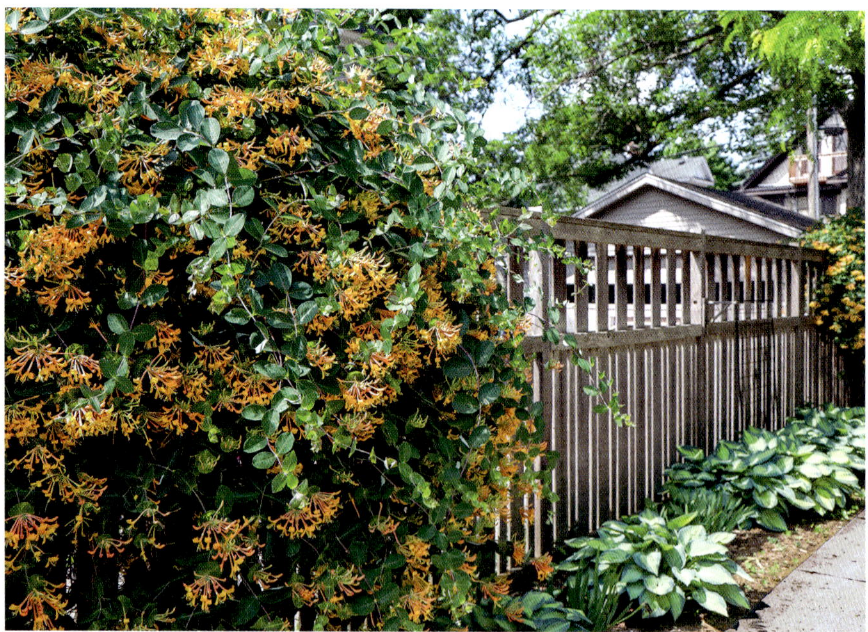

Orange honeysuckle (*Lonicera × 'Mandarin')* softens the fence and adds another layer of privacy.

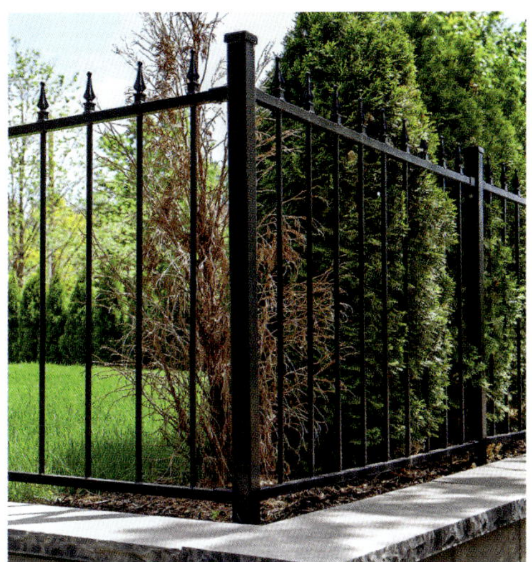

Too many arborvitae create a boxed-in feeling, and losing one affects the whole design.

restrictions and tight spaces, and don't need intense trimming to maintain their original shape.

Don't rule out ornamental grasses for quick privacy. The rustling and swaying beauties can create effective privacy screens. Planting tall—*clumping* rather than *spreading*—grasses in groups can block views and create the desired sense of enclosure. Choosing the right varieties, like feather reed grass, switchgrass, and bluestem, and planting them strategically will help create a natural, appealing privacy barrier.

While you're at it, consider the neighbors. Don't use monstrous plants that will shade out their entire patio, messy plants that will drop excessive leaf litter or other debris, or plants that will need pruning from their side of the property.

To target the right privacy plants for your region, I recommend starting with an online search of botanical garden databases like Missouri Botanical Garden's Plant Finder or commercial sites of the brands you see in the garden center, such as Proven Winners, Monrovia, Southern Living Plants, Sunset Plant Collection, High Country Gardens, and the like. Their websites can be a wealth of information without the obligation to buy. You can plug in your personal parameters and tailor your plant needs for hardiness zone, plant type, mature height, growth habit (like upright or vase-shaped), maintenance level, landscape use (like "good for screening"), bloom time, ornamental characteristics (like fall color and berries), and wildlife value. It's like a dating site for the perfect plant but with better luck finding the right match.

FAVORITE PATIO TREES

Small patio trees provide filtered shade and also help obscure views from upper-level windows. Many of these trees are understory trees, meaning they thrive in the high shade of larger trees, similar to the partial sun to partial shade conditions you'll find with denser housing. Ornamental patio trees, smaller than shade trees, add variety to the landscape, and with open branching and moisture-filled leaves can also qualify as fire-resistant. These trees charm with colorful flowers, intricate leaf shapes, interesting textures, and lovely fragrances. Here are some of my favorites.

Common serviceberry (*Amelanchier arborea*): Zones 4–9
Eastern redbud (*Cercis canadensis*): Zones 4–8
Flowering dogwood (*Cornus florida*): Zones 5–9
Japanese maple (*Acer palmatum*): Zones 5–8
Pagoda dogwood (*Cornus alternifolia*): Zones 3–7
Sweetbay magnolia (*Magnolia virginiana*): Zones 5–10
White fringetree (*Chionanthus virginicus*): Zones 3–9

TRELLISES AND CLIMBING PLANTS

Trellises provide some privacy even before you grow anything on them. Perennial vines like clematis, crossvine, jasmine, American wisteria, Virginia creeper, and honeysuckle are all good choices for a permanent planting, depending upon your hardiness zone. They will need some annual pruning and shaping to maintain their form and continue adhering to the structure. If you are looking for summer privacy, fast-growing annual vines might do the trick: Morning glory, moonflower, cypress vine, black-eyed Susan vine, runner beans, and hyacinth bean are all attractive choices that will invite butterflies and hummingbirds, creatures that are always welcome to stop by without calling.

For greater privacy, raise trellises higher by setting them into a planter box, raised bed, or elevated garden—a series of these effectively creates a living wall. You can easily construct a wider trellis by anchoring one into each of two large containers spaced several feet apart; the vining plants will meet in the middle.

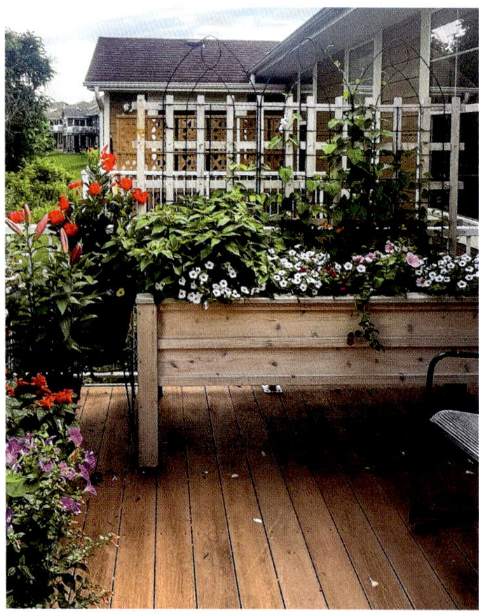

A planter box with trellis provides privacy between neighboring decks. *Photo courtesy of Mary Schier*

If you aren't allowed to plant into the ground, and have limited space for container-based solutions, sometimes a simple row of hanging baskets can distract from what's going on next door and shield you from outside observation.

Your privacy plants will do even more to earn their keep by also blocking wind, buffering unwanted sound, and absorbing dust and pollutants, vital services that will enhance the usability of your outdoor space and extend your home into the garden. A small water feature can also help to limit outside noise and mask your own conversations.

EDIBLE PLANTS FOR FOODSCAPING

Foodscaping, also known as edible landscaping, involves integrating edible plants into ornamental landscapes to create spaces that are visually appealing and provide food.

As I mentioned in the introduction, my grandmother was foodscaping way before the term was invented and before she realized that she was doing it. She grew bananas, berries, citrus, and more, all of it blending into the landscape she fashioned within the bounds of her small lot that was surrounded on all sides by more conventional front yards. I remember riding my tricycle along the sidewalk and pausing to eat strawberry guavas from the bushes she planted smack-dab out front. They looked like any

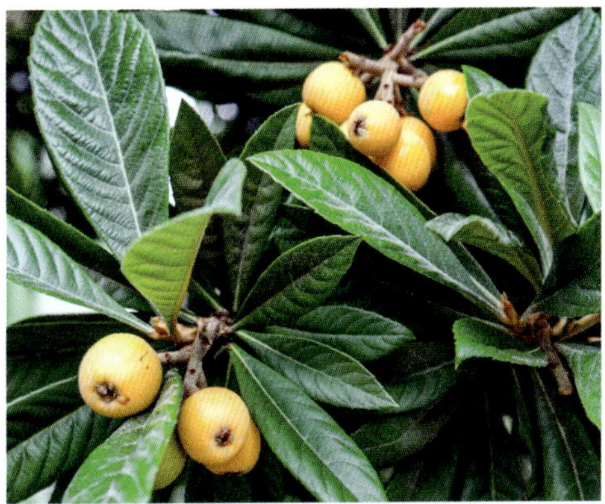

Front yard fruit trees like this loquat are common in New Orleans.

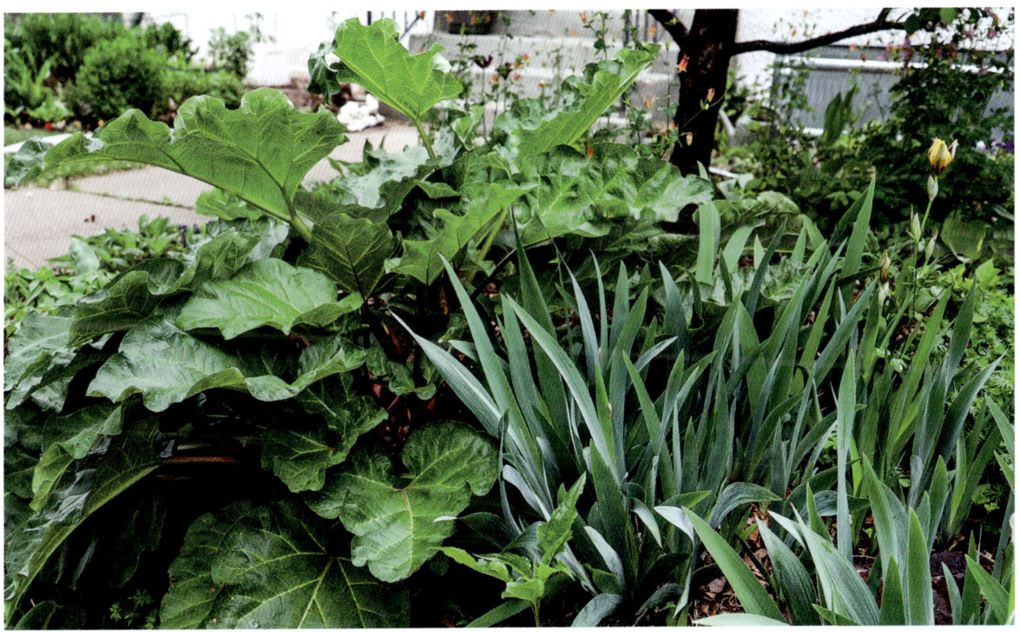

In this front yard planting, rhubarb foliage contrasts with spiky iris foliage for an attractive look.

Okinawa Spinach
You heard of blue zones? These are places throughout the world where people live the longest. One is Okinawa, Japan. And one of the reasons for their longevity includes them sitting around and munching on this delicious plant. I don't know how exactly to describe the crisp and crunchy almost medicinal flavor. It's like you can taste it putting a healing on you.

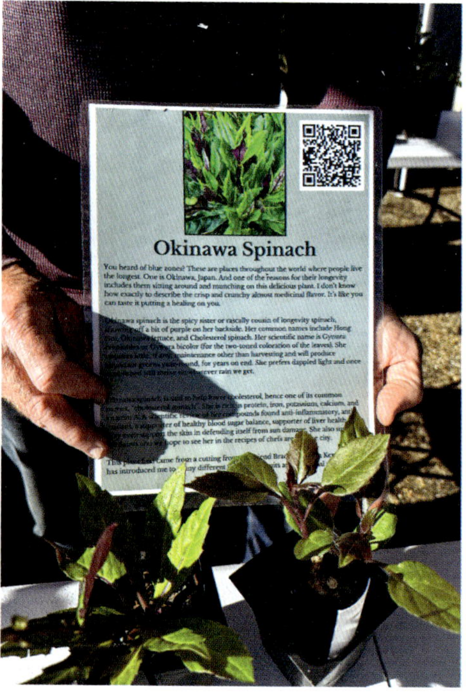

Okinawa spinach is a Blue Zone food, part of a healthy diet associated with longevity.

other ornamental shrub but had the extra value of producing edible fruit. When you grow plants that are both edible and ornamental, blending beauty with functionality in the garden—you've got edimentals.

Wherever there's potential for planting shrubs, it's a game of "plant this, not that." Plant a blueberry bush instead of a burning bush and you'll get fruit in addition to fall color. Other bountiful bushes and small trees that are popular edimentals include currant, gooseberry, pineapple guava, natal plum, pomegranate, dwarf citrus, and bush cherry.

Espaliered fruit trees, such as apple, apricot, and peach, grown against a fence or wall or trellised as a living fence are perfect for small gardens and courtyards. Espalier means "something to rest the shoulder against," and involves pruning and training the branches in a flat plane. This could be an ongoing stand-up project with little need for kneeling.

Edible groundcovers, like alpine strawberry, wintergreen, cranberry, chamomile, and thyme, are a winsome choice and look lovely surrounding pavers and stepping stones. You can substitute grapes, kiwi, hops, or passion fruit for other vines used as a privacy screen and have them do double duty.

Perennial fruits and vegetables need to be planted only once and can produce for many seasons (many have harvestable fruit after the initial two to three years it takes to establish the plants). Rhubarb and artichokes are stunning plants that provide architectural interest with their dramatic foliage. Asparagus and fennel offer an airy contrast with their feathery fronds. Other perennial vegetables include horseradish, sorrel, Good King Henry, and Egyptian walking onions, with even more options in milder climates.

Edible flowers round out the foodscape: anise hyssop, chives, nasturtium, borage, calendula, bee balm, and Johnny-jump-ups offer possibilities for cooking, teas and infusions, cake decoration, and garnishes.

Exploring Perennial Vegetables with Zach George

I first met Zach George at one of my favorite places during winters in New Orleans, the Crescent City Farmers Market, where you'll find me looking for sweet potatoes, pecans, greens, and Ponchatoula strawberries.

Zach's tent held a wide variety of unusual trees and vegetables I hadn't seen before. I was perusing his plants when I spied Okinawa spinach, a Blue Zone superfood. Okinawa spinach (*Gynura crepioides*) is commonly grown and consumed in the Japanese islands as part of the healthy diet associated with the longevity of the population, which boasts a large number of centenarians.

Zach's dad back in Iowa had a garden, but Zach wasn't interested initially. Yet after growing a few tomatoes he started reading about permaculture and edible forest gardens. Later, through his international travels, he discovered subtropical plants and vegetables from all over the world, including many that could translate to the same growing conditions suitable for New Orleans and similar growing zones.

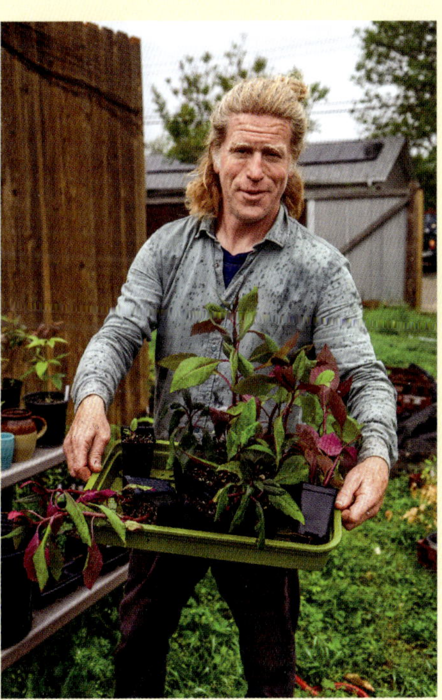

Zach touts the advantages and ease of growing perennial vegetables: "You're not messing with the soil—that keeps the soil alive underneath—and you're not going to be buying plastic pots every year." With Okinawa spinach, as well as longevity spinach (*Gynura procumbens*) and other "spinaches," he finds them vigorous, easy to grow from cuttings, and happy with little supplemental water during the heat of summer.

Zach has taught gardening in local schools, worked with client gardens, and helped neighbors grow things, along with working on his nonprofit, CRISP Farms. His new venture, Gol Che Nursery in the Lower Ninth Ward, promises to bring more of these plants to the people. When I visited the nursery, he pointed to where the greenhouse will go and moved from plant to plant, native and exotic, singing their praises as we passed loquat, beautyberry, moringa tree, and more. It's a whole new world of plants waiting to grow and nourish folks of all ages willing to try the new and unexpected. Referring to his countless uncommon varieties, Zach says: "If I found this much in just ten years, how much more is out there?"

GARDENER SPOTLIGHT

Eric Johnson

Eric Johnson's LinkedIn profile will tell you he's a graphic designer and communication consultant, but I know him as a talented garden writer, speaker, blogger, and photographer. This former theater major uses his blog, Garden Drama, to communicate "the emotional and dramatic impact of connecting to the earth in people's lives."

Eric grew up on a farm where his parents grew corn, soybeans, and alfalfa. He believes the power and independence of producing something of one's own was planted deep within him back then. His parents tended large vegetable gardens with tomatoes, onions, carrots, broccoli, cauliflower, beets, and more. To add color to the farm, his mother planted

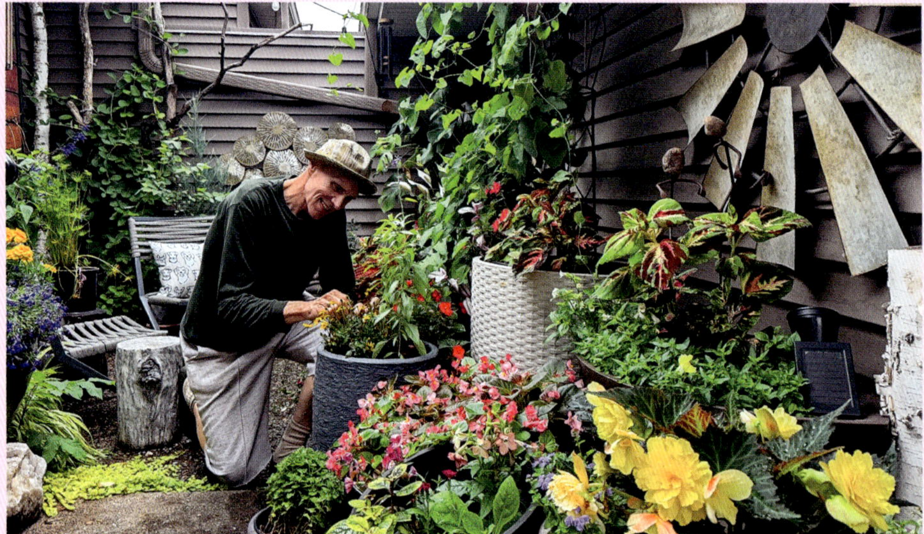

Photo courtesy of Eric Johnson

A LAWN THAT DOES MORE

Many lawns seem to sit there, doing little more than adding the color green, and yet they continually demand time and attention. Maybe your lawn could serve a higher purpose and give back to the (animal) community. Alternative lawn plants offer sustainable and low-maintenance ways to replace traditional grass. Popular choices include clover, creeping thyme, blue star creeper, Corsican mint, and moss, depending upon the amount of foot traffic the lawn sustains.

enormous beds of zinnias, cosmos, four o'clocks, and snapdragons. To this end, he learned, "If you're going to grow things, do it in a big way!"

In college, Eric always grew something at his various rental houses, but in 1990 he bought his first house and began a garden of his own. Over the next thirty years, he slowly removed sod and turned it into a series of garden rooms with hosta beds, a vegetable garden, a mini-prairie, three ponds, a rose garden, an English cottage border, and a potting area.

Eric says that making the decision to leave that garden is one of the hardest things he has ever done. He was nearing 60, and the garden was getting to be too much. He also spends weekends away, and the garden needed two to three hours of care every weeknight after work. It was a lot of joy but also overwhelming. He cried his eyes out on the final walk-through, but he was grateful to know the new owners bought the house partly because of the garden.

Three years ago, he downsized to a townhouse in the suburbs, making sure it had a decent-sized, private patio and an area behind the home where he is able to plant. He also rents a community garden plot nearby that he calls his city garden. Now he has a lush courtyard with clematis, honeysuckle, and Dutchman's pipe, hostas, and other shade plants, plus a small water feature. He always hated containers when he had a whole garden, but now it is the bulk of what he does. "I assemble them en masse and treat them like a garden bed. I will design five containers like they are one swath."

Eric makes many of his gardening decisions based on physical ease, like being able to pull up a stool when he works. He feared downsizing his garden as it represented the passage of time, but he found it opened him up to other aspects of being a plant person. Now he can give more time to his houseplants, orchids and African violets, and they seem to appreciate it.

ERIC'S TIPS FOR DOWNSIZING

- Make do with resin pots versus big ceramic monsters.
- Live with certain plants or plantings rather than feeling a need to always redo and make better.
- Downsizing is a wonderful creative opportunity, and you are able to do less of the grunt work and more finessing.

Lawn alternatives aren't a radical idea anymore. Just down the street, I've been watching a new clover lawn take off (it was seeded with some turf grass). It is lush and green and makes me smile when I walk by. The other day one of our neighbors told me proudly about the bee lawn they are planning.

The University of Minnesota has been working on bee lawns for a while, searching for just the right recipe. For our region, they recommend a blend of Dutch white clover, creeping thyme, and self-heal. But no matter where

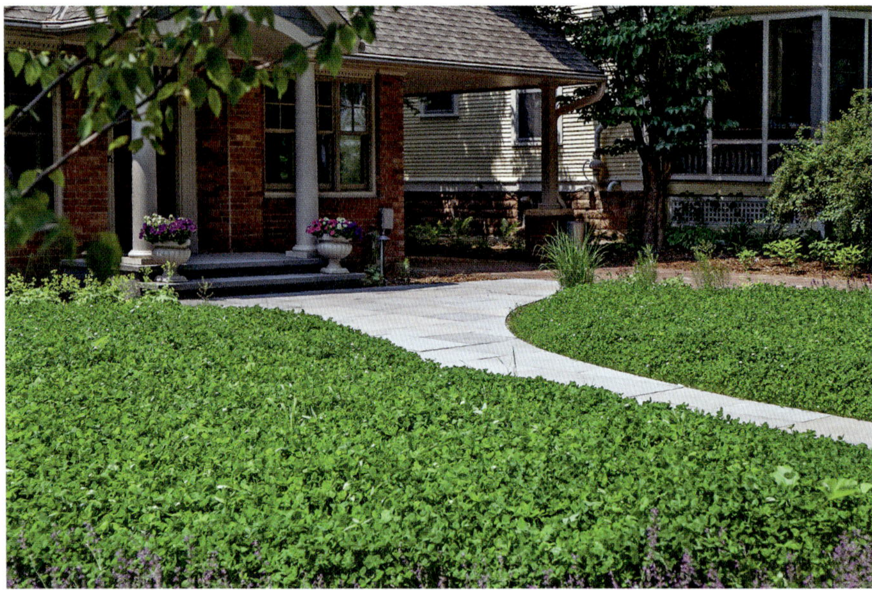

This clover lawn was installed in a new landscape on my block. It gets better-looking every week.

you live, they recommend looking for plants with the following qualities (you can consult your local Extension to find out what works for your area):

- Low-growing and adapted to being mowed
- Flower at low heights
- Tolerant of foot traffic
- Provide nectar and pollen for pollinators
- Moderately competitive, so they can hold their own with the turfgrasses without taking over
- Have a perennial life cycle (living for more than one year) so they are maintained in the landscape with the perennial turf

CHAPTER 6

Smart Gardening Methods

What a great time to be a gardener! It's hard to keep up with all of the ways gardening has been made easier for people of all ages, with everything from innovative products to ingenious growing methods. This is a huge bonus for older gardeners of all abilities looking for smarter, easier, and more enjoyable ways to continue pursuing their passion for plants.

The humble flowerpot has evolved, with new lightweight materials and self-watering systems that allow you to grow a wider variety of plants without the need for digging in the ground. Raised beds offer an improved approach for food growing that goes easy on your knees and back. Elevated and vertical gardening methods enable you to put down the shovel and garden standing up or sitting down with little more than a trowel.

All of this means that however your garden situation changes with age, you can still keep on growing. Moving to a smaller home, townhouse, apartment, or even senior living doesn't have to be the end of gardening; in fact, it might usher in a whole new era.

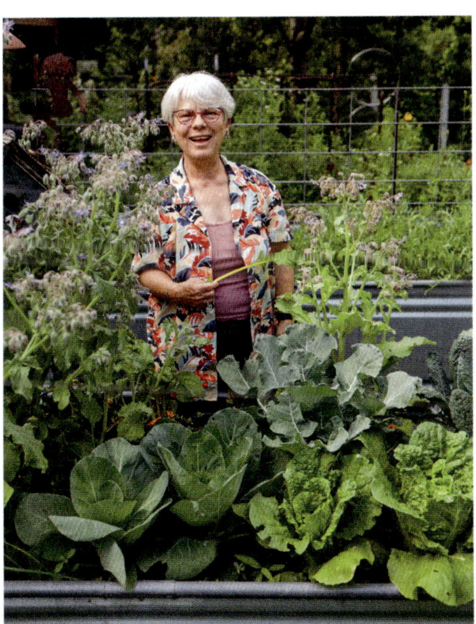

Hennepin County Master Gardener Barb Gasterland uses raised beds that allow her to grow fresh food with ease.

Container Gardening: Pot It Up!

There are so many reasons to use more containers; they're easy, economical, portable, changeable, and, best of all, they bring plants up close and personal to those who can't, or don't, want to bend over to smell the roses, or rosemary, for that matter. There is nothing radical about growing plants in containers; they've been in use for 5,000 years. What I want to know is, When did we start calling them containers? It sounds so industrial. I still love the term flowerpot or, simply, pot.

As for me, my husband likes to say I have a "pot problem." I don't think I have that many. The issue is that with the frigid Minnesota temperatures, almost every pot I use has to go inside the garage for winter, and my dear spouse has to help me empty them and tote them there. I have made some concessions over the years, as the putting away and bringing out of the pots becomes more difficult. So, I've begun "the letting go" and given away most of my big, beautiful, and very heavy glazed pots. I keep one for a dramatic focal point near my kitchen garden, and we (I use that term liberally) have to use a furniture dolly and straps to ferry it up and down the driveway. Someday I will have to let it go, too, or I could pay for help to perform this semiannual task.

LIGHTWEIGHT CONTAINERS

I haven't given up on containers, though. Lightweight containers are such a game changer, and best of all they have come a long way in terms of style, fooling the eye with realistic finishes that imitate terra cotta, stone, or concrete. You'd never know these containers are made of plastic, resin, or fiberglass. I continue to switch out and switch over to lightweight containers whenever I can. Don't discard your older, heavier ones, however; it's easy to find new homes for them through a yard sale or a free curb alert, or you can donate them to a plant sale or garden club.

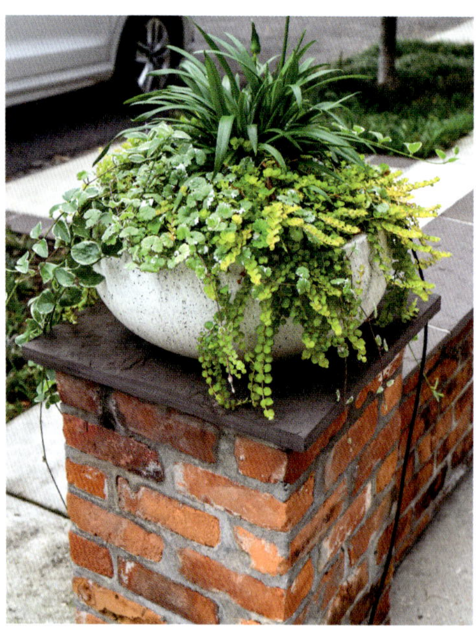

This faux-stone container with drip irrigation is much more lightweight than it looks.

I choose containers made from recycled materials whenever possible. For eco-conscious senior gardeners seeking more sustainable additions for their container collection, Crescent Gardens has introduced a line called Circular

Positive, the first planter of its kind made with a material upcycled from landfill waste (see Resources, page 213). The production of this container diverts carbon and methane emissions to be climate positive—a step beyond ordinary recycled or carbon-neutral materials.

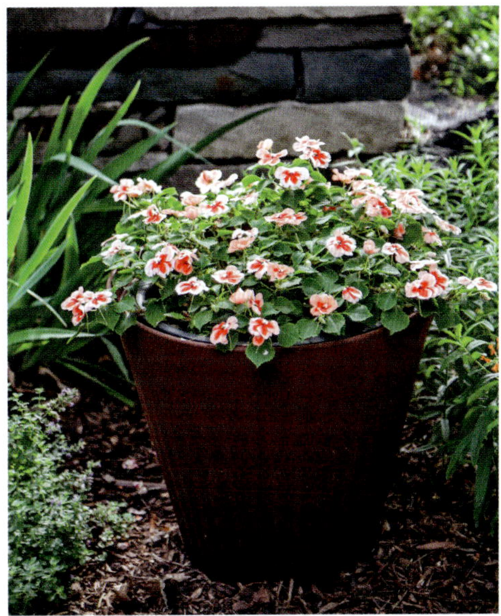

Self-watering Crescent Garden Circular Positive+ (a climate positive container) is made from material upcycled from landfill waste.

Being able to hoist lightweight pots, particularly the huge ones, around the garden without having to ask for help is a big motivator, especially if you're like me and move around pots like some people do their furniture. (A note of caution: When carrying containers around the garden, they can block the view of what's directly in front of you, like a step down or something in the way. Always move deliberately through your garden.) If you prefer to work with a helper, consider the PotLifter (see Resources), an adjustable lifting device that allows two people to carry a pot together, equally sharing the load. What's the old saying, many hands make light work?

Another trick to managing this task is to mobilize your plants by putting the containers on planter caddies, or dollies, with wheels. There are many styles and materials to choose from. Look for sturdy construction and smooth wheel or caster action. Lockable wheels are advised so the planter doesn't get away from you once it's in place (this is especially helpful on sloped surfaces). Caddies allow you to keep your plants ready to move at a moment's notice, to catch some sun, or seek refuge in shade, as well as moving plants temporarily away from frost or storms, or inside for the winter.

Depending upon your location, it's important to know when to bring your containers inside for the winter. This is when you'll truly appreciate the ease and independence of the lighter ones. Even though they're made with resilient synthetic materials, lightweight containers can still suffer damage from cold temperatures and ice accumulation. Be sure your container has adequate drainage holes. Ice forms a layer at the bottom of pots without good drainage, even when they seem dry at the top. Elevate them on pot feet or shim with flat tiles or stones to prevent this from occurring in cold climates. If you have containers with a frost-proof guarantee you can avoid the in-and-out dance as winter approaches.

SELF-WATERING CONTAINERS

Self-watering containers became popular in the 1980s when interior landscaping with tropical plants was on the rise, back when people worked in office buildings and fern bars were all the rage. Remember that?

Today, self-watering containers are so advanced that you can't tell them from a plain old pot. They're a little more expensive than conventional pots, but they're a wise investment for senior gardeners who have physical limitations that prevent them from hauling heavy hoses, or those who travel, especially those who travel a lot—cruise enthusiasts, we're looking at you. They're also a blessing for older gardeners who live in hot, dry climates, and they lend a hand to the forgetful gardener, too. Knowing when to refill is simple: Look for containers with a water-level indicator, or you can insert a thin bamboo stake into the reservoir opening, like you would an oil dipstick, to check the water level.

I cherish the saying, "The best fertilizer is the gardener's shadow." However, in this case, a self-watering container is not far behind, providing consistent water for good root health, while conserving water and reducing overwatering. You'll want to be sure your containers have over-fill drainage holes to prevent waterlogging during big rains. Also, don't use them for cacti, succulents, or Mediterranean herbs like lavender, thyme, and oregano.

Self-watering hanging baskets take the drudgery and danger out of watering your Boston fern or other hanging favorite. However, you still have to fill the reservoir, and they can be hard to reach. When maneuvering a watering can or the hose up to a hanging basket, it's a literal slippery slope; I usually end up wetter than the plant. But if you ask a nimbler, younger person to climb a ladder to install a retractable pulley with a carabiner clip, you'll be able to easily lower the pot to water it at a comfortable height, then hoist it back up using the pulley and hanging rope or wire. The carabiner clips the pot securely to the rope but allows you to remove it easily.

Gardening in Grow Bags

Grow bags are great for any gardener, but they're a real boon for people living in townhouses, condos, and apartments, or anyone wanting to garden in small spaces like patios, decks, balconies, or even a front step or stoop. They can be a godsend for the older gardener since they are lightweight and portable and they're easy to set up so you can start growing immediately.

They're also helpful in situations where there is limited storage, contaminated soil, septic tanks, poor drainage, or weed pressure. But be sure to get the kind with handles.

Grow bags prove their worth when you see what they do for your plants. The roots of plants grown in plastic pots reach the edge and start to circle. You've all pulled out a plant and found that tight, root-bound mass at the bottom. When roots reach the edge of a grow bag, the root tip is exposed to the air (hence the term "air pruning") through the breathable fabric. The root dries out and stops growing, signaling the plant to develop new, branching roots. The result being dense fibrous roots within the bag that absorb moisture and nutrients more efficiently, making for a healthier plant. In addition, while plastic containers really heat up in hot weather (having a negative effect on roots), grow bags stay much cooler so plants are less stressed.

Grow bags are a relatively new planting container. They were reinvented and improved upon by a tree farmer in the 1980s. Today's iterations come in all sizes, styles, and colors and can accommodate a wide assortment of plants, flowers, herbs, and veggies: beans, broccoli, eggplant, kale, carrots, onions, greens, chard, and more. There are even types for growing potatoes that come with a viewing window!

For most flowers or veggies, use at least a 5-gallon (19 L) grow bag; the bigger the bag the less watering you'll do. Fill them with regular potting soil or a container mix; don't use heavy garden soil. Use a liquid organic fertilizer to feed your plants as directed. Because of their permeability, grow bags will dry out faster than regular containers. As with other containers, grouping plants together in grow bags will simplify watering. If you have a lot of grow bags going you can hook them up to a simple drip irrigation system for more consistent watering.

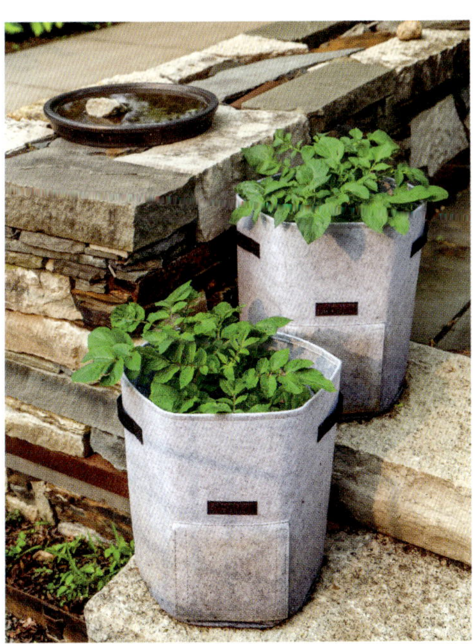

Potatoes planted in grow bags.

Grow bags are reusable and washable. You can simply hose them off, or even wash them in a machine with cold water. Then fold and put them away for next year. If you plan to reuse them as is, be sure to refresh part of the soil, and watch out for insects and disease that could carry over from the previous season. You

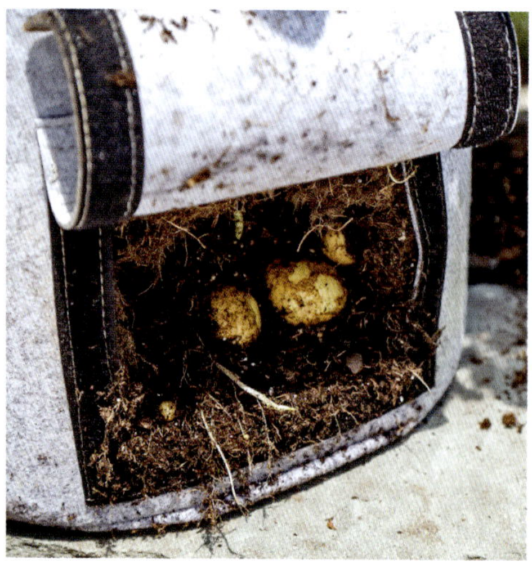
Potato grow bag with a "viewing window."

can place grow bags on tables or benches for an easier reach; just make sure to put something between the bag and the surface to prevent staining.

Grow bags are made from different materials like PET felt made from recycled plastic bottles that are collected, compressed, shredded, and melted down to create granulate, or plastic flakes. Others are made of landscape fabrics or geotextiles. Look for those labeled as lead-free and BPA-free. In general, grow bags will last from four to six years, depending upon use and exposure to weather. Once they are worn out, cut them up and repurpose the pieces for mulch, hanging basket liners, weed suppression, or other uses.

Up Your Game with Raised Beds

Raised beds aren't revolutionary anymore, but if you've resisted getting on the raised bed bandwagon, now's the time to make the leap. They can make gardening possible for years beyond the bending and stooping phase of life, to name one clear benefit. Raised beds are a big reason for my kitchen garden's success. Sure, I've got lots of sunshine on that side of the house, but it's the soil I've been able to build in those beds that makes the magic. They make it a joy to play in the dirt. Once you've gardened in raised beds, you might never look back.

Let me count the ways I love them.

- Raised beds warm up faster than the ground does in the spring, allowing for earlier planting and a longer growing season. I gain as much as two weeks on either end of the growing season.
- You control the soil composition in raised beds, ensuring it's rich in nutrients, well-draining, and free of contaminants. This can be a saving grace if you live in a flood zone where heavy metals could contaminate your ground soil.
- Raised beds allow for better drainage, preventing waterlogging and root rot, which can be a problem in clay soil.

- They allow for better aeration and root development, leading to healthier and more productive plants. This makes for a high-yield harvest in limited space.
- The soil doesn't get compacted by foot traffic because you never need to step into the beds to reach all of your plants.
- You'll have fewer troublesome perennial weeds, and the weeds you do have will be easy to remove in looser soil.
- They can deter some pests.
- They look great.

There are a few cons to raised beds, for those of you keeping score. Raised beds act as a large container, so they dry out faster. The taller the beds, the more frequently you'll need to water. However, this can be remedied with drip irrigation or a gridded irrigation system (see Resources, page 213) that also functions as a square-foot gardening guide.

In cold climates (Zones 3–4), you'll want to stick with annual crops and flowers since raised beds aren't insulated from the cold like inground beds. In a raised bed, perennial plant roots will freeze quickly instead of undergoing the gradual process that helps a plant move toward dormancy.

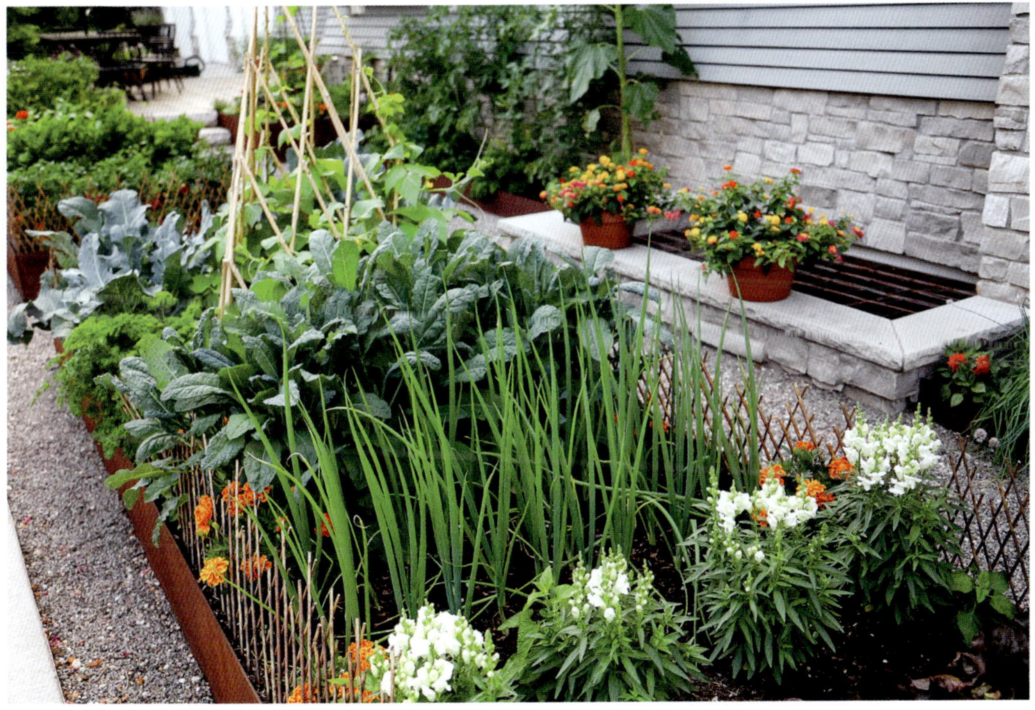

The raised beds in my kitchen garden are made of Corten steel, which has a natural weathered patina.

RAISED BED SIZE AND DEPTH

Think twice, and maybe a few more times, before building (or buying) and placing your raised beds; they aren't easy to move. Multiple smaller beds might work better than a single enormous one. Make sure you are near a water source or can bring water there without added hassle or expense. If you use more than one bed, be sure there is enough path space between them for a mower, cart, wheelbarrow, or just maneuvering around—at least 2′ (.75 m) in width.

The most common size of raised bed is 4′ × 8′ (1 × 2 m), which is largely determined by standard lumber dimensions. An ideal width is 3′–4′ (1 m) to allow access to the center from both sides, so there's no need to step in the beds. A narrower bed limits your planting options. You'll want to factor in planting space if you use blocks or pavers; their width can take up a few more inches of planting area in the bed—valuable growing space if you have limited room for growing. Stake it off and walk it to get a feel for it first.

Different situations call for different heights: 12″–18″ (30–45 cm) is considered ideal, but you might want to go to 36″ (91 cm) to foil rabbits and other pests. To avoid excessive bending, aim for somewhere between 24″–30″ (61–76 cm). What you want to grow determines the depth: 8″ (20 cm) is the minimum; 12″–18″ (30–45 cm) is adequate for crops like lettuce, greens, kale, cucumbers, herbs, strawberries, and even zucchini; for tomatoes you'll need 15″–18″ (38–45 cm).

RAISED BED MATERIALS

Cedar is the gold standard when it comes to decay-resistant, long-lasting wood. There's also oak, hemlock, black locust, and redwood, any of which could be harder to source. Pressure-treated wood is the most decay-resistant of the standard wood options. It has gotten less toxic over the years, but it is still made with toxic chemicals that can leach into soil. If you want to go this route, you should research further on your state's Extension website. Never use older treated lumber or railroad ties, which contain highly toxic creosote.

Galvanized steel is an attractive option with lots of different sizes and designs available. Note that zinc (used for galvanizing steel to add corrosion-resistance) might leach out of this in highly acidic soils. Steel beds that have been dipped in special eco-friendly coatings (like Vego Garden) are gaining in popularity.

My raised beds are made of Corten steel, or weathering steel. Corten steel is considered an eco-friendly material due to its high durability, extended lifespan, 100 percent recyclability, and low maintenance requirements. Mine are longer than typical beds, as they were designed to conform

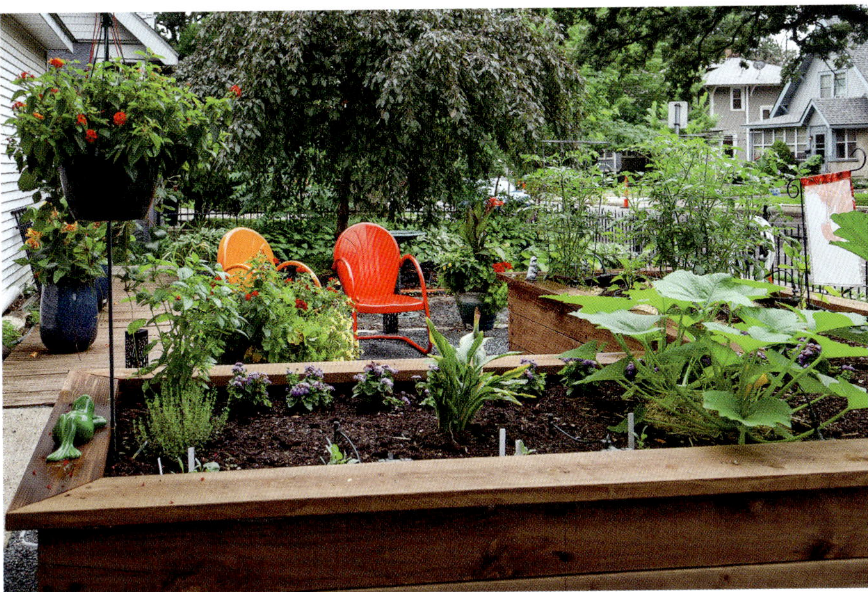

This L-shaped cedar raised-bed garden creates both a nice alcove for sitting and more growing space.

to our long driveway for maximum planting space. My only regret is not having the steel edge rolled at the top; the edges are sharp making them uncomfortable to lean against.

SOIL FOR RAISED BEDS

Garden centers, lumber yards, and other landscaping supply companies now carry blends of soil specifically formulated for raised beds, and some are certified organic. To make your own blend, the recipe is simple: two-thirds topsoil and one-third compost. You can buy it in bags for smaller beds, but if you're going big, buying soil materials in bulk and having them delivered is the most painless way to get your raised beds up and going. I refresh my beds with a few inches of manure and compost each spring to revitalize the soil and top up what has sunken down over the winter.

You should do a soil test every two to three years. Consult your local Extension office for soil testing procedures (some garden centers do this, too). You want to be sure that the soil has the right nutrients before you plant (and that you're not over-applying amendments). It can take a while to get your soil balance right when first using raised beds. Phosphorous can build up in the soil with excessive fertilization. Heavy feeders, like tomatoes, squash, peppers, melons, and cucumbers, can deplete the soil by the end of the growing season. Rotate your crops every three to four years (just as you do with conventional gardens) to avoid pests and diseases.

Vertical Gardening Grows Up

When space is limited, sometimes the only way to go is up. Vertical growing is one of my favorite gardening methods, and I'm always on the lookout for more ways to do it. The ideas are endless and allow for so much innovation and creativity—you might say the sky's the limit.

The main benefits of vertical methods for older gardeners are less bending and kneeling, fewer trip hazards, maximizing your gardening real estate, fewer to no weeds, and added visual appeal. For food growers, it means cleaner crops, increased yield, and an easier harvest. And with a little imagination, it can be really affordable. The benefits to your plants are just as desirable: better air circulation (so less fungal disease like powdery mildew), less access for ground-crawling pests, and increased sunlight. Win-win!

VERTICAL VEGGIES

People are always amazed at how many veggies, flowers, and herbs I squeeze comfortably into the raised beds along my driveway. Much of that is due to vertical growing. Not only does it increase my yield; it also fits with my goal of bountiful and beautiful. Vertical structures offer what I call punctuation points, showcasing vegetables that might otherwise blend into the background.

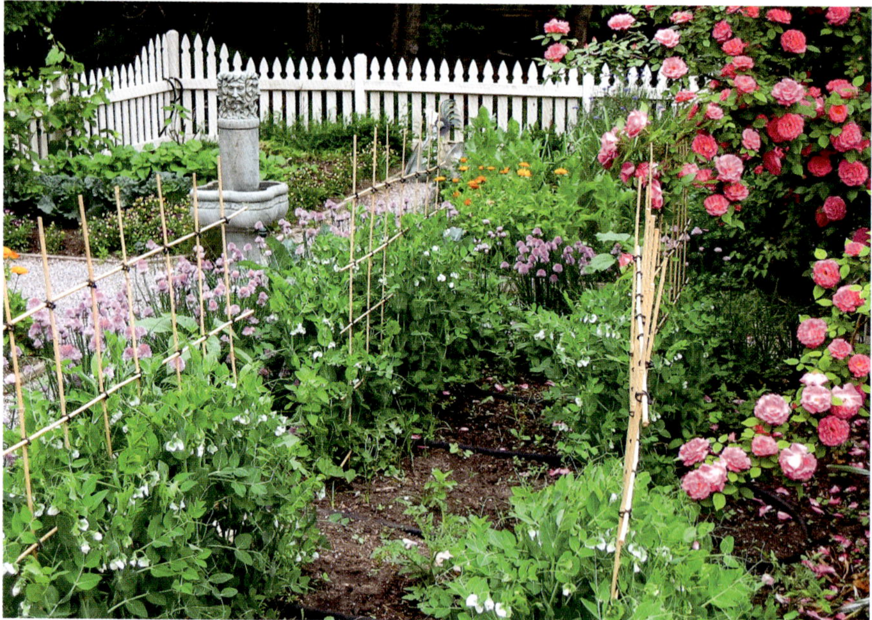

Peas growing on handmade bamboo trellises in my old Kansas kitchen garden.

There are purpose-built supports galore if you have the budget: trellises, tripods, expandable teepees, A-frames, arbors, arches, and simple cages. If you want to go posher, you can use *tuteurs* (French for "trainer") and obelisks most often reserved for climbing roses and other fancy plants. Imagine a cherry tomato vine clambering over a classic tuteur painted a sumptuous shade of blue.

For economical and eco-conscious solutions there are just as many options. With a bit of ingenuity, you can fashion cattle panels, chicken wire, chain link, metal headboards, gates, and other upcycled materials to hold up any number of climbing vegetables. Simple trellises of twine or string held with stakes or T-posts also work well for peas, beans, and other lightweight crops. Who will know once they are covered with gorgeous veggies?

When you're thrifting, be on the lookout for potential plant supports. And those old rickety ladders you promised to swear off for safety reasons would make an interesting trellis or plant shelf or, better yet, two connected by a crossbar.

I like to make an easy grid-style trellis from thin bamboo stakes found at the garden center. To make them, I arrange the stakes crisscross on a table or flat surface to the size I want (leaving one edge longer to push into the ground or container) and bind them at each intersection with a black zip tie, trimming the ties neatly when I'm done.

Some cautions: I use galvanized U-pins to anchor my bamboo trellises and teepees in the event of sudden wind gusts during storms. Take note of any wind-tunnel effects that occur around your home or outbuildings during weather events, so your crops don't sail away. Remember to match the weight of your crop to the stoutness of your support. Keep in mind the depth of your raised beds when placing the supports; heavier trellises might need to go deeper in the ground.

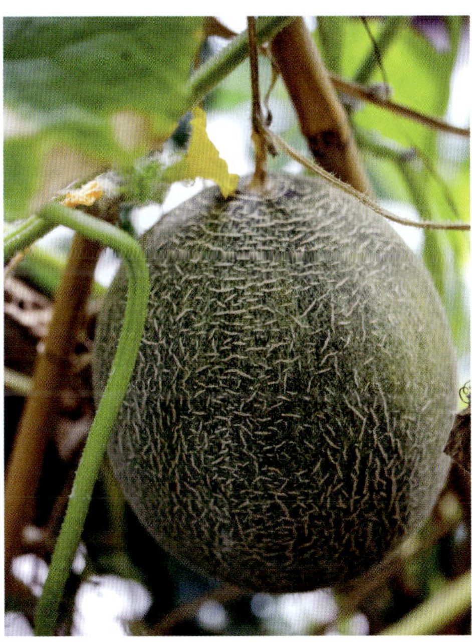

A 'Sugar Cube' melon dangling from an A-frame trellis.

I grow all the usual suspects vertically in my kitchen garden: pole beans (I refuse to stoop anymore for bush beans), peas, cucumbers, and tomatoes. I take it further and grow melons (my all-time favorite being 'Sugar Cube' cantaloupe) on a simple

A-frame. I love how they hang down like Christmas ornaments as they mature, then they fall off when they're perfectly ripe. I can grow a second season of lettuce beneath the A-frame in the shade of the foliage before melons form.

I always challenge myself to grow something new. Last year it was the Cuca melon, or mouse melon, an interesting addition to summer salads. It quickly climbed along the empty spots on my bean teepee where a baby rabbit infiltrated my pretty willow fencing and nibbled the beans off at the base. It's good to improvise a succession crop when one fails for whatever reason.

I have no room for roaming and unruly squash. So up we go. I grow 'Climbing Honey Nut' baby butternut squash on a trellis, using no more than bread ties to keep them ascending. This year, I'm making space for a new variety of yellow summer squash, 'Rise and Shine,' which climbs rather than squats (so it doesn't take up too much precious real estate). A green zucchini called 'Incredible Escalator' does the same. You'll hear that 'Trombocino' climbs, too, if you can keep up with it; the huge, silvery leaves will give you a run for your money. One of these sprinted across my patio and circled around when I turned my back. I occasionally found one of the curled squashes nestled in my landscape like a napping cat. I encourage you to experiment and see what else you can grow up. Always look for ways to stretch your gardening imagination.

Indeterminate, or vining, tomatoes obviously need sturdy supports like the traditional cage, or more inventive devices—the bigger, the stronger, the better. But smaller plants with large fruits, like eggplant and bell peppers, can

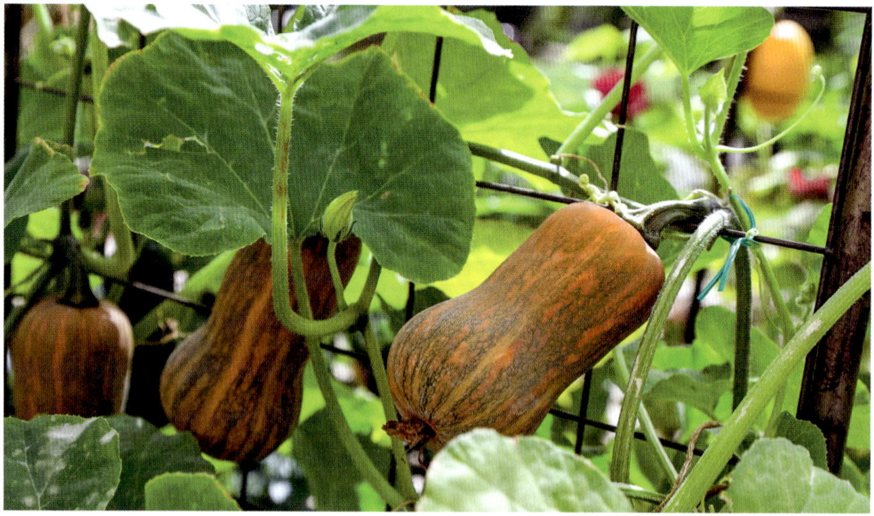

'Climbing Honey Nut' butternut squash growing vertically on a panel of welded wire fencing.

benefit from a little help, too. Placed in a short cage or discreetly tied to a trellis, they're less prone to toppling over, and the better to show off the colorful fruits as well. Sometimes I coordinate my colorful peppers with red-painted cages for a jazzy note. I crisscross tall bamboo hoops to brace my broccoli and cauliflower plants when they lean too much toward the sun. The hoops offer support and a decorative accent at the same time.

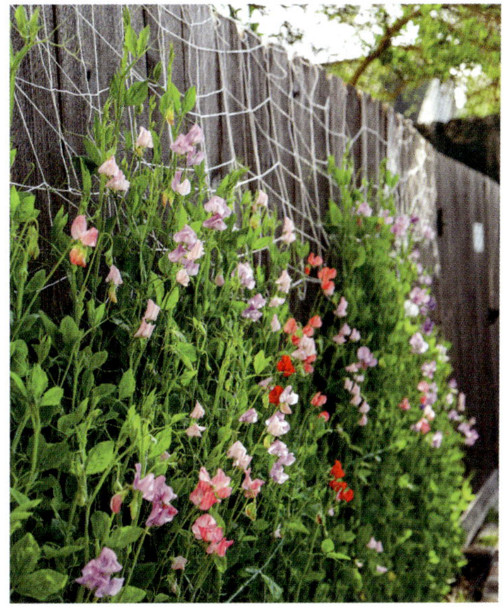

Sweet peas adorning a fence in a tight space.

FLOWERING VINES

Flowering vines derive and provide all the same benefits as vegetables when grown vertically. Easy to tend, they thrive in their elevated state and become stunning additions to our gardens. Fast-growing annual vines started from seed and grown vertically offer an exclamation point to flower beds and a spot of color in the kitchen garden, all while attracting pollinators. The orchid-colored blooms of my hyacinth bean plants are striking, but it's those bronze leaves that give the vegetable beds a certain *je ne sais quoi.*

Here are some delightful flowering vines to try.

Black-eyed Susan vine (*Thunbergia alata*)
Cathedral bells (*Cobaea scandens*)
Cypress vine (*Ipomoea quamoclit*)
Garden nasturtium (*Tropaeolum majus*)
Hyacinth bean (*Lablab purpureus*)
Spanish flag (*Ipomoea lobata*)
Sweet pea (*Lathyrus odoratus*)

Wonderful Wall Gardens

Pretty as paintings, wall gardens are living, carbon-dioxide-breathing collections of plants that offer a big dose of green in a very small footprint. They're perfect for those with limited space or limited mobility or for someone like me who is always scoping out the next blank space that needs a plant. No bending required.

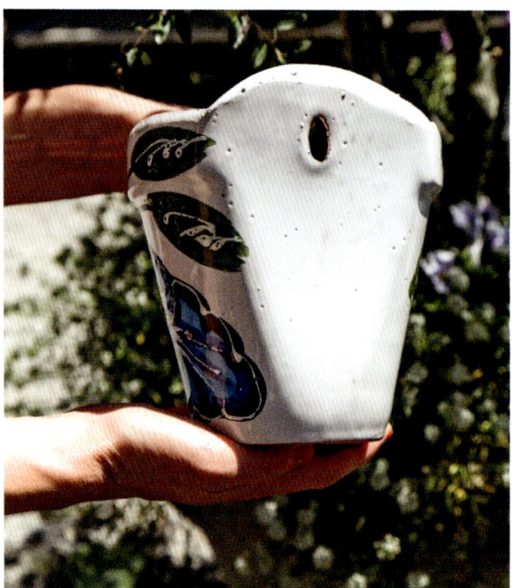

Wall-mounted Spanish-style pots are perfect for herbs, geraniums, and other water-wise plants.

WALL-MOUNTED PLANTERS

Wall-mounted planters or pots are self-explanatory. Picture those Mediterranean gardens that fill an entire wall with mounted pots of colorful geraniums. The pots, like orzas and tinajas, are made with a flat side and a hole for hanging. Whether a single container or a grouping, this type of wall garden gives off a shady courtyard or sunny patio vibe. You can find hundreds of styles of planters, according to the look you want, or you can upcycle something you have around the house. There are also purpose-made containers that attach directly to a wall, many of them self-watering. Another wall-mounting option is to use flowerpot rings that attach to the wall with brackets and hold pots that are easy to slip in and out of the rings.

Beware that smaller pots dry out quickly. On hot, sunny walls use appropriate plants like cacti, succulents, geraniums, or other water-wise varieties. On the other hand, if your planter wall is your only garden space, you might enjoy the ritual of watering and tending the plants frequently.

LIVING WALLS

Living wall, or picture-frame-style, gardens usually consist of a plastic module of individual lined planting holes or a series of pockets made from recycled or industrial felt, like those from Woolly Pocket or WallyGrow (see Resources). WallyGrow bags are designed to absorb water and nutrients and feature a clever watering channel that directs water to the roots, promoting healthy growth and reducing the frequency of watering. The breathable front panel allows for better air circulation, helping to prevent problems like root rot.

Even wood pallets work for living walls. Depending upon your available space, you can combine multiple sections to create dramatic wall-mounted landscapes. Most systems are easy to put together, but you might need help attaching them to the wall.

Be sure to look for a system designed to prevent wall damage from seeping moisture. If you go the homemade route with a wooden pallet, you'll have to mount it in a way that it stands out from your wall at least a few inches. Otherwise, look for wall gardens that have a built-in reservoir (for indoor use) or built-in drip irrigation. These systems are designed to be watered from the top, allowing moisture to percolate down. It takes a while to get the amount of water right to reach all the way to the bottom.

For an easy DIY version, make a simple, inexpensive wall garden from an over-the-door shoe organizer. Just be sure you aren't worried about the wall or fence it sits against. You can tack up plastic sheeting behind it first to minimize moisture damage. Place your plants in the pockets and carefully fill in with a potting mix or a lightweight soil-less seed starting mix (you'll need to add a liquid organic fertilizer in this case.) This method will require more frequent watering as the season warms up.

It's important to use the right soil mix for any living wall system. A soil-based mix with organic matter and all the right nutrients to support healthy plant growth can become too heavy. In that case, use a lightweight soil-less mix made of materials such as coconut coir, Rockwool, or perlite, and feed the plants with liquid organic fertilizer as needed.

Choose plants suitable for your location's sun exposure—shade for tropical houseplants or sun for succulents, and so on—and give the plants room to grow. You can start with easy plants, like herbs, or common container plants like begonias, impatiens, sweet potato vines, or coleus, then expand your horizons. A living wall is a living tapestry; experiment with flower color, leaf shape, texture, contrast, and trailing effects.

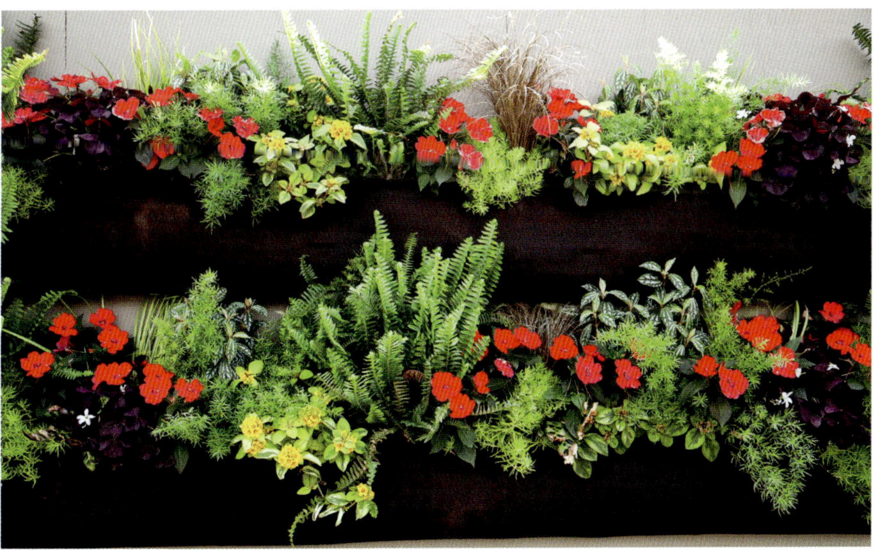

WallyGrow bags planted with New Guinea impatiens, aluminum plant, hoya, purple oxalis, ferns, grasses, and sedum.

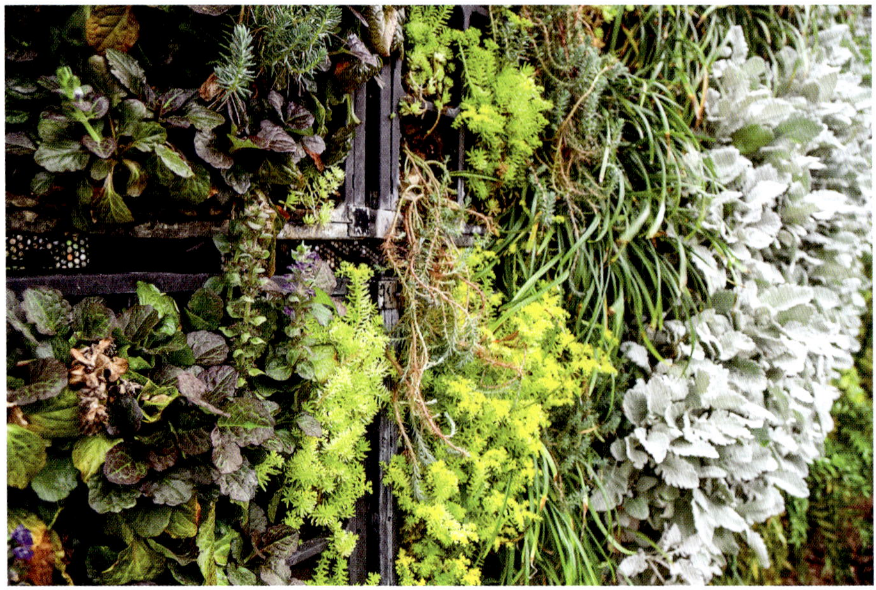

Sedum, ajuga, dusty miller, and other plants in a wall module planting.

Note that plants in wall planters, just like in containers, do not adjust to or withstand cold temps like inground plants do. A plant that is normally hardy to Zone 5 should be considered more a Zone 6 or even 7 when growing aboveground. Take this into consideration before attempting to overwinter your wall.

Here are some plants to try for different living wall situations.

Sunny ornamental walls (6–8 hours of sun):

Blue fescue (*Festuca glauca*): Zones 4–8
Blue oat grass (*Helictotrichon sempervirens*): Zones 4–9
Cuban oregano (*Coleus amboinicus*): Zones 9–11
Dusty miller (*Senecio cineraria*): Zones 8–10
Mexican daisy (*Erigeron karvinskianus*): Zones 6–10
Plumbago (*Ceratostigma plumbaginoides*): Zones 8–11
Rock rose (*Portulaca grandiflora*): Zones 9–11

Shady ornamental walls (tolerates morning sun):

Bugleweed (*Ajuga reptans*): Zones 4–9
Coral bells (*Heuchera*): Zones 4–8; named cultivars might vary
Ferns: Zones vary by species and variety
Heart leaf bergenia (*Bergenia cordifolia*): Zones 4–8
Japanese spurge (*Pachysandra terminalis*): Zones 5–9
Sedge (*Carex*): Zones vary by species and variety

Siberian bugloss (*Brunnera macrophylla*): Zones 3–8
Smaller hosta varieties: Zones 3–9

Sunny edible walls (6–8 hours of sun):
Basil
Chives
Cilantro
Dwarf cherry tomatoes
Oregano
Sage
Strawberries
Thyme

Shady edible walls (morning sun):
Alpine strawberries
Arugula
Dwarf runner beans
Lamb's lettuce or mesclun
Lettuce
Mizuna
Parsley
Red giant mustard
Spinach

Stack It Up: More Ways to Garden Vertically

Once again, when pressed for growing space, sometimes the only way to go is up. Shelf gardens and plant theaters allow you to grow a number of plants in the same space as a bookshelf. Vertical planters (growing towers) and elevated gardens can easily fit on a deck or patio.

SHELF GARDENS

Shelf-style tiered structures, such as the Gronomics vertical garden bed, offer lots of growing area for small spots like balconies and decks. They take up only a few square feet of floor space while providing 15–20 linear feet (4–6 m) of planting space. These are ideal for gardeners with little room to exercise their green thumbs. Very little bending is required to tend this type of garden. The price may be off-putting at first, but consider it an investment in your health and happiness.

For those of you with arthritis or limited strength, look for a unit that comes preassembled (see Resources.) Some include an easy-to-use drip watering system. You might need help setting it all up, but once it's in place you'll find it a handy and enjoyable way to grow edible crops, like salad greens, strawberries, and herbs, along with flowers for butterflies. There's nothing quite so gratifying as growing fresh food steps from your kitchen.

PLANT THEATER

Let your special plants take the stage. A plant theater is a beloved, traditional English gardening concept, featuring either a tiered plant stand or a shallow wall-mounted shelf, with three to five rows for display. The most well-known is an auricula, or primrose, theater with individual flowers potted in patinaed terra cotta. At alternate times, spring favorites like snowdrops, violas, and muscari might have a turn, followed perhaps by pelargoniums. The idea is to showcase your best specimens or a particular collection. The display then rotates with the seasons. An American version might include succulents or cactus as the weather heats up.

PLANTING TOWERS

I'm excited for my first go with the Greenstalk vertical planter (see Resources). I've been lusting over photos of them, overflowing with strawberries, herbs, salad greens, and annual flowers. I love the idea of utilizing my patio's airspace and harvesting strawberries out the back door, but the most satisfying part will be when I thumb my nose at the audacious rabbits that have become braver and more brazen with every season.

Growing towers vary in design and are created with stackable modules—planting pockets—made of food-grade plastic. They come with a reservoir system for watering. The Garden Tower 2™ features built-in composting using worms; you can make your own organic fertilizer with kitchen scraps. How's that for sustainable gardening in small spaces?

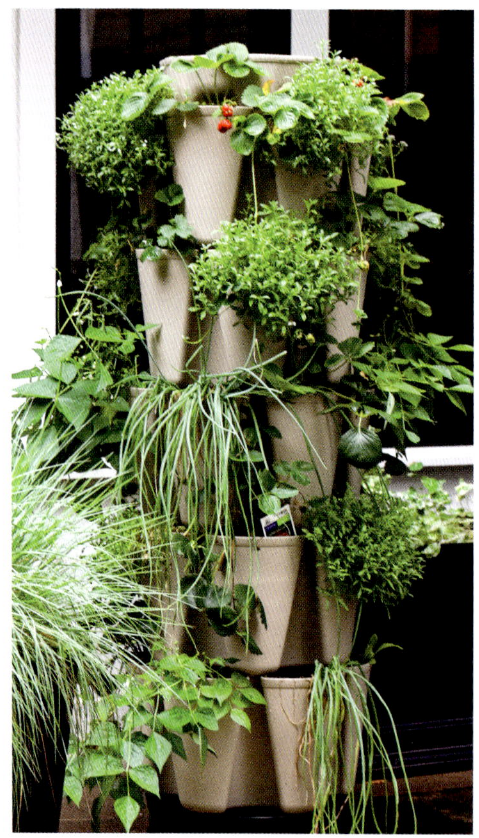

Greenstalk vertical planter with green beans, shallots, alyssum, and strawberries.

There are lots of instructional videos online showing how to assemble the planters. However, you might want to enlist the help of a friend or family member. I found placing the very top module a bit challenging. You'll want to make sure the planter is sited on a hard, level surface, sheltered from high winds. Once you've assembled the planter and added a soil mix, you can start by sowing seeds or directly planting into the individual growing pockets. Some come with a spinning base or wheels so that you can turn your tower as the sunlight moves, or easily roll it inside in bad weather. I really like that this is a gardening solution for all levels of ability, and what a fun project to do with the grandkids.

ELEVATED GARDENS

Think of it as a garden on legs that does all the heavy lifting for you. Elevated garden beds are popular with all ages but give an extra boost to seniors. In this case, the numbers are important: most elevated gardens are around 29″ (73 cm) tall—just right for easy planting, tending, and harvesting, with no bending or kneeling, just the fun parts. At 8″ (20 cm) deep they have plenty of depth for the roots of most annual flower and garden crops. The overall dimensions are around 40″–50″ (101–127 cm) long and 24″ (61 cm) wide; this means the planting area is accessible from either side.

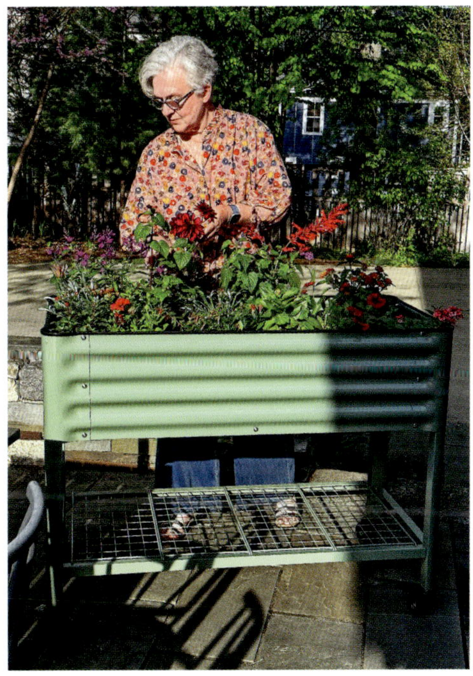

Thanks to the casters, I can move the Vego Garden elevated bed planted with hummingbird flowers to catch the sun, or whenever I want to sweep that area.

An elevated bed is big enough for growing a culinary-themed mini-garden: a single tomato plant, plus peppers, oregano, and basil for a pizza garden; a bush cucumber, hot and sweet peppers, onions, and dill for a pickling garden; or a tea garden with lemon balm, bee balm, lavender, stevia, and spearmint (contain mint inside a small pot within the bed so it doesn't take over). Add marigolds, alyssum, or violas to make it pretty and attract pollinators.

Elevated gardens come in a number of styles and materials, including wood, metal, and plastic. I'm enjoying the Vego Garden

GARDENER SPOTLIGHT

Larry Cipolla

If we listed all of Larry Cipolla's accomplishments as an author, speaker, and Master Gardener, we would run out of space—he is a busy guy who, to date, has volunteered over 6,000 hours as a Master Gardener. He teaches a wide range of topics related to vegetables and herbs and specializes in hydroponics. His gardens have been on numerous fundraising tours and featured in television programs, newspapers, and periodicals. He even developed his own organic heirloom Italian paste tomato; I've grown 'Cipolla's Pride,' and I can tell you it is one heck of a tomato.

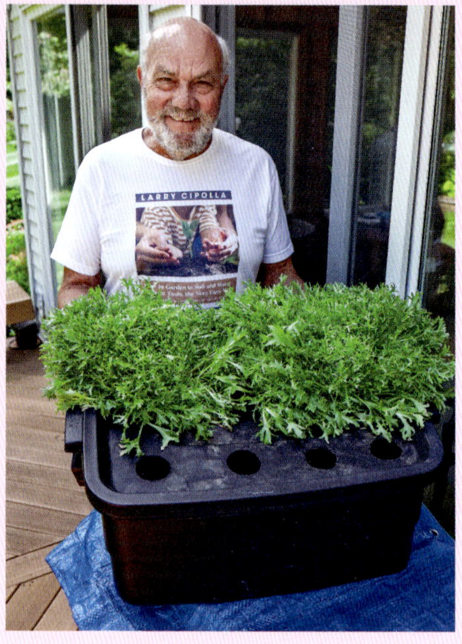

As a lifelong gardener and lifelong learner, Larry's goal is to encourage people to integrate hydroponics with soil-based gardening, whether you're a first-timer or a seasoned gardener. His intent is to help people garden year-round, whether they live in a detached home, condo, apartment, or senior high-rise. His passion is to encourage people to become more independent and more self-reliant in order to take control over what they eat.

Larry first saw hydroponic growing systems on a business trip to Singapore in 2010. People were growing tomatoes (very

elevated garden bed. It's good-looking, well-constructed, and easy to assemble—a good investment for long-term gardening. It's also perfect for a hummingbird haven (as shown on this book's front cover).

Wedge-shaped and desk-style elevated garden beds are wheelchair accessible, allowing people of all abilities the opportunity to tend a garden of their own and on their own terms. A standout example is the Wheelchair Accessible Raised Garden Bed from Gardener's Supply Company that provides ample clearance for wheelchair users. It is designed for a wheelchair to fit comfortably underneath and allow users to tend even the farthest corner without uncomfortable or dangerous overreaching.

close together) in active systems using tubes and electric pumps. He started pondering the idea of designing a system for people with limited space, and without using electricity. Fast forward—he participated in a trial with the University of Minnesota to evaluate a passive system using 10-gallon (38 L) totes.

Larry has gone on to refine and simplify his design so that it can be done with minimal tools and supplies—a system he calls, "Set It and Forget It." If you are interested in learning more about hydroponics, I highly recommend his book, *Hydroponic Gardening: The Very Easy Way*.

Larry praises hydroponics for making his gardening life easier. No spring soil prep; just fill the buckets with water, hydronic fertilizer, and plants. No mulching. No weeding. No soil disease. No bags to haul. No winterizing.

To make his soil-based gardening easier, Larry, who is eighty-one, has downsized from a larger garden and converted his original garden space to raised beds and elevated beds to accommodate his aging knees and hips. Among the benefits he touts, there's no more rototilling, and he now uses mostly hand tools. He composts plants at the end of the season. In fall, he grows a cover crop or uses straw to minimize weeding in spring. He practices botanical rotation (according to plant families) to prevent insect damage and disease. He loosens only the top 2″–3″ (5–7 cm) of soil in spring before planting. He credits the changes he has made—moving to raised beds and hydroponics—for dramatically reducing his labor and need for equipment.

LARRY'S TIPS FOR YEAR-ROUND HYDROPONIC GARDENING

- Take control by growing what you like to eat, which means fewer trips to the store to buy vegetables and herbs.
- Harvest only what you intend to eat that day—less food waste.
- Using hydroponics avoids pesticides and herbicides.
- Growing with hydroponics indoors, you can garden without weather worries from frost, snow, hail, heavy downpours, and high winds.

Easy Hydroponics

No soil, no problem. Grow fresh salad greens year-round, letting water do most of the work. Hydroponic actually means "working water," and these gardens have been used since the ancient days of Babylon; now NASA hopes to use them to grow potatoes in space. But don't worry; this simple setup will work just fine on your balcony or deck. While yours might be a small operation, you'll get faster growth and higher yield for the space allotted than with conventional gardening.

A passive deep-water hydroponic system doesn't require complicated tubes or pumps. You can buy ready-made snap-on, wide-lipped plant

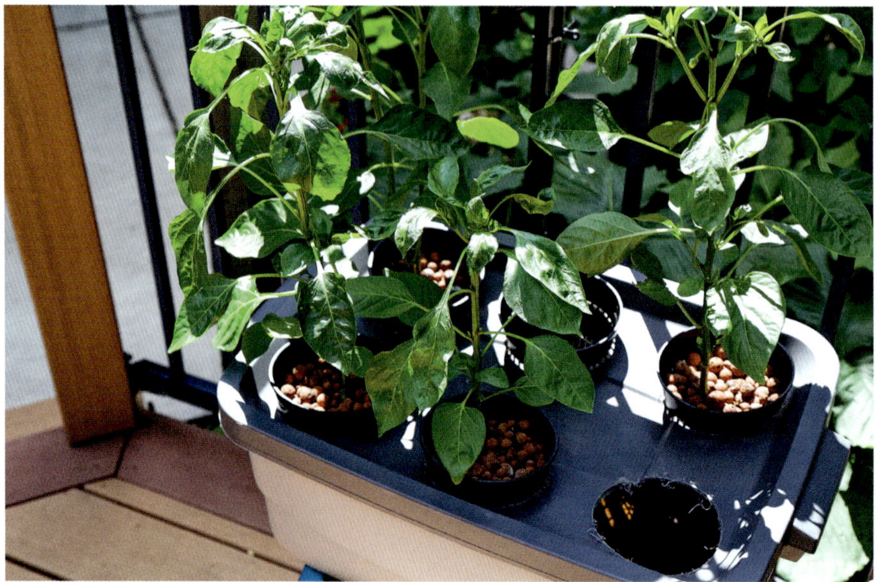

Peppers grow in a simple hydroponic system made from a rubber tote.

baskets (WLB) for use with 5-gallon (19 L) food-safe buckets, eliminating the need for drilling. These are great for growing single tomato plants or even peppers or cucumbers. Grocery stores and bakeries often give away 5-gallon (19 L) food-safe buckets after a single use if you want them in quantity. Help save them from the landfill and give them new purpose.

Multiple plants can be grown in rubber totes using the same principles. However, you'll need to drill holes in the lid (the size depends upon the size of the plant baskets) for the number of plants you want to grow, keeping in mind spacing requirements. You'll also need the seed or seedling, plant baskets, substrate (growing medium), and nutrient solution to add to the water.

Along with fresh salad greens, you can grow parsley, basil, cilantro, chard, mustards, and Asian greens in this easy-to-use system. For indoors, use basic fluorescent shop lights with a sturdy metal or resin rack and you'll be harvesting fresh food all winter long. Diving into hydroponics is a great exercise for the brain and might open up a whole new world of ideas to you for small space gardening.

CHAPTER 7

Smart Tools of the Trade

When I think back on my first garden, a planting bed off the back door of the rental house where I lived during college, I marvel at how much I did with so little. Besides strawberries, beans, and lettuce, I grew lots of flowers, like sweet peas and cosmos—anything I could start from seed. I was working two part-time jobs and going to school full-time; money and time were tight. I remember using an old butter knife for lots of tasks, a versatile tool if you have nothing else and are young and nimble.

At this point in life, I have quite a few tools at my disposal, but I still fall back on my favorites. They are like old friends that get the job done. That said, I try to stay open to new ideas, and part of that is to actively seek out more tools that make gardening easier and more comfortable. And there are plenty to choose from, so many it can be overwhelming.

Older gardeners should look for tools that offer ease of use, comfort, lightweight materials, and features that minimize muscle strain. Tools with these characteristics are described as ergonomic—designed to be comfortable, safe, and efficient to use. Most quality garden tools today incorporate ergonomic design, but there are lots of specialized tools that go the extra mile to accommodate aging gardeners.

Perhaps most important, before you head out there to break in your new tools, make sure to outfit yourself with the right protective gear—gloves, footwear, kneepads, sunscreen or sun-blocking clothing, and, if necessary, tick protection. Always remember that your body is the most vital tool in the garden. Prevention really is the best medicine!

Note: See the Resources section for sources for specific tools and brands mentioned in this chapter.

Trowels

The hand trowel is one of the most used gardening tools. It's an essential tool for planting, transplanting, weeding, and breaking up soil. Because it is used so frequently, comfort and efficiency are critical. We lose grip strength as we grow older, and arthritis can weaken our hands even more so. Hand tools are so personal and might be unique to our grip and our gardening style, and when we find one that we like, we don't want to give it up. But if you've been using the same one for years, it could pay to look at how these tools have evolved.

Before you even start digging, get a grip—it's the most important part of the trowel. The ideal handle diameter for both women and men is 1.3″ (33 mm). Hold the trowel and check to see if your thumb overlaps your other fingers, if it does, the handle might be too small.

According to a study in the *Journal of Hand Therapy*, when using a tool with the optimum handle diameter, the muscles exert the minimum force needed to hold the tool and perform gripping activities.[1] The right design also protects the hand's underlying joint structures and reduces the risk of developing cumulative trauma associated with repetitive tasks done with your hand in an unnatural or awkward position. In addition to grip diameter, a rubberized or padded handle can enhance grip strength and is especially important for wet conditions.

New ergonomic trowel designs are angled to keep your hands in a neutral position, neither flexed nor extended. The distinctively curved handle of Natural Radius Grip Trowel has been covered in numerous gardening publications and featured on *The Today Show*. One of the trowels in my arsenal is from Corona. It has a long, narrow blade for deep digging (helpful

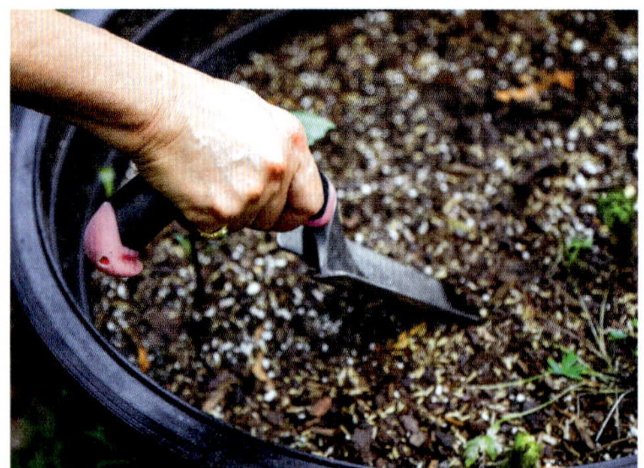

An ergonomically designed trowel with a curved handle reduces wrist strain.

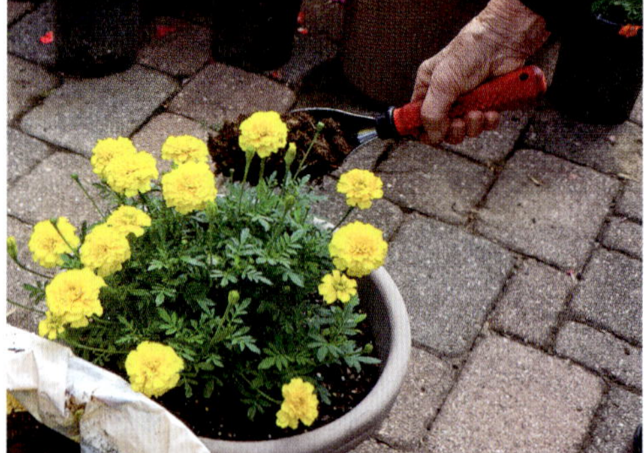

The blade of this trowel is shaped like a scoop and follows the curve of a container to reduce spillage while potting plants.

for planting tomato seedlings) and an angled profile with a gel handle to reduce hand fatigue. It features an anti-slip thumb riser on the top of the handle and a hook-shaped finger guard on the underside for better control. When I want a traditional trowel with a smaller, wider blade, I fall back on my DeWit with the old-style but comfortable ash handle.

Besides the classic design, trowels come in various styles for specific uses to make different jobs easier:

- Transplant trowels have long, narrow blades for working in confined spaces; they might also come with a depth gauge, which is particularly helpful when planting garlic and bulbs.
- Scoop-like trowels are handy for planting in containers; I like my serrated Original Soil Scoop™ because its shape follows the curve of the container, so I can add soil with less mess.
- Heart-shaped trowels are good for hard or rocky soil.
- Fishtail trowels are effective weeders.

Specialized trowels that have upright grips perpendicular to the tool place the hand into a natural fist position, making it easier for anyone with arthritis to use. They are designed so you can plug in a support cuff for extra help. The cuff increases leverage and allows the forearm and upper arm to assist. You might not find these tools in garden centers or big box stores—look online for "adaptive gardening tools" in both gardening, arthritis, and medical supply categories, such as the series from Peta Easi-Grip.

Shovels

The shovel is the workhorse of the garden, so it's important to get the right one. If you have room in your garage or shed, you might want several for different jobs. The long-handled shovel with a rounded point and angled shaft is an all-purpose tool, best for heavy work, such as digging holes for trees and moving compost, soil, and mulch.

The act of shoveling uses many muscles, in the back, shoulders, arms, core, and legs. A long-handled shovel keeps your body in an upright position. The handle should be chest-height to reduce back strain, especially for tall people. Most important, a lightweight shovel reduces fatigue that comes with repetitive use on a big project. The lighter the shovel, the easier time you will have digging. A padded handle that fits your hand naturally reduces the need for extra pressure and protects against blisters. If your shovel handle isn't padded, you can slip a section of foam pipe insulation onto it.

Shorter shovels with a D-handle and narrow blade, sometimes called border spades or transplant shovels, are meant for accuracy—working in tight spaces in garden beds, lifting and dividing perennials, slicing roots, removing large weeds. They can be easier to use for a shorter person, giving more control than a long-handled shovel. The D-shaped grip helps to ease hand fatigue. A square-bladed shovel with a D-handle, also known as a transfer shovel, is designed for loading, moving, and cleaning up piles of material. It's also great for scraping dirt, mulch, and mud from sidewalks and driveways.

Augers

An auger is a corkscrew-like attachment that you use with a standard power drill. It often allows you to skip the shovels and trowels and bypass a lot of potentially back-breaking work. If you have adequate balance, stamina, and grip strength, an auger can make digging holes much easier and faster. Not only that, while digging the hole the auger breaks up the soil and aerates it, creating better drainage along with improved moisture and nutrient absorption. It can therefore be argued that an auger makes for a healthier plant.

Augers are best for making precisely spaced holes and making multiple holes quickly, which is perfect for planting grass plugs, starts, small transplants, and bulbs. For this purpose, use a 2″ × 7″ (5 × 18 cm) auger attached to a 3⁄8″ (.9 cm) or 1⁄2″ (1 cm) cordless drill. For an even speedier process, plant with another person —one person drills while the other one drops the plant material. You can add a handful of compost or manure into the hole at the same time, and the loosened soil is easy to backfill.

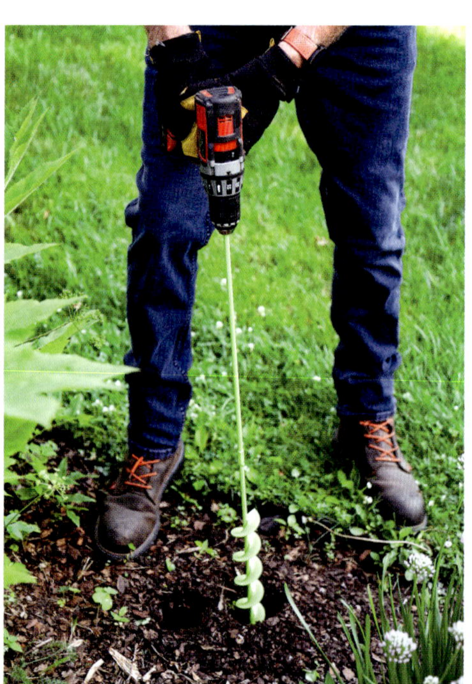

Augers are especially useful when multiple small holes are needed for planting bulbs, plugs, and seedlings.

Always check for utility lines before digging deeper holes. Make sure to wear protective clothing while using the auger, including safety glasses or goggles, sturdy gloves, and closed-toe shoes or boots. Here are a few tips for working with augers.

- Make some practice holes if you're new to this.
- Know the desired hole depth.
- Don't force it; let the tool do the work. A slow up-and-down motion works best.
- Adjust the drill clutch to slow down the speed so it doesn't twist out of your hands, adjusting to the soil type and condition.
- Keep the auger clear of roots and debris.

Rakes

Raking is one of those tasks that seems easy but can strain the muscles with all that repetitive motion. Look for a rake that's versatile—for clearing leaves, flowers, weeds, and grass in the garden and on paths. The Fiskars Ergonomic Rake has a lightweight aluminum handle, strong plastic tines, and a firm, comfortable grip with a nonslip handle.

I don't mind raking leaves; I rake lots of them into my planting beds, a woman's version of "lazy man's mulch." We have plenty more where those came from, and the city requires them bagged for the compost program. The Radius Gator Grabber helps with that task. It's a back-saving cleanup tool that helps lift leaves, brush, rubbish, and more without bending or straining. It has a telescopic handle that can be adjusted to suit any task.

Weeding Tools

You've heard all the quotes about weeds—how they are simply plants out of place, plants whose virtues have yet to be discovered—and it's all true. I'm sure lots of people wonder why I let wild violets proliferate in my landscape; it's because I think they are adorable, and they have value as a larval host plant for fritillary butterflies. Who's to judge? Well, you. It's up to you to decide what grows in your garden and, in the meantime, you'll need a good weeding tool.

HOES

Just like shoveling, weeding while standing up reduces strain on your back. Anytime you can do the job standing rather than on your knees, go for the standing option. There are a number of hoes that will keep you upright while eradicating weeds. The best ones for weeding in open areas are the Dutch hoe and the scuffle hoe. A Dutch hoe, also known as a push hoe, features a flat, sharp blade that's angled forward, so it can be pushed through the soil to slice weeds just below the surface. By contrast, a scuffle hoe (aka stirrup hoe, oscillating hoe, hula hoe, action hoe) has a looped, double-edged blade that's used in a back-and-forth motion.

For effectiveness and versatility, there is the Skidger Xtreme Weeder, a souped-up sort of scuffle hoe. It has pointed edges that are sharpened inside and out for both pushing and pulling, and it clears weeds quickly and easily. It weeds beneath drip lines, under fences and gates, and between plants, and it extracts weeds from lawns and groundcover. It also creates furrows for planting and irrigation water.

A conventional hoe is meant to draw or pull soil or organic material toward you, and when you weed, the soil piles up with the weeds. Thanks to its hollow blades, this doesn't happen with the Xtreme Weeder; the soil is sifted back into the area you are weeding. These hoes are perfect for ridding your gardens of young annual weeds, which then can be left on the surface to decompose.

STAND-UP WEEDERS

There are a number of stand-up weeders on the market, with slight variations of style and mechanism. My stand-up weeder, from Walensee, is satisfying to use—you know that feeling, when you get all the root of some stubborn weed. Best of all, no stooping is necessary. These tools are most effective with deeply rooted plants and those with long taproots, like dandelions, plantain, dock, and thistles.

They are simple to use once you get the hang of it. Position the prongs over the center of the weed, step down on the foot pedal, then twist, tilt, or use the lever to loosen the roots, and lift. Some have prongs that grasp and then eject the weed, while with others you have to shake the weed loose.

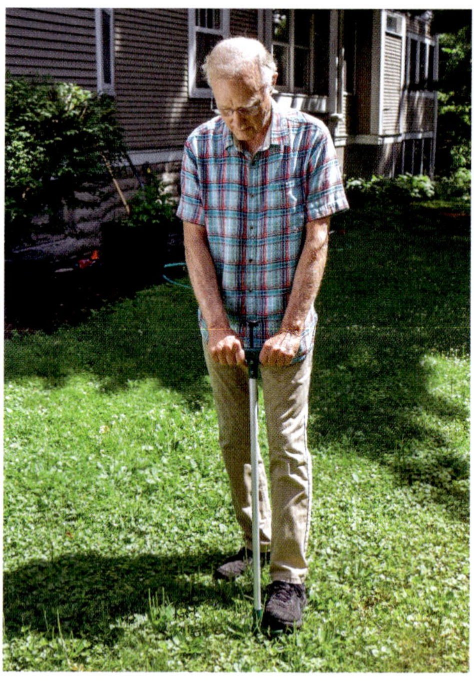

The stand-up weeder lets you target dandelions and other taprooted weeds without having to kneel or bend.

HAND WEEDERS

Using a stand-up tool is always better than bending and kneeling, but there are times when you want to get down in the dirt and up close and personal to confront those suckers, spreaders, and clumpers. Weeders are like trowels in that we all have a particular style we are accustomed to using, but it pays to try out different kinds from time to time—you might find a better way to deal with pesky plants.

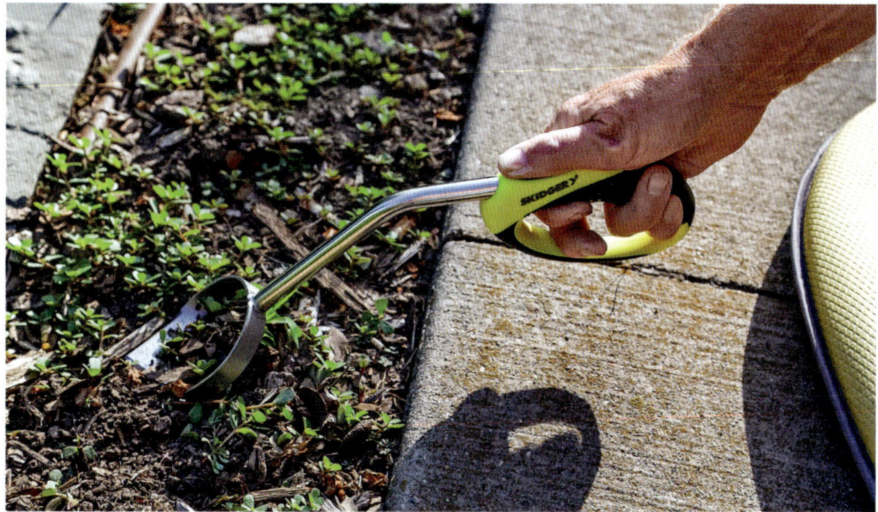

The Wicked Little Weeder scrapes out annual weeds cleanly and has a pointed tip that goes between plants with ease.

There's the traditional dandelion fork we all know, a tapered wooden handle leading to a long stemlike blade that ends in a V-shape, ideal for leveraging a weed by its central taproot. New and improved versions of these are more lightweight and more ergonomic, with rubberized handles for a better grip. Some, like the DeWit Weedpopper, have a half-moon metal rocker on the underside that provides extra leverage and reduces hand fatigue and arm strain. Others also feature the fist-style adaptive grip by Peta Easi-Grip that keeps your hand in a neutral position.

My new favorite weeder is the Wicked Little Weeder from Skidger. This is a handheld version of the Xtreme Weeder. It has a stainless-steel blade with a V-tip that cuts through roots and stems, a double-sharpened blade that works with push-and-pull motions, a rubberized grip for hand comfort, and an ergonomic design to make weeding easier. The best part is the story behind Skidger: Both of these weeding tools were invented by the company CEO's 70-year-old mother! He started the company just to share his mom's innovations.

You might want to use a hybrid trowel-weeder, with a wide, V-shaped blade and a serrated edge that can be used for anything from dividing plants to cutting thick stems to planting bulbs. There are also hand weeders with hoe-like blades that can shave and scrape weeds. Some have flat blades, while others have more aggressive-looking pronged blades for attacking tenacious weeds.

Many people swear by the CobraHead curved weeder and cultivator, which was recently awarded the GardenComm Member Approved seal of approval. Its forged-steel blade is styled after a plow part: a single cultivator tine. The ergonomic handle works for both right-handed and left-handed people. Just as a plow works, you can dig into the soil with this "steel fingernail" and pull back, keeping your hand in a natural fist to dislodge deep-rooted weeds, or turn it sideways and scrape shallow-rooted weeds. You can also use it to break up soil and make rows for planting.

The most-talked about hand weeder is the *hori-hori*, which is Japanese for "dig, dig." It's a serious -looking tool with a wide, knife-like blade, one side of which is often serrated. Maybe it's just a bad-ass version of that butter knife I used back in college, and it's just as

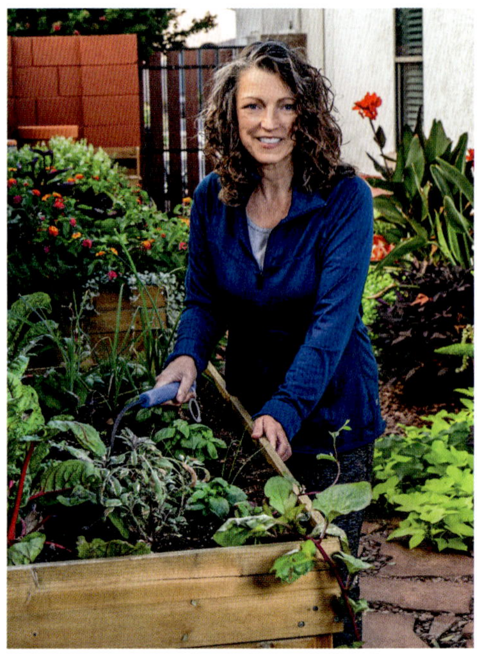

Shawna Coronado using her CobraHead to cultivate raised beds. *Photo courtesy of Cindy Dyer*

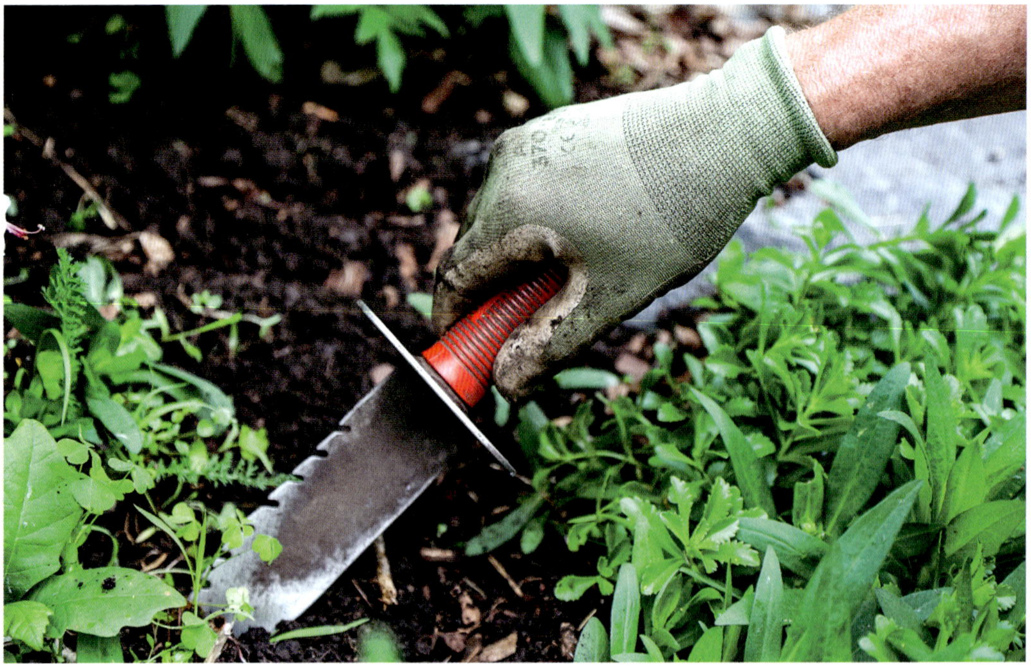

The hori-hori slices, digs, weeds, and splits; it can also be used for sowing, planting, and transplanting.

versatile. Lots of people claim this as their favorite all-around tool, one with myriad uses, from digging weeds to cultivating soil, transplanting, cutting twine, and slashing tough plant growth.

I have some reservations about the basic hori-hori being used by seniors. The basic straight handle (often wooden but sometimes hard plastic) isn't designed for people with diminished hand strength or other conditions. However, there are "deluxe" versions from A. M. Leonard, Corona, Fiskars, Radius, and Lesche that have a more rounded, rubberized handle for a better grip, as well as a guard to prevent your hand from slipping. As with any sharp tool, stay safe and keep your hori-hori secured in a sheath or separate compartment while carrying it. Never put pointed tools in your pocket.

Another useful tool is the crack weeder, a long-handled stand-up tool with a sharp wedge-shaped blade that you can pull down the sidewalk or driveway to get those impossible-to-pull specimens that defy logic and flourish in the tiniest of crevices.

Pruners

My pruners are the Felcos with the iconic red handles. I've had them for at least twenty years, and they are still going strong. Talk about an excellent return on investment. That's not to say there aren't other pruners out there offering great features and good value. Your hands change as you grow older. Hand strength weakens, and arthritis causes pain that wasn't there before. So, it may be time for a new pair. Here are some things to consider when choosing pruning tools.

HAND PRUNERS

The most important characteristics of a hand pruner are: blade quality; a comfortable, ergonomic design; a strong spring mechanism for easy blade opening; a reliable locking system. A good pair of pruners should feel like an extension of your hand, simple to use and able to deliver a clean cut over and over without straining your hand. The head of the pruner should be angled so that you can hold it in a neutral position with your hand neither flexed nor extended.

Hand pruners come in two basic types: bypass and anvil blade. Bypass are the most popular. They have two blades that slide past each other like scissors to cut cleanly through plant materials. This makes them ideal for shaping and trimming plants. An anvil blade mechanism crushes stems as it cuts, which can injure delicate plants and bruise plant tissues, potentially allowing disease to enter. Anvil style pruners and loppers are best used for dead wood. For both styles, look for blades made of carbon steel.

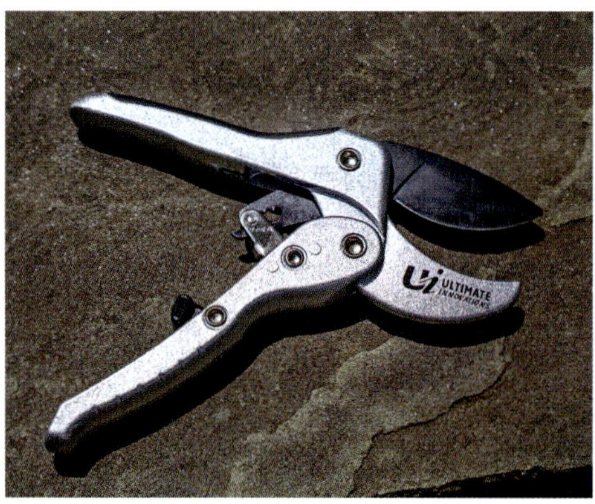

These compact ratchet pruners from Gardeners Supply Company work well for people with smaller hands.

A pruner's grip should be designed to fit comfortably in your hand, spreading pressure evenly and reducing the risk of blisters or friction. Rubber handles offer more comfort. Pay attention to how far the handles spread when fully open. If it's too wide for your hand it will require extra effort with each cut, provide less control, and feel uncomfortable as you work.

Unlike when you use a pair of scissors, the strong spring mechanism of pruners helps the blades open and close easily after each cut, reducing effort and fatigue. Pruners with a ratchet mechanism go even further. They work by using a series of clicks and releases to gradually increase force, making it easier to cut through thicker branches. As you squeeze these pruners, the ratcheting mechanism locks the blades in place, allowing you to release the pressure and squeeze again. Each squeeze-and-release motion moves the blades farther into the cut, providing progressively more leverage until the branch is severed. Where you might have had to use two hands before, ratchet pruners can do it with a few calculated movements.

If you're in the store you can handle pruners to see how they feel. If you're looking online, some brands will offer statistics to help you select the right one. Felco offers a variety of pruners, and you can choose specific cutting diameters, length, hand size (and right- or left-handed), and weight. As I'm a big-boned girl I was able to go with a larger hand size. These pruners have interchangeable parts so they can be repaired when broken or worn out—extra points for sustainability.

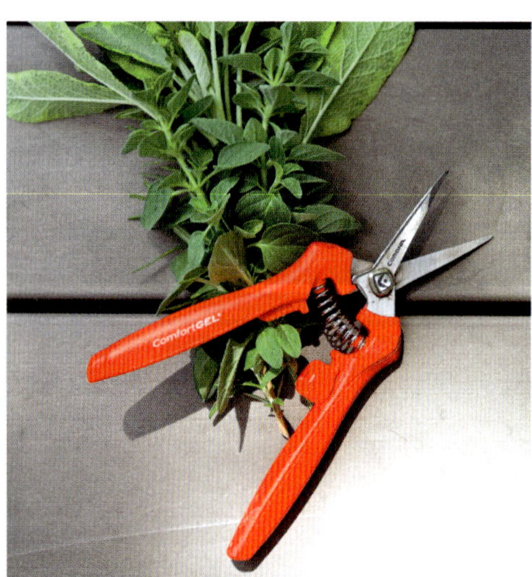

Corona snips are handy for harvesting herbs.

There are pruners with an enclosed grip on one side that helps keep the pruners from slipping, and others that feature a palm handle meant to spread out

Keeping Your Tools Clean and Sharp

I carry alcohol wipes to clean my tools between plants, like tomatoes, so as not to spread disease. You can also dip them in isopropyl alcohol to sanitize them, with no need to soak. Another method is to soak tools for ten minutes in a 10-percent solution of bleach, which is obviously less convenient. Also, bleach is corrosive to metal, while alcohol is not.

Sharpening your tools between uses, or even as you work, will make lighter work. Small handheld sharpeners are convenient to carry in your pocket and are simple to use. A few passes with a sharpener make your blade like new.

pressure. Some pruners have adjustable blade tension. These are all worthy features to try, since everyone has uniquely shaped hands and personal work styles. Finally, make sure the locking mechanism works well for you so you can easily lock them to carry them safely between uses.

POCKET SNIPS

Sometimes called secateurs, I like these for refined work, like harvesting herbs, deadheading delicate stems, and cutting or trimming flowers for bouquets. You'll want all the same ergonomic features of pruners, such as sharp blades, comfortable handles, and a strong spring mechanism. The more pointed the blade, the more precise the cut. Some come with open scissorlike handles for better control. I use three kinds for all types of garden and kitchen tasks—one with an open handle, one with a locking mechanism, and my favorite (from Corona) that uses a small leather loop to keep the blades closed.

CORDLESS PRUNERS

If it can be done with a power tool instead of a hand tool, my husband is right on it, so of course he likes our cordless pruner. He's not so keen on gardening and is generally disenchanted with horticulture from having to rogue corn and walk beans in his farming youth. He especially detests digging potatoes. But he helps me more lately, and I'm grateful. So, go ahead, Dear, and fire up the electric tools.

Cordless hand pruners offer benefits, such as reduced fatigue and faster cutting, but also have downsides, like higher cost and sometimes heavier weight. They can be more efficient for large pruning jobs, while manual pruners are better for smaller, precise tasks. As always, you should only use power tools if you have adequate balance, strength, and stamina as well as good vision.

Some cordless pruners have a physical safety lock that functions like a kill switch that needs to be engaged before the trigger can be activated. Others have a trigger lockout feature that requires a specific action, like pressing the trigger twice quickly, to activate the pruner. Some pruners might also use beeps or lights to indicate when the safety switch is engaged or disengaged. Be sure to wear safety glasses and protective clothing when operating power tools.

Watering Tools

The first couple of times you water at the beginning of the season, it's actually fun. You're outside, and the sun is gently shining, the birds are singing, and the water droplets sparkle with tiny rainbows. Fast-forward to mid-July and you are so over it. Dragging hoses around the garden in the hot sun is pure drudgery. But lightweight hose technology keeps improving, and now there are lots of alternatives to hauling around heavy hoses.

LIGHTWEIGHT HOSES

When my father-in-law gave me an expandable hose, I silently scoffed. I figured it was a gimmick straight off the home-shopping channel. Forgive me, Joe. It quickly became one of my most treasured gardening tools. Sure, the original one he gave me eventually burst and flailed around, thoroughly soaking me. But I was hooked on the concept's good features, and I have found better quality versions since.

Expandable hoses can change size in length or diameter when the water is turned on. My favorite is the former. My hose has an inner core that can stretch to more than twice its resting length. When the water is off it shrinks and melts into a puddle like the Wicked Witch of the West. It is so light and easy to put away. But I must warn you, there is a catch: You can't leave the nozzle in the OFF position while the water is still flowing; the pressure is too much for this hose's particular construction.

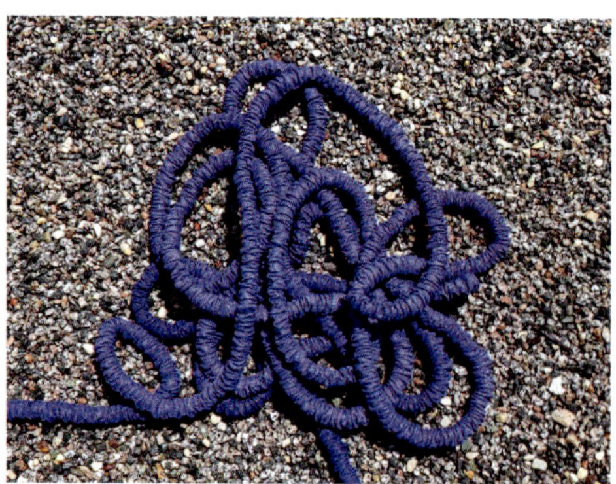

This expandable hose shrinks into a puddle once you're done watering.

The Flexilla hose, a popular brand, expands in diameter. It has an inner core made of rubber or plastic that ensures flexibility and durability. It also has zero memory, which allows the hose to lie flat

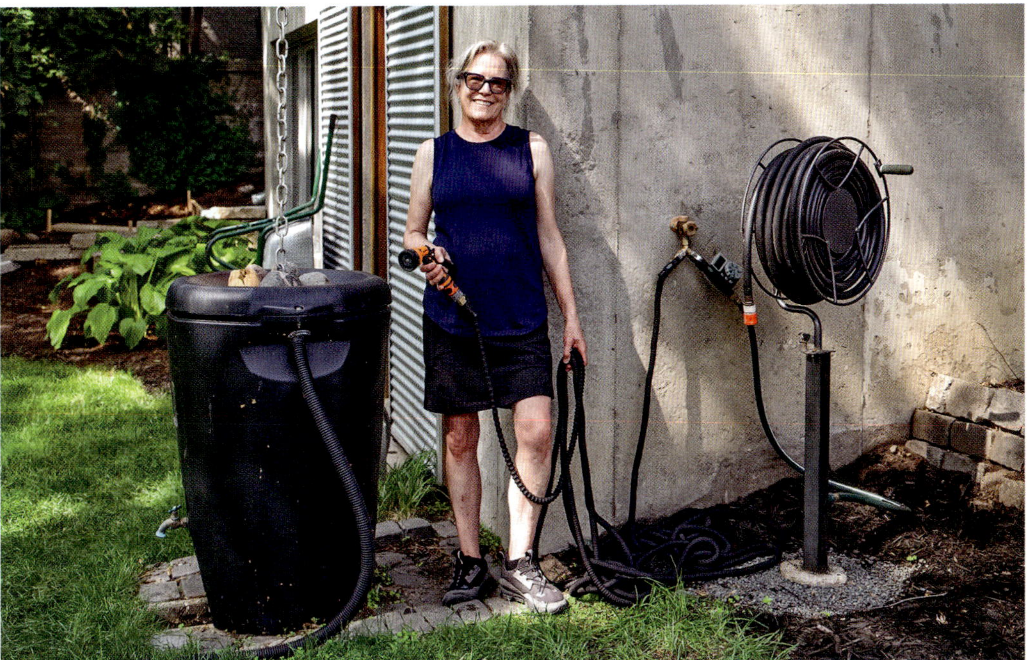

Landscape designer Cory Barton manages watering with her expandable hose, standing hose reel, and rain barrel.

and ensures that sprinklers stay put without twisting and turning over. This also makes it easy to put away and store.

All of these expandable hoses depend upon sufficient water pressure to make sure water flows adequately. If you have low water pressure, conventional lightweight hoses might be your best option.

WATERING WANDS AND NOZZLES

For those of us who experienced vinyl the first time around, I'm beginning to sound like a broken record. Whether you prefer to use a watering wand or a nozzle, the criteria is the same. Just like with other tools, it should be easy to use and comfortable in your hand, with features that reduce hand strain, all while providing good control. It should also come with spray patterns that fit your purpose. I have a regular multipattern wand for general use, as well as a "rain" wand that allows for full flow and delivers a soft spray pattern for watering young seedlings and transplants.

I like Dramm watering wands, which allow your arm to rest in a natural position while you reach high or low. The lever for turning on the water exerts less pressure than a conventional trigger-style nozzle, and I can lock it in place. I also like the precise aim; I can water at the base of a plant knowing I'm watering the roots instead of simply spraying foliage. These wands are

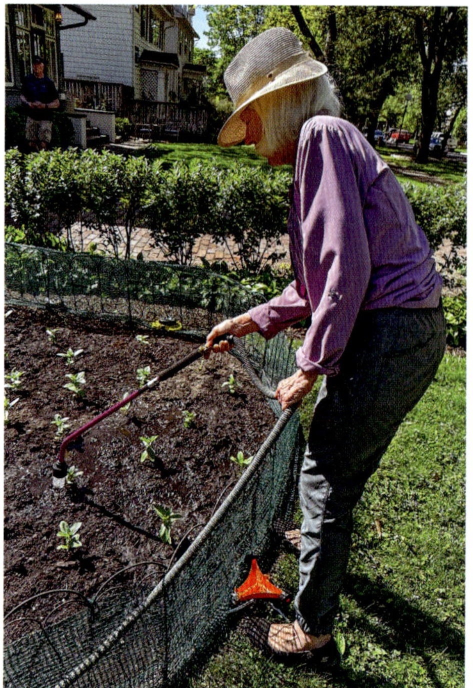

Donna Hamilton uses a watering wand to reach her zinnia seedlings over the bunny fencing.

particularly good for watering hanging baskets.

An adjustable, telescopic wand, such as the one from Gardener's Supply, works well for tough, potentially dangerous spots, such as sloped areas. You can extend the wand's reach to water while staying on solid, flat ground.

Nozzles with a thumb control, such as the Melnor® RelaxGrip®, are another great watering tool for seniors, as they eliminate the need to squeeze continuously. Check for brands and styles of watering tools with this feature and others deemed arthritis-friendly and certified by the Arthritis Foundation Ease of Use certification program. This program recognizes products designed to be easy to use for people with arthritis and other physical limitations, including gardening tools. These tools are independently tested and evaluated by experts and people with arthritis.

SMART WATERING

I may live in the Land of 10,000 Lakes, with water everywhere, but it's still embarrassing to see your sprinkler going in the middle of a rainstorm. That doesn't happen anymore because we have a smart watering app that knows better.

Despite choosing the right (resilient) plants for the right place, you might still need an irrigation system. It can protect your investment in maintaining a mature landscape or help to establish a drought-tolerant landscape until it weans itself from supplemental water. The raised beds in my kitchen garden act like enormous containers and rely on a small but consistent amount of water to produce healthy plants and plentiful fruit.

I now use a smart watering app that helps us use the least amount of water for the best results. The old digital control box for our irrigation system, installed a dozen years ago, with its confusing mixture of odd- and even-day cycles and buttons never made sense. With my Rachio smart watering app (connected to our Wi-Fi), I'm able to customize each garden zone for plant type, soil type, topography, and sun exposure. The scheduling process is user-friendly for regular watering times, or I can do a "quick run" on a particular zone. And I do it all from my phone.

You don't even need an irrigation system to take advantage of smart watering technology. The Rachio Hose Timer (connected to your Wi-Fi through a small indoor hub device) lets you create schedules and control outdoor faucets, allowing you to run soaker hoses or yard sprinklers from your phone.

The app is connected to weather data so it will skip watering (and let you know) if it's too cold, too windy, or raining. It tells me how many gallons of water I've saved. I'm the first to hesitate to allow too much technology into my gardening experience, but this saves water, time, and worry—embrace it.

Tools to Help with Toting, Lifting, and Hauling

It never fails. When I have a quick gardening task to do, I grab a couple of tools and head down to the front yard only to realize I need more things to complete the job. Walking back up the driveway, I tell myself that at least I'm getting in my steps, and the health app on my phone will praise me. But doing that too often means my energy budget goes to the wrong activity—endless back and forth instead of tending my plants. I'm trying to be better about toting all my tools in the same load. To that end, I have a new tool caddy with shiny red wheels and rubber tires from Gardener's Supply. It has a bucket with a tool apron and an extra can for weeds and debris. Everything all in one spot, and it follows me around.

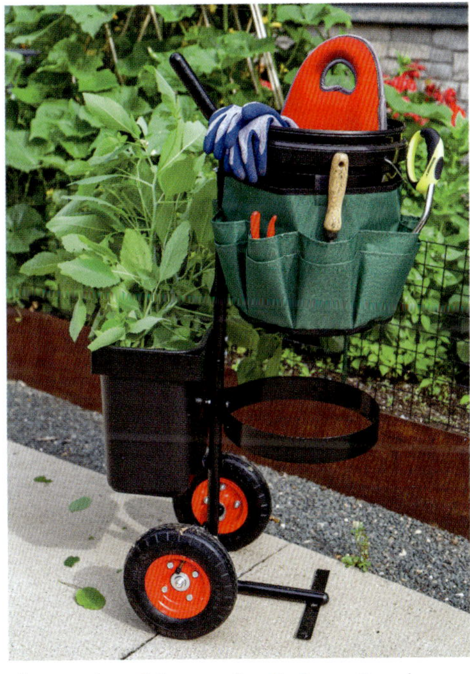

This tool caddy on wheels from Gardener's Supply Company carries everything I need, including weeds.

Whether you have a simple bucket, a tool apron, or a fancy wheelie tote keeping your tools at the ready, if your stuff is right there you won't put off a task, like tying up a floppy stem or pruning an errant branch. This results in a

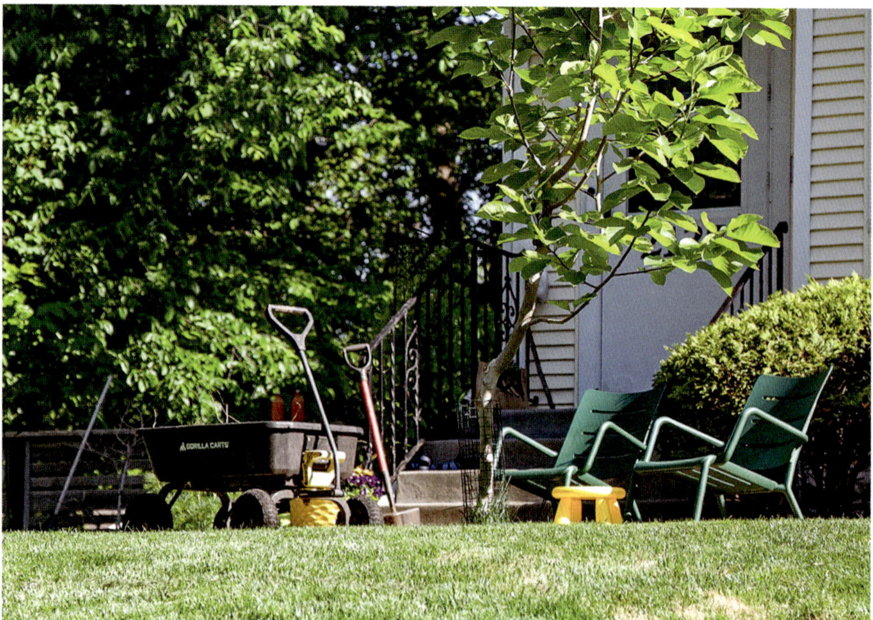

A wide-based garden cart like the Gorilla Cart is safer than a wheelbarrow for seniors.

more focused approach to your gardening. You won't lose your tools among the plants. Your tools are safely secured to avoid injury. Most important, you'll save that strength and stamina for where it counts: your garden.

When it comes to hauling tasks, it's time to ditch the three-point wheelbarrow. They are difficult to maneuver and prone to tipping. You know that feeling, that point of no return when you lose control and lose your load. That twisting and spilling motion can cause you to lose your balance and risk a fall. There are easier, safer ways to transport gardening supplies around the yard.

When I was younger, I used to haul plants and heavy bags around the yard with a vintage red wagon with squeaky wheels. I liked the look. But now I have my eye on a Gorilla Cart, a poly tub garden cart with dumping capability, like your own personal dump truck but smaller and quieter. It has four wheels and an extra-wide base for stability. These garden carts are lightweight and easy to use, with pneumatic tires to handle uneven terrain or just your lawn. They have a quick-release mechanism so you can dump out loose soil or mulch exactly where you want it. Even if you don't have something to dump, they are great for hauling plants and bags from the back of your car to the yard.

If the dump cart seems like overkill for your small garden, or is over your budget, a lightweight collapsible wagon might just be your speed. It will still haul a couple bags of potting soil or a flat of plants. You'll be able to use it for other things, too, like hauling picnic supplies to the park with your grandkids.

If you're not ready to give up your heavy pots, get help. The Small Red Potwheelz Garden Dolly is one of many ready to go. It can maneuver easily around corners, over thresholds, and in tight spaces. You'll reduce the risk of injury to yourself and damage to your pots and plants. It has balancing rear casters that allow for easy handling while moving or pausing, along with flat-free tires and a tilting handle for storage. And such a jazzy color!

Knee-Savers

You can't talk about weeding and many other garden tasks without a discussion about kneeling—specifically, how to make it more comfortable and less painful. I like to use kneeling pads, but my husband (when he finds himself helping in the garden; much appreciated, Honey) prefers wearable knee pads. Kurt, another important man in my life who takes care of jobs in the garden beyond my ability and prunes like an artist, wears stylish overalls with built-in knee pads.

I don't use just one kneeling pad. No, I line up several and do what I call the "knee pad shuffle," moving on my knees from one pad to the next, then moving the pads farther along, over and over along the garden edges. This makes it so I don't repeatedly have to get up and down, which aggravates my vertigo. I drag my lightweight weed basket along with me as I go.

There are kneeling devices meant to save wear and tear on knees and make getting up easier. A popular option is the garden kneeler, or kneeler and seat. It has a small, bench-like seating surface and two upright sides (with some designs, these fold down for compact storage). You can flip it upside down and the seat becomes a close-to-the-ground kneeling surface. The sturdy sides, with horizontal handle sections, are there so you can give yourself a boost when it's time to stand up.

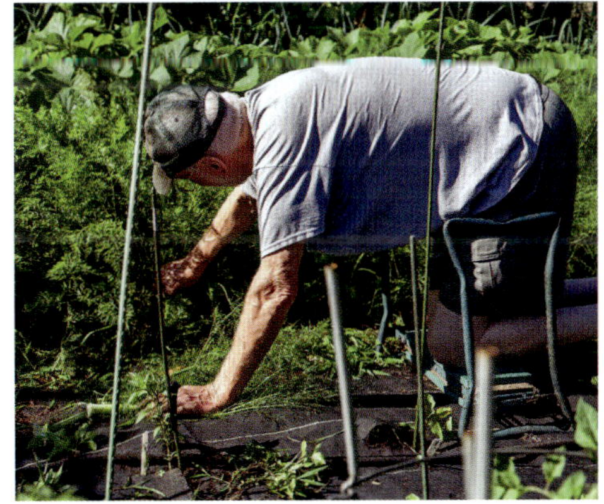

Jeffrey Loesch uses a kneeler to thin carrots in his plot at Dowling Community Garden in Minneapolis.

To avoid kneeling altogether, the ROCKr gardening seat is designed with a concave base that provides maximum freedom to allow you to reach, bend, and move. The base rocks, so your body and how you move control where the seat moves. Keep in mind that you do need the stability to get up and down from the 14″ (35 cm) height of the seat.

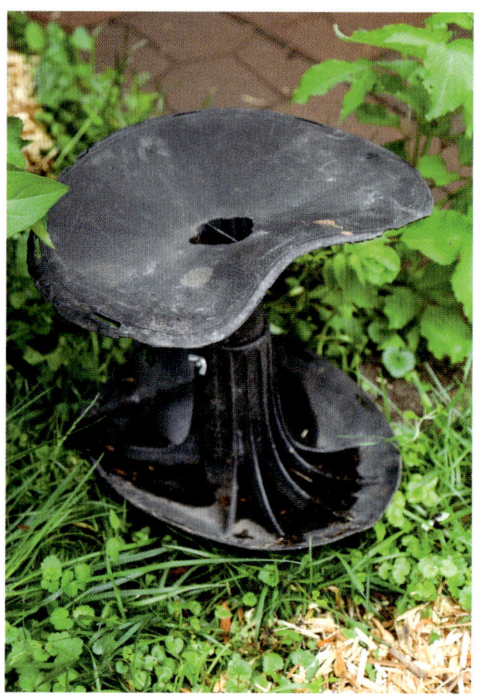

This well-used ROCKr seat has seen some weeding action.

Gloves

Once upon a time, I almost pruned off my index finger. Since then, my hard-and-fast rule is: gloves on whenever I pick up the pruners. Our skin thins as we age, so scratches and cuts can become serious wounds, leading to infections. Many of us are on blood thinners, making a simple cut quite dramatic. Protecting your hands, (wrists and arms, too) from things like thorns, branches, and jagged rocks goes a long way toward preventing these types of injuries.

There's a glove for every purpose and style: leather, nylon, rubber-coated, cloth, and latex, to name a few. That doesn't include all kinds of long-sleeved gloves (called gauntlets) for working around stickery plants, like the dastardly thorns on my Meyer lemon tree. Glove choice is very personal and unique to your gardening tasks; you might need several types to cover all of your routine jobs. You wouldn't want leather gloves to sow seeds, and you don't want cute cotton ones to prune roses. And if gloves don't fit properly and feel good, you probably won't wear them. Rather than looking online (where the endless supply of reviews can be confusing and overwhelming), go to the garden center or hardware store and try lots of them on to get the best idea of what's right for you.

Look for gloves with these qualities:

- The right size, fit, and comfort (and padding, if needed)
- High-quality materials and construction
- Grip (sometimes gloves need breaking in to test the grip)
- Waterproof, if needed
- Breathable
- Thorn-proof, if needed
- Good value
- Long-lasting

Wearing proper gloves protects you from any number of risks in the garden, but one you might not think of is tetanus. A tetanus shot often hurts more than the wound that necessitates it. But getting tetanus is far worse and can prove fatal if not treated promptly. The weakened immune system of older adults makes us more susceptible.

Tetanus, sometimes referred to as lockjaw, is caused when the bacteria *Clostridium tetani* enters a wound, typically via a puncture, cut, or burn. Because this bacterium lives in soil, manure, and dust, it's especially important for gardeners to get a tetanus booster every ten years, as recommended. That's a long time between shots, so ask your doctor if you're current the next time you visit. Meanwhile, if you suffer a dirty or severe wound, check with your healthcare provider to see if another tetanus shot is warranted. Wearing gloves whenever you're gardening will lessen the chances of hurting yourself and needing another shot.

Footwear

Clogs are the footwear of choice for many gardeners. They are great for slipping on and off as we go inside and out. You can hose off the rubber ones. And they're stylish. That said, I haven't been wearing them as much recently. I feel like I'm betraying my Dutch ancestors (who probably wore them in the tulip fields) when I report that clogs aren't always considered a good choice for gardening, especially for seniors. They lack proper ankle support, have poor traction on uneven surfaces, and might not provide adequate protection from sharp objects like gardening tools. In some cases, clogs can immobilize your toes into an unnatural extended position, causing foot pain and other issues. Sometimes you just slip out of them when you don't intend to.

Like with gardening gloves, this is a personal decision, and you might be happy with that muddy pair of sneakers you keep by the back door. However, if you're in the market for safer gardening footwear, look for shoes that are comfortable, provide ankle support, and have a deep tread for better traction and stability. If your garden has areas with brush or woods, ankle boots or wellies will better protect your lower legs. If you garden in wet areas make sure your footwear is waterproof.

Power Tools

Power tools can be a blessing and a curse when it comes to using them once you hit a certain age. Is there a cutoff age, like 65, when you lose your power tool license? Not quite; it really depends upon your individual situation.

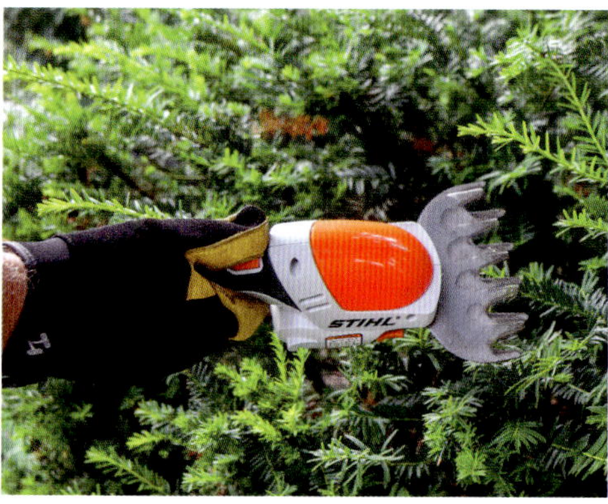

Cordless trimmers in action.

On one hand, large power tools, like hedge clippers, pole saws, and chain saws, can make light work out of a tedious or difficult chore, such as shaping a hedge, pruning branches, or cutting up a downed tree. In this regard, power tools help to preserve your independence and sense of self-worth, giving you the confidence that you can still handle chores around your house and garden.

On the other hand, power tools can be dangerous to operate in many situations, especially if you have issues related to aging, like limited mobility, vision problems, cognitive decline, or medications that cause dizziness or lightheadedness. Power tools are also heavy, which can make them unwieldy and hard to control, not to mention powerful—even the ever-helpful power drill can injure your wrist (or break it) if the thing it's turning gets stuck, causing the drill itself to spin with great force.

You'll want to be honest with yourself: Do you have adequate strength, dexterity, and coordination to handle power tools safely, or is it time to hand them off to outside help or a younger family member?

If you decide to continue using power tools, look for battery-powered, lightweight versions that are powerful enough for the job but easy to maneuver. Cordless tools take away the tripping hazard. Most important, any tool should have a kill switch that shuts off the tool immediately when it senses the absence of constant pressure on the control. Beyond that, it's recommended that you never use power tools when you're alone.

Ladders

When my father-in-law was in his seventies, he fell off the roof. I don't remember if he was fixing a shingle, cleaning the gutters, or what. I do remember that he was lucky enough to fall into a flower bed and make a semisoft landing in a lush patch of ferns and ditch lilies. We were lucky to have him for two more decades, but if . . .

You'll have to weigh the risk versus the benefit of climbing ladders as you age, depending upon your individual health, your physical and cognitive condition, and any medications you take. Keep in mind that there's an increased risk of ladder falls as you age due to decreased mobility and balance. Even falls that result in minor or moderate injury can still have a negative impact on your quality of life. Gardening will be that much harder if your arm is in a cast or your shoulder is in a sling. Don't lose a gardening season!

If you are determined to use a ladder, look for these features in any ladder you use:

- Stability—a large frame with a wide sturdy base to lower your center of gravity
- Wide, slip-proof steps
- Lightweight, easy maneuverability
- Legs that lock firmly in the open position
- A tool tray to minimize trips up and down
- Handrails, if it has more than five steps (and maybe reconsider if it's more than five steps)
- Easy folding for transporting and storage

Most ladder falls occur from not properly securing the ladder, overreaching, or setting the ladder on an unstable or uneven surface. Be sure to double-check the stability of the ladder before climbing on it. And stay in the middle of the ladder and don't stand on the top step. Wear nonslip footwear and avoid using a ladder during bad weather. Don't combine power tools and ladders; that's a bad mix. Have someone spot you if possible.

Sun Protection

Along with all the great vitamin D generated by your time outside gardening, the risk of skin cancer goes up. That's not news, of course, but the topic of sun protection can be confusing given the number of sunscreen options on the market and the many recommendations from experts. Finding the right sun protection, and using it regularly, will make all the difference in avoiding the three kinds of skin cancer carcinomas: basal cell, squamous cell, and, the most dangerous, melanoma. Consistent use of protection is the key.

Most of us already have cumulative skin damage from years of sun exposure. As a fair-skinned teenager growing up on the beaches of Southern California in the 1970s, one of my biggest concerns was getting a tan. I had no idea I should be concerned about getting wrinkles, sunspots, and worse. Sunburn, after all, was the price you paid for that golden glow. If I had only known.

There are two types of ultraviolet rays: UVA and UVB. UVA is the one that penetrates and damages the thickest part of your skin, causing premature aging, wrinkles, and spots. UVB rays cause sunburn and redness. The best sunscreen is a broad spectrum one that contains ingredients that reflect UVB rays and block the absorption of UVA rays. It should also be

Avoiding Pain and Injuries in the Garden

Gardening is a low-risk hobby, but with any physical activity comes risk. These types of common gardening activities can result in strain or injury:

- **Lifting:** back injuries, muscle strains
- **Digging:** back injuries, shoulder problems
- **Weeding and planting:** overuse or strain on muscles, tendons, nerves in hands, wrists, and shoulders; repetitive strain injuries, carpal tunnel syndrome, tendonitis
- **Tools:** cuts and lacerations, hand and wrist injuries

Whenever you work in the garden, try to rotate your tasks. Fellow garden writer Toni Gattone has great advice, which she calls the "20-20-20 rule." She urges older gardeners to switch their activity and focus every 20 minutes to avoid repetitive strain on one set of muscles. I just say, "Mix it up!"

One more thing: When you're out in the garden, always keep your phone nearby, preferably in a pocket—just in case.

THE RIGHT MOVES FOR A HEALTHY BACK

Lower back pain is one of the most common complaints among gardeners. In these photos, Jacq Hauser, a Certified Personal Trainer specializing in corrective exercise and senior fitness, demonstrates the right and wrong postures for preventing back pain. (She's also an Extension Master Gardener so she knows both worlds.)

- **Kneeling:** Use a half-kneeling position to enable your forward leg to support your lower leg.
- **Reaching:** Always stabilize your back before reaching for heavy objects. Take a deep breath and pull your navel toward your spine. Continue to breathe normally. Then, press your shoulder blades down. You should feel your chest rise slightly. Maintain this posture while you reach for and pull the object close to your body.
- **Lifting:** Always station your body as close as possible to the object you are lifting. Stabilize your back as described for reaching. Push your hips back to lower yourself toward the object. Do not bend over at the waist; instead, bend your knees and keep your hips back. Lower yourself as much as necessary to reach the object. Finally, push through your feet and legs to come to a standing position.

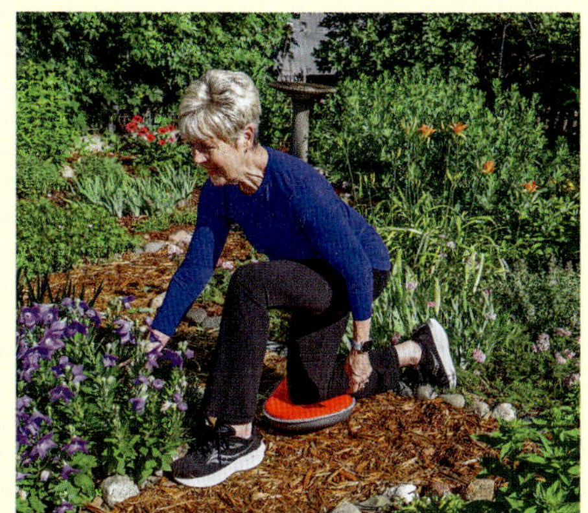
Correct posture for kneeling.

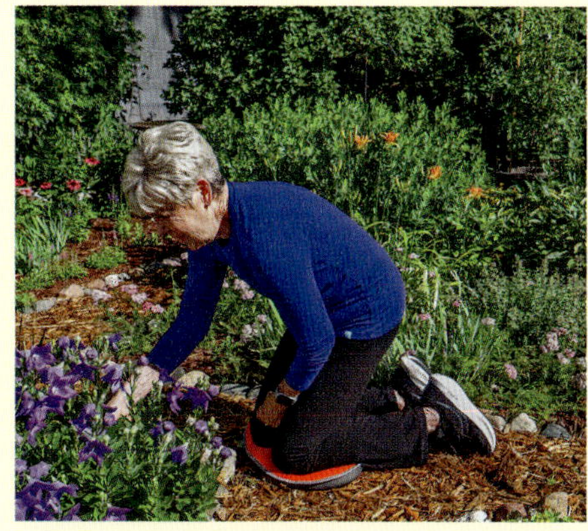
Incorrect posture for kneeling.

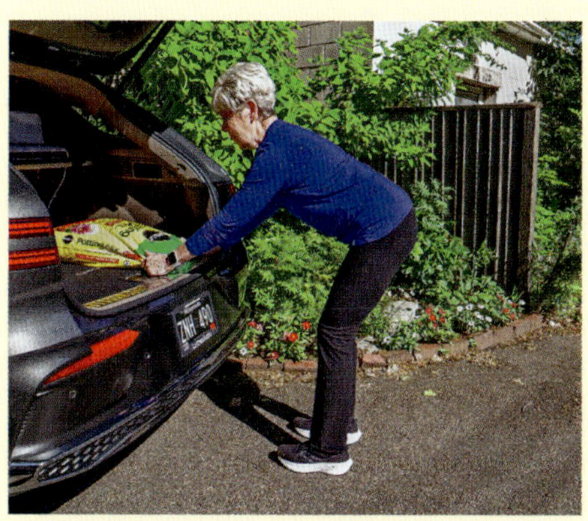
Correct posture for reaching.

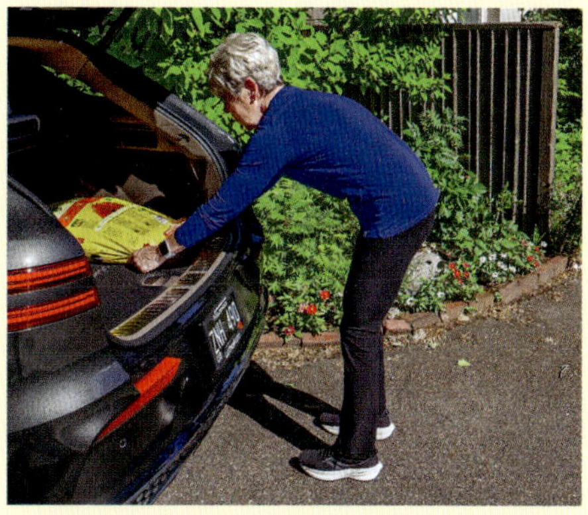
Incorrect posture for reaching.

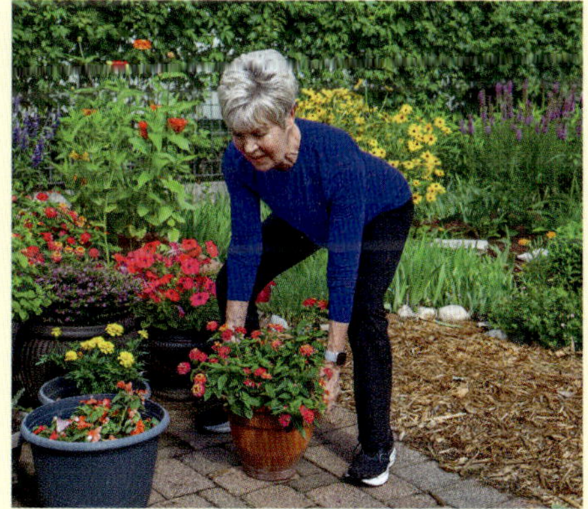
Correct posture for lifting.

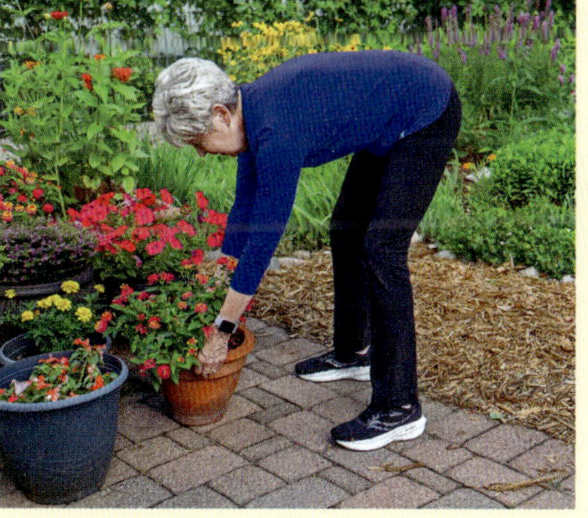
Incorrect posture for lifting.

water-resistant—but it still needs to be reapplied every two hours, and more frequently if you're sweating.

You need a different SPF (Sun Protection Factor) according to your personal history and time in the sun. The American Academy of Dermatology (AAD) recommends SPF 30 for daily use. An SPF of 30 means that when used it will take thirty times longer to get sunburned than if you didn't use it at all. The AAD recommends applying one ounce of lotion (they compare it to a shot glass) for complete coverage.[2] If using a spray-on sunscreen, your skin should glisten to indicate full coverage; with stick-type, make sure you wipe or roll it in both directions for assurance.

Unfortunately, many chemicals found in sunscreens find their way into the ocean and damage coral reefs. Look for reef-friendly sunscreens, and double-check to make sure they don't include the following ingredients:

- Oxybenzone
- Octinoxate
- Octocrylene
- Homosalate
- 4-methylbenzylidene camphor
- PABA
- Parabens
- Triclosan

Even with careful application, dermatologists will tell you that it's hard to apply sunscreen with adequate coverage over every exposed part of your body. And lots of people dislike and sometimes avoid using sunscreen because of the greasy, sticky feeling. Count me as one of them. Here's where UPF (Ultraviolet Protection Factor) clothing comes in. UPF clothing uses dense, tightly woven textiles that absorb and scatter UVA and UVB rays. UPF clothing with a rating of 40–50 can block 98 percent of those rays, better than most sunscreens.

Nowadays, there are lots of companies selling UPF clothing in a multitude of stylish and comfortable options—shirts, long-sleeve tops, blouses, hoodies, sleeves, rash guards, pants, skirts, buffs, swimwear, and more. UPF clothing life varies by manufacturer, fit, and wear. New laundry detergents are coming onto the market that can extend clothing life and actually add protection. But you'll still have to use sunscreen for exposed areas.

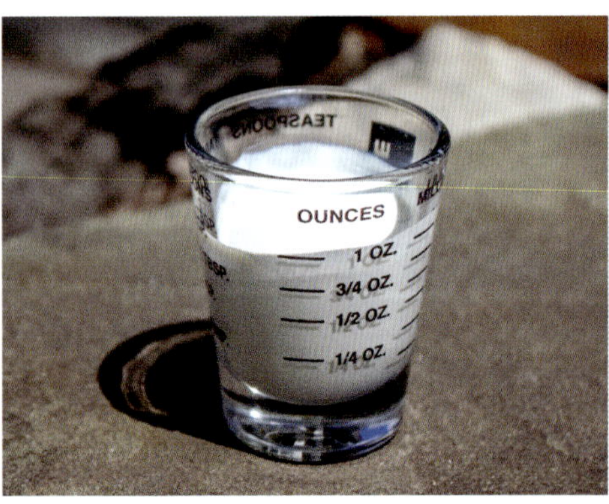

The AAD states that, at a minimum, most adults need about one ounce of sunscreen, roughly the amount to fill a shot glass, to fully cover skin not covered by sun-protective clothing.

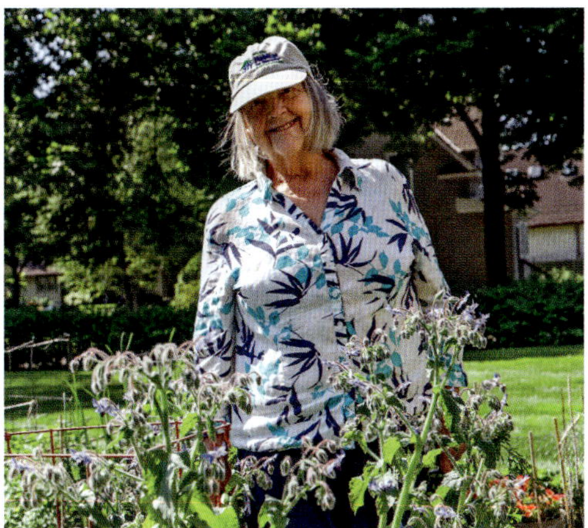
Hennepin County Master Gardener Doris Wickstrom wears a hat and long sleeves to protect against sun damage.

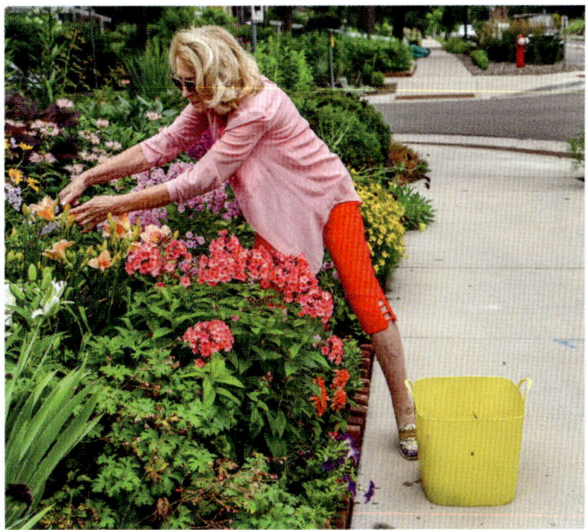
Hennepin County Master Gardener Sandra Mangel advises, "Sunglasses, sunscreen, and sturdy shoes."

I've started wearing UPF tops whenever I can. UPF clothing is especially beneficial for gardeners who:

- Are sun-sensitive
- Have darker skin (which makes skin cancer harder to detect)
- Live at higher elevations
- Use medications that increase sun sensitivity
- Live closer to the Equator

Besides using sunscreen, the AAD urges you to avoid exposure from 10:00 a.m. to 4:00 p.m., when UVA and UVB rays are the strongest. They also recommend using sunscreen lip balm and wear sunglasses and a wide-brimmed hat. Gardeners will do well to heed all of this advice.

Heat and Hydration

As gardeners age, heat becomes more of a problem. According to my doctor, our internal thermostat starts to fail as we grow older, making adjusting to changes in temperature, especially sudden ones, more difficult. One reason for this is that our sweat glands decrease production as we age.

Obvious but true: It's important to stay hydrated, particularly when we are actively gardening. Staying well hydrated helps cognition, decreases joint pain, increases energy, and regulates body temperature.

Water or electrolyte drinks are the smartest choices. Avoid alcohol, caffeine, and energy drinks because they increase urination, which leads to dehydration. Be aware of medications that have a diuretic effect, making it

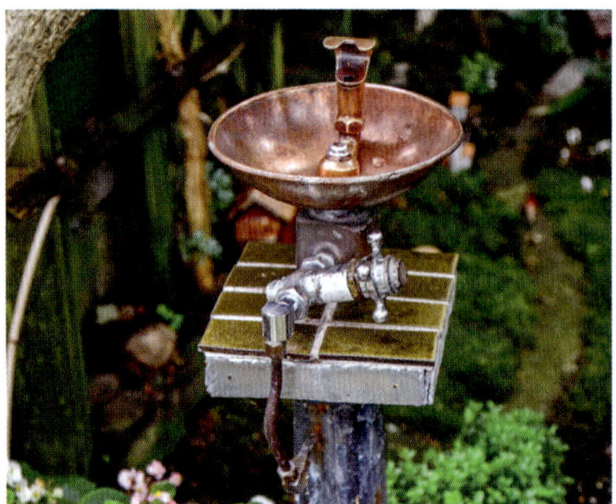

If only every garden could have a drinking fountain like this one!

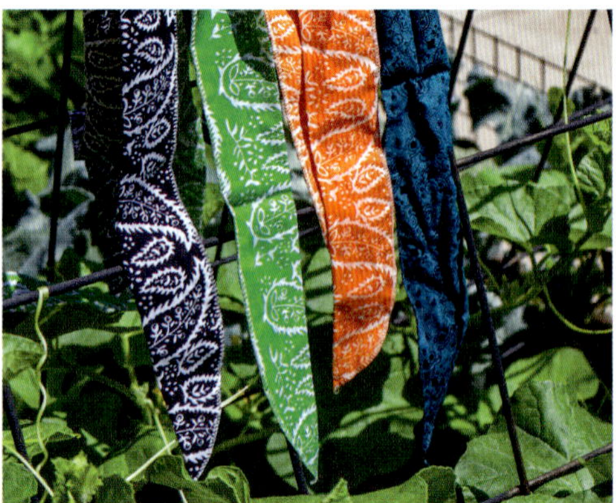

I rotate through this collection of cooling scarves on hot days.

even more important to hydrate. Leave that glass of wine (its higher alcohol and sugar content elevate the problem) until day's end in the garden, when you can sit back and appreciate your efforts at the same time.

To help combat heat, take care to wear loose-fitting, lightweight, light-colored clothing while tending the garden. In addition, I like to wear a cooling bandana, one of those neck scarves that can be soaked in cold water and frozen. Try to garden during the cooler parts of the day, and remember to take breaks and seek out shade when possible. In fact, shade gardening sounds more and more inviting lately.

Tick Protection

Writing about ticks gives me the heebie-jeebies. These little bloodsuckers have been the reason for many a gardener to give in and give up. Such is their pervasive annoyance and potential danger. They are most likely encountered in forests, undergrowth, tall grasses, and leaf litter; in other words: nature. Unfortunately, though, in many cases they inhabit our gardens, too.

Ticks are arachnids that feed on the blood of deer, mice, small wild animals, birds, and humans, jumping from vegetation (such as a blade of grass or a branch) and onto their host. When they attach to feed, they transmit different bacteria that cause vector-borne diseases. The most commonly known is Lyme disease, but there are many others, including anaplasmosis, Heartland Virus disease, tularemia, alpha-gal syndrome, and Rocky Mountain spotted fever. Different species of ticks are found in regions across the US. They are more prevalent with rainfall and tend to decrease during dry spells.

It can be challenging to avoid ticks in the garden, especially in tall grass, wild (or rewilded) areas, or vegetation left standing over the winter. But there

GARDENER SPOTLIGHT

Dee Nash

Dee Nash gardens in Oklahoma on 1.5 acres (.2 ha) where she lives "in a log cabin between the woods and the prairie." A longtime garden blogger, she is also a garden coach, writer, and author. I first met Dee at the 2012 Garden2Blog Summit hosted by P. Allen Smith. At the time, we were all shiny, fresh bloggers excited about this new way of communicating our passion for plants. To this day, Dee's award-winning blog, Red Dirt Ramblings, remains a knowledgeable, reliable voice, providing hands-on advice and encouragement for gardeners in Oklahoma and beyond. You can also listen to her podcast, *The Gardenangelists: Flowers, Veggies, and All the Best Dirt*, cohosted by Carol Michel.

Like many of us, Dee is a lifelong gardener thinking about her gardening future. She recently decided to downsize her expansive gardens. With help, she has begun removing six large beds, and after that plans to reevaluate before doing more. These beds were her least favorite and hardest to get to, and best of all their absence won't change the overall look of her main garden.

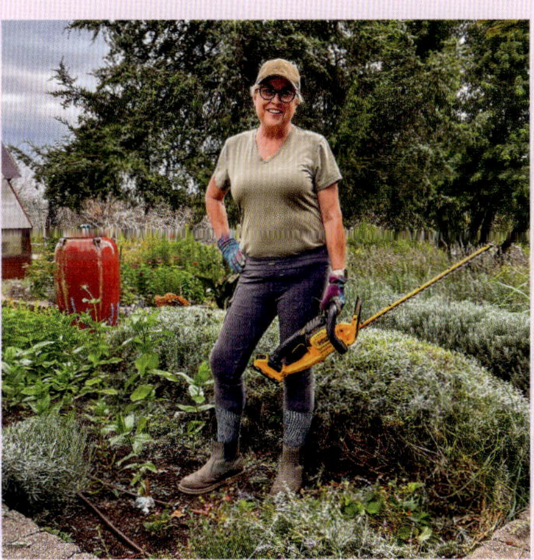

Dee Nash, dressed for dealing with ticks with treated clothing, and double-sided tape around her socks. *Photo courtesy of Dee Nash*

She has moved and saved plants that she loves, like resilient peonies and tough, beautiful, pink muhly grass, while clearing out aggressive plants like *Rudbeckia* 'Goldsturm.' In her back garden, a formal layout, she is eliminating more beds and moving the fence up. She has planted low-maintenance trees and shrubs in her borders. So far, she has reduced her garden and workload by one-fourth.

Dee is also motivated to downsize after being bitten by Lonestar ticks and acquiring a condition called alpha-gal syndrome, or AGS. AGS is a serious, tick-borne allergy, also known as red meat allergy. Besides red meat, other products derived from mammals, like dairy, gelatin, or medications, can also trigger reactions.

Dee explains that ticks tend to like the shady areas of her garden because they can't control their body temperature and that is why they're prolific under her trees where it's cooler. In her wooded areas, she has arranged it so that she now goes through them only once or twice during the growing season. She has pulled out her hostas and other plants that visiting deer like to eat. Because deer are tick vectors, anything she can do to have fewer deer in her garden the better.

Whenever she works in the garden, Dee wears permethrin-bonded clothing. She also wears socks over her pants legs and seals the socks with double-sided tape. Along with her great gardening advice she has now become an advocate for AGS education, hoping to help others avoid or better navigate this horrible condition.

For Dee, downsizing is about knowing when to let go. As she says, "I don't want to be a servant to the garden; I want to enjoy my time out here." As she goes about the process mindfully, being more selective about what she grows, she feels a new sense of creativity. After gardening since her teens and for thirty-six years on this Oklahoma plot, she says, "People change. Gardens can, too."

DEE'S THREE TIPS FOR DOWNSIZING THE GARDEN

- Don't be afraid to do it.
- Use more structure: trees, shrubs (like flowering native shrubs like chokecherry, viburnum, and spicebush), grasses, even art.
- Hire help when you need it; find someone you trust, and then treat them like gold.

are numerous ways to minimize the risk of exposure. These range from using tick repellents to wearing separate clothes for gardening (that you remove and treat when you come into the house), repellent-treated clothing, or even a full-body tick suit.

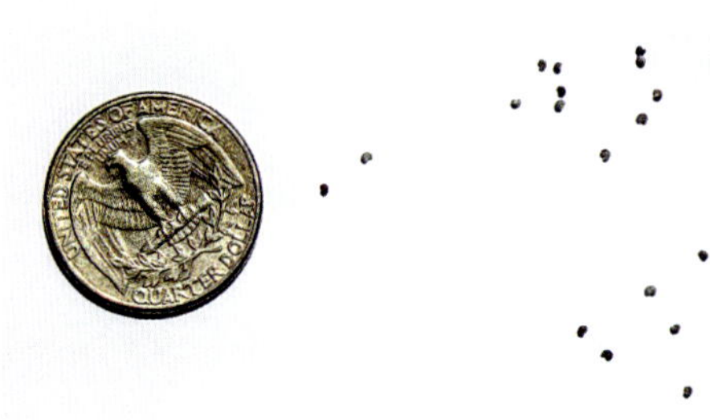

Nymphal deer ticks are the size of a poppyseed.

Checking for ticks right away after potential exposure is crucial. It takes twenty-four to forty-eight hours for ticks to transmit pathogens, so the aim is to detect and remove them as soon as possible. It isn't always easy to check every place on your body by yourself, so it's best to do this with a partner. If you are alone, a mirror can assist in the process. And you'll literally want to use a fine-tooth comb to go through your scalp; ticks like to hide in hair, and some species are extremely small.

Because tick species and associated illnesses vary by region, it's best to consult health authorities in your area (such as your state's health department) for relevant details about tick seasons and distribution, risks and prevention, and detection and removal methods. You can also find instructions on safely removing ticks by visiting the websites of the Cleveland Clinic or Mayo Clinic and searching "tick removal."

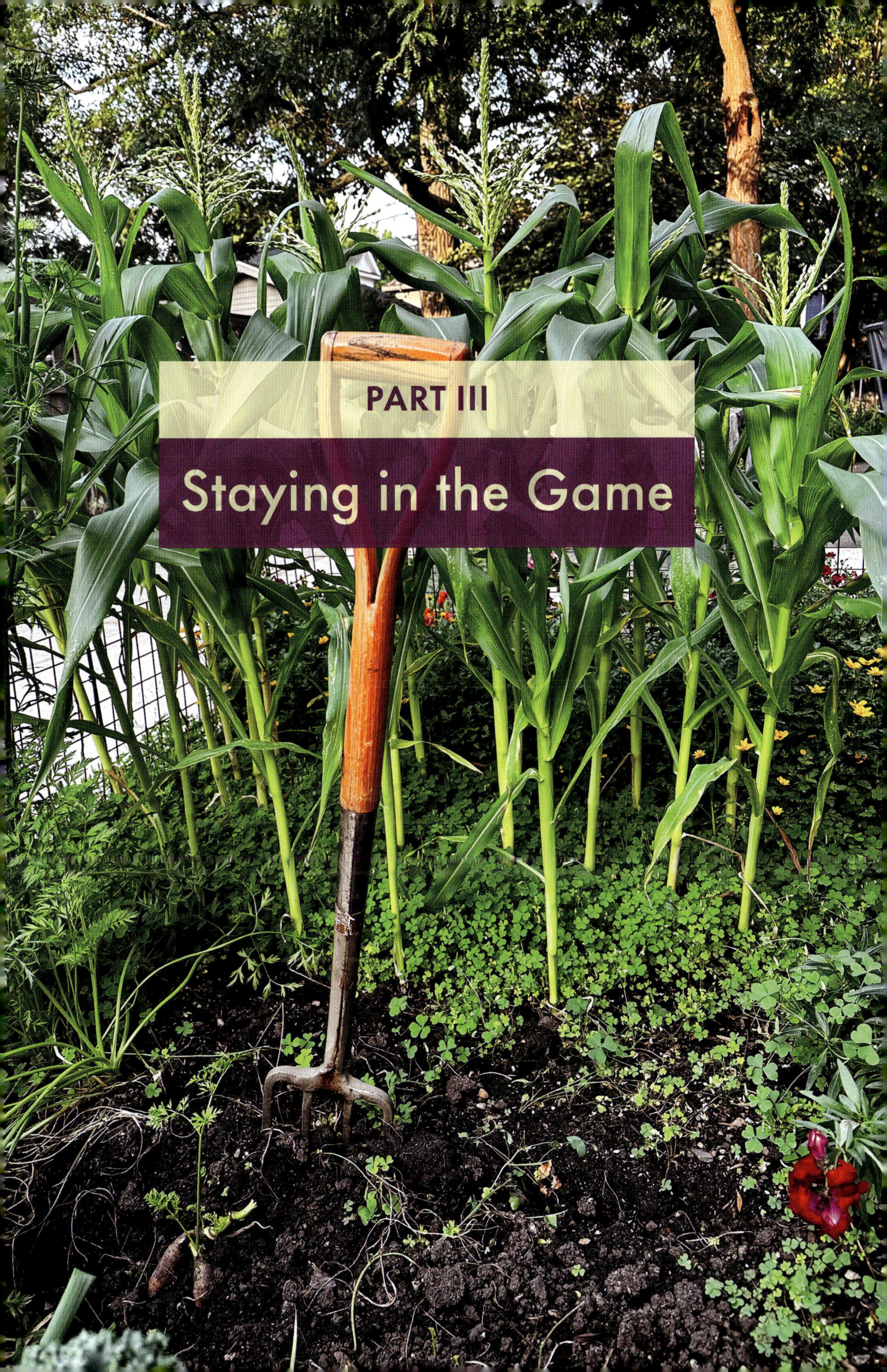

PART III

Staying in the Game

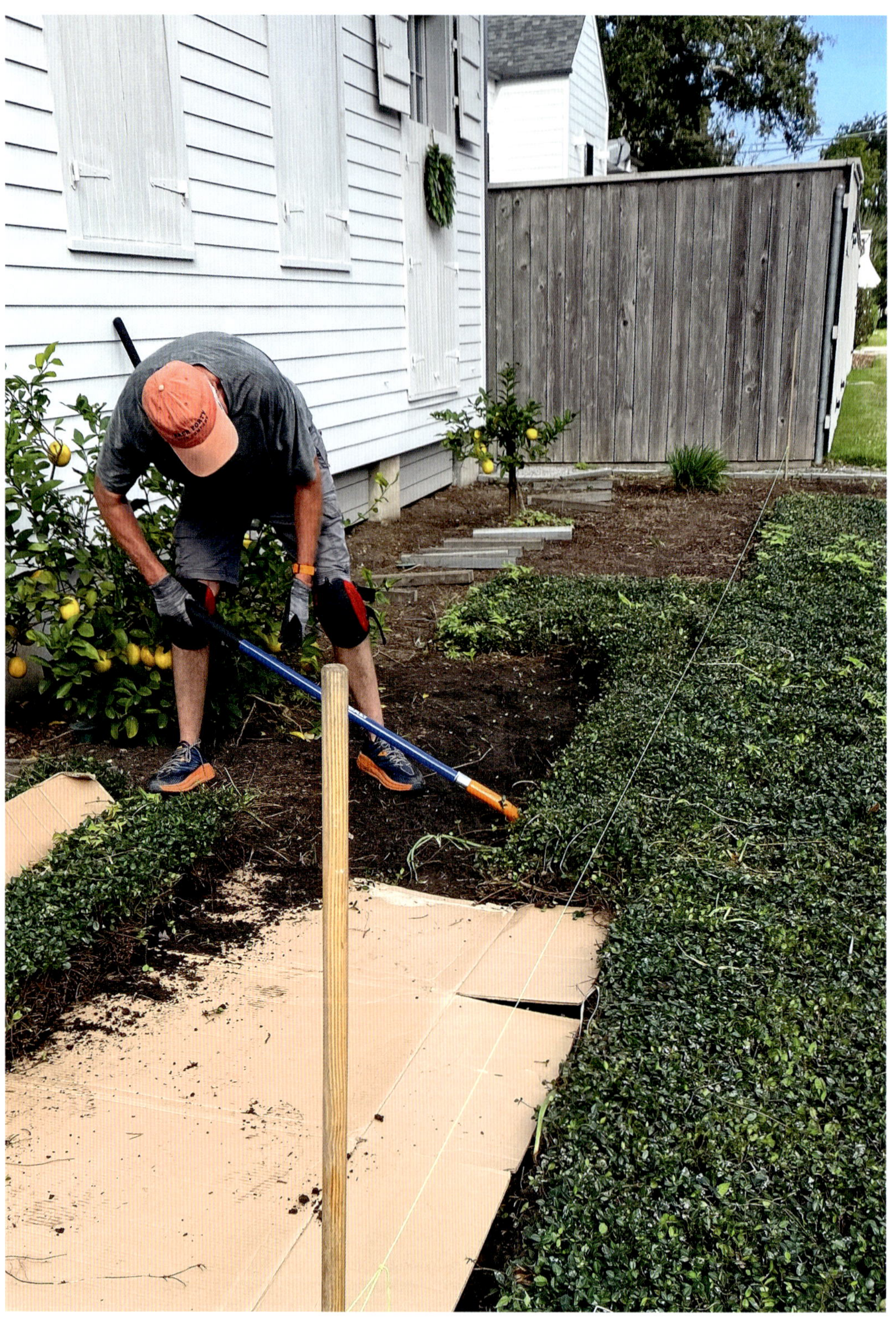

My husband helping me to rearrange the groundcover in New Orleans.

CHAPTER 8

When and How to Get Help

It's hard to ask for help. I know. It can feel like giving up in a way. The idea of paying someone to do what you're used to doing yourself can hurt your pride, and your pocketbook. Furthermore, we like how we do things and can't always trust another to do it with the same care or precision, or on the same timetable.

For a long time, I had trouble with the idea of hiring help when needed. It felt like giving up ownership of my garden. If someone else pruned my honeysuckle or planted a viburnum, was it still my garden? I've made peace with that now. There are times when I just can't get around to it all. Whether for lack of time or unexpected health issues, life happens. I also no longer feel like it's cheating; it's prioritizing. It leaves me time and energy for the fun part, and after a lifetime of gardening, I think I've earned it. So have you.

As we age there are plenty of legitimate reasons to ask for help, no matter our fitness level. For starters, we don't have the same strength, stamina, or balance as before. Yet how do you decide when you are capable of the task at hand? You can start by simply asking yourself some questions: Can I break down the work into manageable chunks? Can I do it safely? Can I space it out over several sessions? Will I know when it's time to quit for the day?

If you decide that it's best to get help with a task or project, or to farm it out entirely, the next step is to identify the best person or people to recruit or hire. That, as it turns out, can be a simple process, too.

Getting Help from Family, Friends, and Neighbors

First, look to those closest to you for help. If your family lives nearby they might be more than willing to take over some gardening activities. Adult children and grandchildren can join forces for the big seasonal cleanup while you sit back and point. Think of it as team building. In the process,

Helpful Workarounds

There are easy ways to lighten your load and maintain independence; one of the simplest is buying products in smaller packages, such as a 16-quart (15 L) bag of potting soil instead of a 25-quart (23 L) bag, or a 1-cubic-foot (.02 m^3) bag over a 2-cubic-foot (.06 m^3) bag. This might cost a bit more, but so does a hospital bill and time away from your garden.

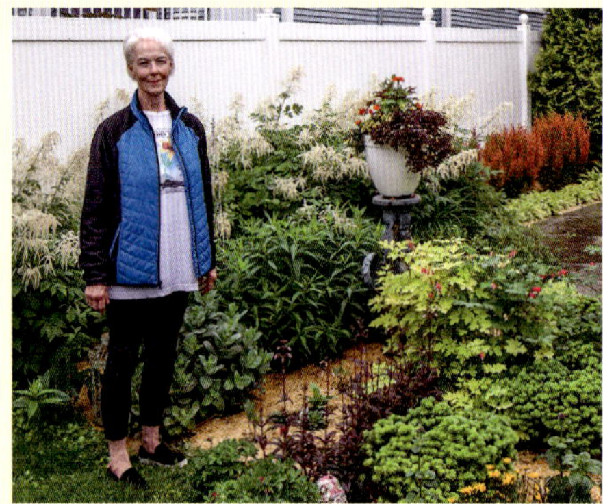

Jeanne Morgan uses lightweight seed mulch instead of heavy bags of wood mulch.

During a recent garden tour in Saint Paul, I visited a charming little garden where I recognized a fellow gardener after my own heart. Jeanne Morgan was seated under a tree in her backyard, perusing a book about native plants while she awaited tour visitors. As I walked through the small but unique space, I noticed she had a different kind of mulch than usual. Jeanne explained to me that she couldn't handle heavy bags of mulch anymore, so now she uses seed mulch, the lightweight straw mulch used for seeding grass. The bags and straw pieces are smaller than that of baled straw or conventional mulch. She likes that it has tack and stays in place. That is due to a bonding agent, a plant-based "tackifier" like guar gum that makes it stick together. And it's biodegradable.

For those trying to go peat-free, lightweight, sustainable coconut coir can be the answer. In the past, the husks left over from coconut harvesting were considered

you can hand down valuable gardening knowledge and perhaps inspire a future love of gardening. Provide pizza at the end of the day and lavish compliments on their hard work.

In the summertime, neighborhood teenagers are always looking for small jobs to do, like mowing and weeding. You can point out the most common weeds and have them ask you for a plant ID before they pull out the questionable ones, or they might pull out their own phones and ID them for you! Hiring two at a time makes it social for them and helps their day go faster.

Look to neighbors when you need to remove, divide, or thin out plants, and offer free plants to those willing to dig. Put out the word on Nextdoor.com (the online neighborhood network) or in a neighborhood newsletter, or post a sign in your front yard with the date and time of the event, which

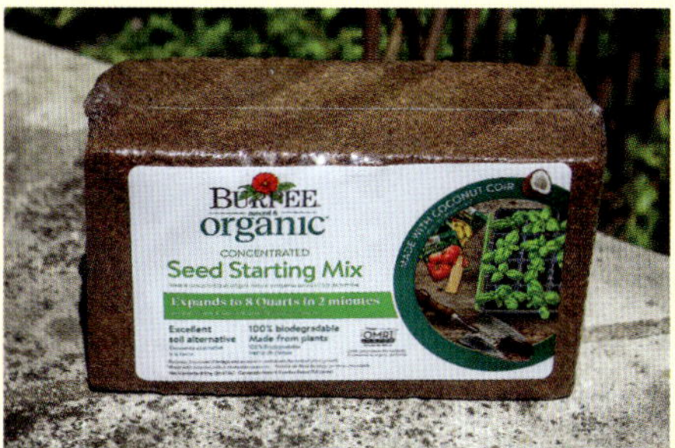

Coconut coir in an expandable brick makes it possible to transport 8 quarts (7 L) of potting mix with little effort.

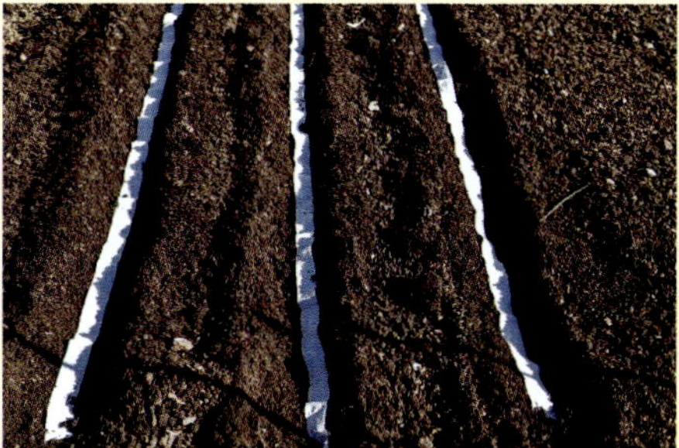

Seed tapes for carrots make straight rows with proper spacing without the need for nimble fingers.

a waste product, and all of the material, from the husk to the inner shell of the coconut, was discarded. Now it has many applications in gardening and home products. Coconut coir compressed in bricks or blocks, and weighing 1–10 pounds (.5–5 kg) depending upon the product, expands with water and can be used as a seed-starting mix, potting soil, soil amendment, specialty substrate, and more. Conceivably, you could carry your potting mix home in your handbag!

Seed tapes can be a big help for people who have difficulty with bending and kneeling as well as handling tiny seeds for their vegetable gardens. Common varieties, like carrots, beets, onions, radish, lettuce, and herbs, can all be found in seed tape form. It saves time and energy twice—first in the sowing (just lay the tape down on the soil or in a shallow furrow depending upon the variety) and second because the seeds are evenly spaced so little to no thinning is needed.

plants will be available, and any other pertinent information. If you're feeling ambitious, make it a potluck or provide drinks and snacks. Young homeowners starting out will be grateful for free plants and you can pass along growing advice at the same time. You'll get the work done and make friends as well.

Help can also be reciprocal. Swap out gardening skills with a friend; you might be blessed with an eye for pruning while they prefer weeding or deadheading (some people actually enjoy it). One of you can start seeds for planting in their space and then you share the harvest. Visit each other's gardens and determine which special talents or aptitudes you might barter to make lighter work for both of you.

You might even want to enlist or pay a gardening buddy in a casual arrangement, someone to work alongside of you to get chores done faster

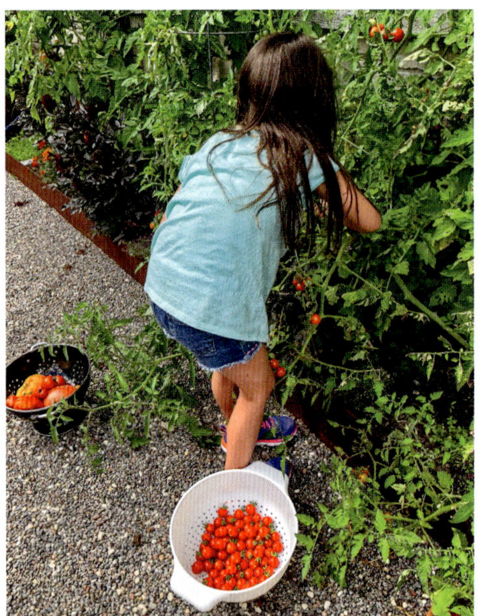

My nephew's daughter, Violet, is the best cherry tomato picker!

and be of immediate help when you need it. You can rake while they bag the leaves or fill the compost pile, then switch places to spread the physical effort equally.

Finding and Hiring Professionals

Sometimes all you need is sheer muscle, while other times you need a competent person with gardening experience. For big jobs, like installing a new garden or making over an existing garden, you'll want professionals with relevant expertise. Knowing the level of help you need can save you time and money, and help you make sure the job gets done correctly.

Muscle is needed for strenuous physical jobs like clearing brush, hauling bags of mulch, pushing wheelbarrows, turning soil, and moving rocks—no gardening experience required. When it comes to more specialized tasks, like pruning trees, trimming shrubs, and cutting back ornamental grasses, more plant knowledge is needed. Plus, it's a repetitious job; you might be able to prune or trim a few stems or branches at one time, but doing it over and over is when you risk exhaustion or injury. You'll want someone for this work who is both patient and diligent.

It's worth paying for an arborist when it comes to maintaining the health of your trees. Trees are the most valuable part of your landscape, so much so that insurance companies have a formula for calculating tree replacement costs. Other things you can't put a price to: beauty, shade, sentiment—and don't forget how much they mean for pollinators and wildlife, food, nesting sites, and shelter. Regularly check your trees for signs of pests, disease, decay, and damage, as well as safety concerns, and consult an arborist with any significant concerns.

When it comes to damaged trees or tree removal, you don't always need an arborist, but you do need an experienced (and properly insured) tree care professional. Felling trees and even pruning large limbs is arguably the most dangerous work associated with home ownership, and if something goes wrong, it potentially exposes you to significant liability. That's why you want to hire only licensed, insured, and experienced pros for this type of work. One more tip: Get several bids from both big and small operators, as prices for tree care can vary dramatically for the same project.

Once you know the kind of help you want, the search begins. Ask for referrals from friends, neighbors, and local professionals. Cruise the neighborhood to see if there are regular crews maintaining a yard you admire. Go analog: Community newspapers still have classified ads in the back for landscape design and maintenance companies. When looking online, beware that the shiniest website might not mean anything more than having a good web designer. Read the reviews and read between the lines.

When a potential individual or company representative visits your property it might be advisable to have a friend or family member present for a second opinion. Do a gut check. Beyond the expense and expectation of work done, does this person show respect for your wishes? Are they courteous, and do they listen? Will you feel comfortable having them on your property? Ask about their last job and how it went—are they hesitant or happy to talk about it? Depending upon the size of the job it might be a good investment to do a background check or verify the company credentials with the Better Business Bureau. If you don't feel sure

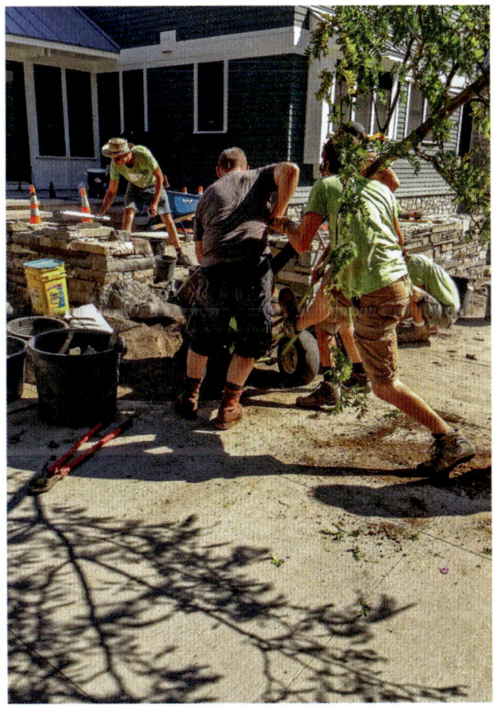

Landscapers planting a large tree for my patio.

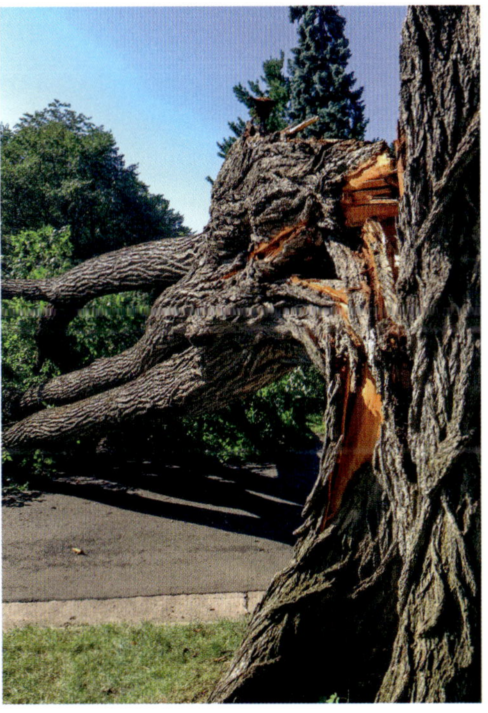

Fallen trees are best taken care of by professionals.

about them, keep looking. Get multiple quotes and don't be afraid to negotiate within reason.

Once you have someone lined up, make sure the lines of communication are clearly drawn. Get it all in writing, specifying these criteria:

- Scope of the job, and what completion looks like
- Quality of workmanship—using sustainable materials and practices
- Timeline from start to finish, allowing reasonable delays for weather and supply chain issues
- Budget, overruns, and deal-breakers
- Method of payment—deposit, half up-front and half upon completion, or all upon completion?
- Expectations about daily schedule, work hours, noise, dust, and debris removal

If applicable, take pictures to document the process as work progresses. And if any concerns, doubts, or a desire for change arises, address this with your contractor right away. It's better to stop and regroup than to have regrets.

Working with Landscape Professionals

I would be remiss if I didn't state the case for consulting with a landscape professional. Just as some people have the talent, skills, and energy to remodel their own kitchen, others are able to redesign and build a garden without outside help. However, most of us will turn to the pros for complicated jobs. Landscape architects and designers not only offer their expertise but also a fresh set of eyes.

Help from these landscape specialists can range from a one-time, one-hour consult to guide a DIY project to turnkey design and installation services and project management. In any case, they can be worth their price when you consider that it's a one-time cost for an enduring investment in outdoor enjoyment that enhances and possibly lengthens your good years. According to the American Society of Landscape Architects (ASLA), "Homes that have been professionally landscaped can fetch 15 percent to 20 percent more at the time of resale than homes with less attractive landscapes."[1]

To know whether you need a landscape architect or a landscape designer you should know what each one offers. A landscape architect is licensed by the state and possesses a higher level of technical knowledge, with experience in structural design, grading, drainage, and infrastructure. Some only design parks, commercial sites, and public spaces, while others do those and residential work. When assessing your property's problems and possibilities, they see the landscape as a series of systems. For example, a single design might expand your living space, lower your energy bills, and make your irrigation system more effective. They can also seek out the best contractor to do the actual work.

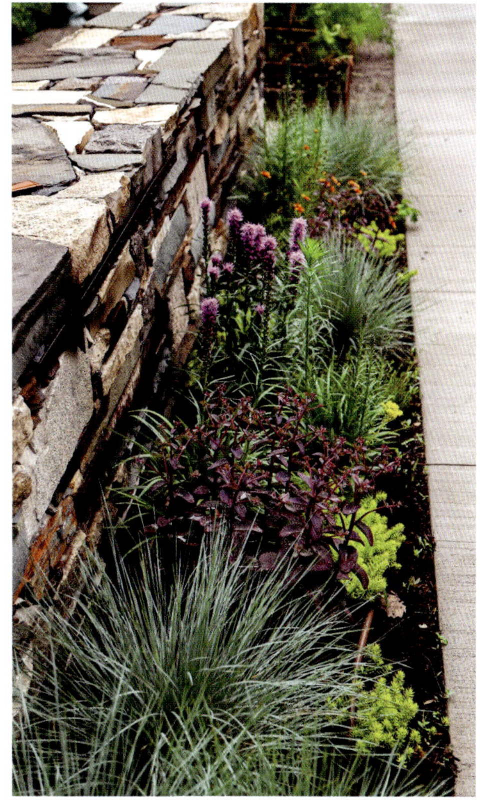

An imaginative plant palette by a landscape professional.

A landscape designer focuses more on plants and aesthetics, helping to design a cohesive landscape plan, curate a plant palette, and source plants that might not be readily available to the public. In some cases, they might also be experienced at hardscape design, or be connected to a company with this expertise. A landscape designer can also help if you are only wanting to tweak an existing landscape or do a small fix. Both landscape designers and landscape architects bring a fresh perspective with an aim to improve the design and functionality of outdoor living spaces and maximize usability.

Thomas Kerby, the landscape architect whose keen eye was behind my Minneapolis landscape plan, explains, "A landscape architect can offer a more comprehensive review and design to a client's landscape. They may see an opportunity to build a stronger connection between the home and landscape with architectural features, such as adding an entry from a kitchen that opens the garden to a client who cooks or build upon the architecture of the home and reflect it into the garden. Landscape architects can also work with city zoning and permitting to ensure any design elements will meet all building codes for city and state."

He advises, "To make the most of the time at a landscape consult I suggest clients define a particular area within their landscape to focus on. It offers the time to form a clear direction for the area with greater detail and then suggest how this area can work into the other parts of the landscape."

GARDENER SPOTLIGHT

Donna Hamilton

In the summer, I work from the porch on my laptop, and as I'm writing I can see my neighbor Donna Hamilton, more than 10 years my senior, working in her yard across the street—mowing, raking, watering, planting, and weeding. She puts me to shame with her impressive efforts. The former designer then gets in her car and drives to her second garden a few miles away and does it all again.

Yet she doesn't think of it as work. "When I'm gardening, I can get lost in time. A half-hour becomes two and half. I spend a lot of time planning and envisioning. It's almost like an artwork," Hamilton says. "The garden requires all my attention, so I'm released from daily concerns."

She thinks of the yard across our street as a landscape to maintain while the other is a true garden. That one is located behind her studio, a building that housed her stylish Christmas décor business for over twenty years. Now retired, Donna and her husband, Bryce, have reinvented the building as an art gallery and gathering place, and the garden remains a stunning feature. However, it began as a parking lot. They dug it up, and over time the garden took shape, in the form of a central bed surrounded by borders on four sides, bursting with colorful annuals and perennials. You might say it's picture perfect.

That's because Donna's favorite garden chore is primping and weeding, making things look good. She likes buying flowers and tools, but not so much the digging and planting. And now that she's older she likes planting in pots. Until very recently she did all the work by herself. After hiring help for spring and fall cleanups, she realized maybe she might like more help.

After several attempts, she landed on a solution that is ideal for her. Through a friend of a friend, she found Barb O'Meehan, and now they tackle the work in tandem, weeding and zhuzhing things alongside each other until it suits Donna's liking. She is grateful that Barb knows how to garden and even comes up with ideas that Donna wouldn't have thought of. During these companionable but paid sessions they have a great time because they enjoy being together, and the social aspect makes the work go quicker. Donna loves how "the whole process is so comfortable."

Donna is glad for help nowadays. She says she could do it all, but then there

Tom currently has a client who wants to age in her home and is having an Accessory Dwelling Unit (ADU) built in her backyard for family to visit now, and for her to stay in once it is necessary. He is developing a plan that will work with her desire to keep gardening as long as possible (such as with raised bed areas) and eventually pulling in more sensory aspects, like fragrant plants, once she is not able to participate actively but still wants to would be no time for all the other things that make her life rich and rewarding, like painting, traveling, and socializing.

DONNA'S TIPS FOR FINDING THE RIGHT HELP

- Keep your ears open all the time in case you hear about someone who does good work; or you might see someone working at a neighbor's house.
- Make sure they follow instructions; you don't want to use that time teaching someone the job instead of doing it yourself.
- Communicate with your help partner about your priorities; Donna especially likes it when Barb helps her clean up the edges and feels that if the edges are neat and tidy the rest of the garden will look good.

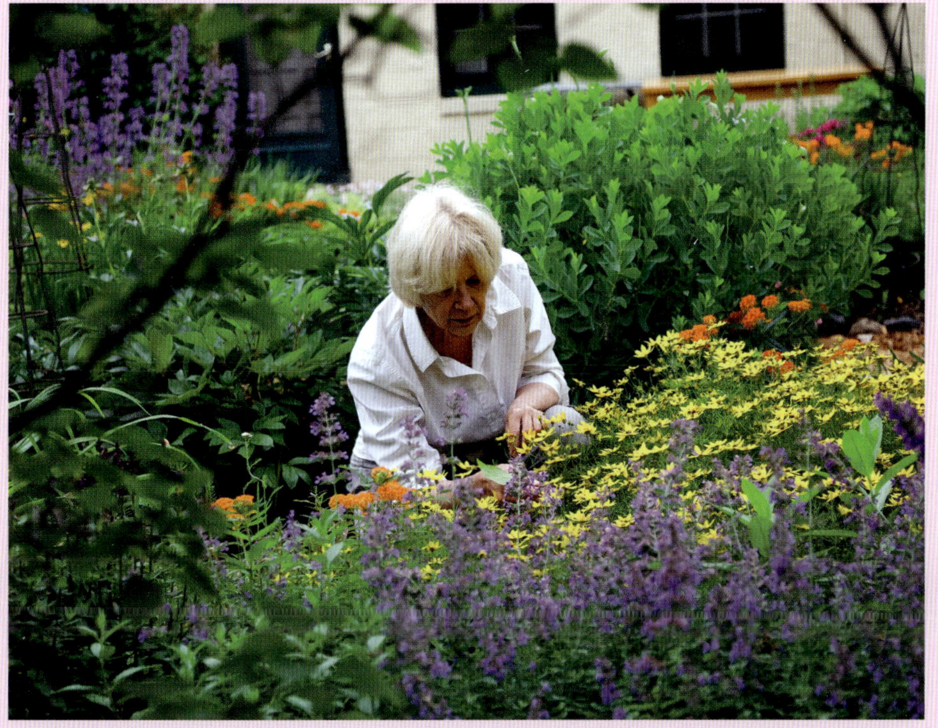

appreciate the garden. He finds smell to be a very powerful trigger for memory and imagery.

As for himself, although he is younger than this target audience, Tom is already creating garden areas that require less stooping and knee work, incorporating more woody plants and natives to minimize deadheading, watering, and fertilizing. His goal is to create a more layered garden that

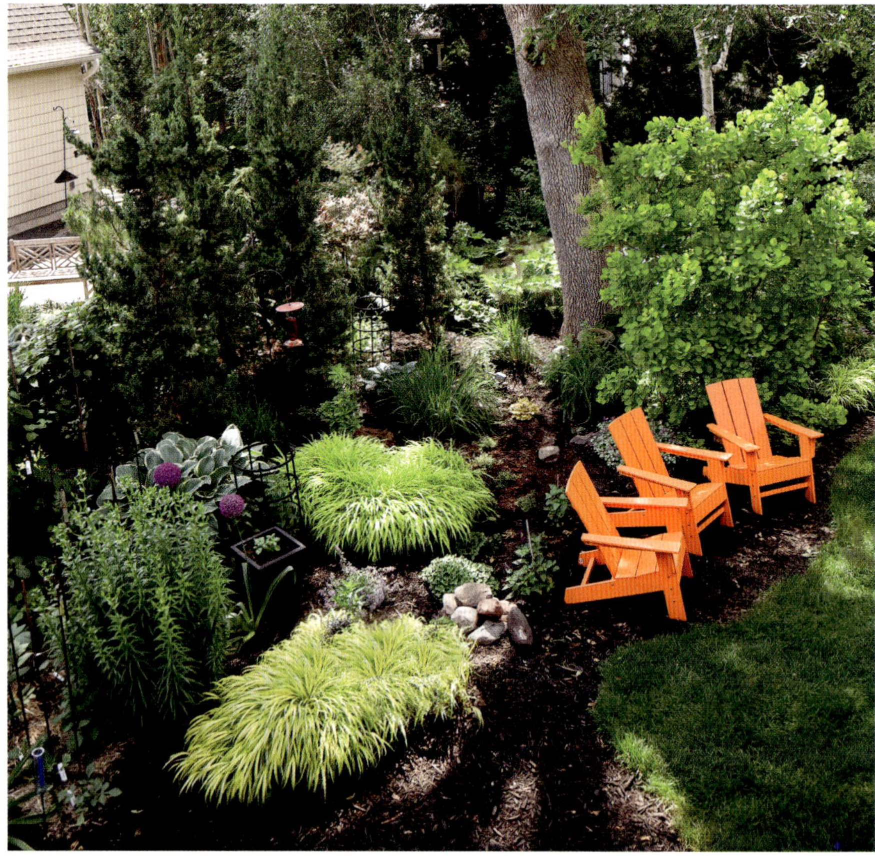

Landscape designer Cory Barton's inviting backyard retreat.

will fend for itself during drought, heat, and cold. He is also using containers or raised bed areas as site features within garden beds to allow easier gardening for seasonal plants.

"I have transitioned my own garden to a more native palette of perennials and shrubs with more diversity to plantings. My garden has become more of an evolving landscape that changes with our unpredictable weather patterns. If we have a drought, I have plantings that can do well during those periods. I also use a lot more containers to grow vegetables and seasonal annuals."

CHAPTER 9

Remembering, Forgetting, and Recordkeeping

It happened recently; it was a busy day, and I was out front planting a new shrub (before the rainstorm predicted for that evening) when I realized I needed my pruners to clip a few bent stems. I walked back up the driveway and through the garage door, and then I stopped in my tracks. I stood there and stared, my mind a total blank. I looked around for a clue as to what I had come for and finally saw the red handles of my Felcos peeking out from my tool bucket. Oh, yeah.

I'm sure you can relate, and, trust me, it's nothing to worry about. (We'll talk more about it in this chapter.) The larger point is that we all forget things—faces, phone numbers, Felcos, you name it. And gardens are especially fertile ground for useful facts that nevertheless wither in our memory. How soon should I start the sweet peas? Where did I buy those prize tomato plants? Which bed got the crocus bulbs and which one got the daffodils?

Trust me on this, too, as I speak from experience: Both you and your garden will benefit from better planning and organization—from mapping beds, marking plants, noting bloom times, seed locations, planting dates, and more. The next time you can't remember a certain plant, or someone asks about it, you'll say, "Wait a minute, it's right here in my garden planner!"

Wisdom Moments

When was the last time you went from the laundry room to the kitchen and forgot what you came for? Once people reach a certain age, they start to worry about memory loss, and each incident of forgetfulness plants a tiny seed of concern. In this case, there's no need to panic; you're not losing the thread. The name for this phenomenon is the "doorway effect." It's a common occurrence experienced by people of all ages.

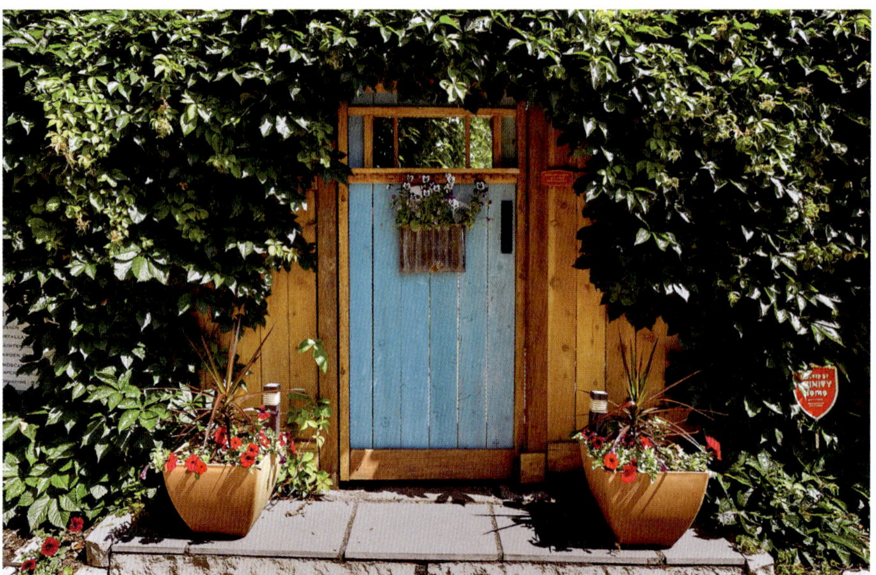

The "doorway effect" happens when you cross a physical boundary.

It is also called the "location updating effect" because it happens when you cross a physical boundary. It's not the doorway per se but rather the transition to a different environment. Entering a new space, your brain, which is nothing if not a supercomputer, reboots. It's a good thing. Your brain compartmentalizes every new context to make it easier to retrieve information when capacity is limited, especially if your brain is in a situation where it's working extra hard.

There are other times when a Latin plant name is on the tip of your tongue, or when you can't remember the garden center where you bought that really nice coneflower—it's so frustrating. I always compare it to a filing cabinet stuffed tightly with folders. It's hard to find the right one and harder to pull it out. This can be a simple case of memory overload; it's a real thing.

As explained by Charan Ranganath, University of California, Davis memory researcher and author of *Why We Remember*, "Although we tend to believe that we can and should remember anything we want, the reality is we are designed to forget. We naturally forget older memories our brains deem less important in order to make room for newer, more valuable information." Memory is a competitive process, according to Charan.

These benign memory glitches are sometimes called "senior moments," but they are not limited to older people, although the aging process can, and does, affect one's memory. I agree with Dr. Matthew Kaplan, professor of Intergenerational Programs and Aging at Penn State, that the term is ageist. He offers a more positive alternative: "wisdom moment." According to

Matthew, this phrase generates images of competence and draws a connection with an older adult's sense of completeness, meaning, and virtue tied in with their life experiences and reflections.

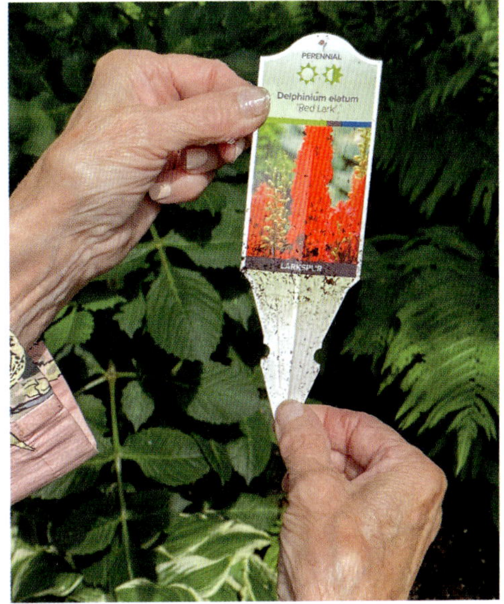

Sandra Mangel holds the plant label for a new delphinium; she had it readily available to show me the name of this variety.

Information overload can be more pronounced when someone is stressed, trying to multitask, or not getting enough sleep. Women going through menopause are more susceptible due to fluctuating estrogen levels that can exacerbate the effect. Besides stress and anxiety, it can cause attention and concentration problems. The suggestions for avoiding memory overload are notably similar to some of the key benefits of gardening: exercise, healthy diet, adequate rest, and meaningful friendships.

To apply these solutions to your garden routine, here are some practical measures you can take:

- Break up tasks into smaller chunks
- Take breaks and hydrate
- Do a digital detox (and don't compare your garden to others)
- Practice mindfulness and meditation
- Use strategic information management

That last suggestion sounds like it came from the board of directors of a multinational conglomerate! In plainer terms, get it together. Your garden, that is. This is where you start the mindful, meditative, and downright practical process of recordkeeping for your life of gardening.

The Rewards of Recordkeeping

Mention recordkeeping and gardening in the same breath and I can hear your response loud and clear: "I garden to *get away from* paperwork." However, some type of record will help you keep track of all the statistical aspects of gardening, allowing you the freedom and brain space to enjoy wonderful memories of your glorious morning glories and other fabulous plants. And it will make you a better gardener.

Everyone has their own organizational style, suited to their own temperament. This might be reflected in your garden. As English poet Alfred Austin wrote in *The Garden That I Love*, "Show me your garden and I shall tell you what you are." I wrote this book on a laptop, though behind the process is a carefully curated system with stacks of yellow legal pads and a flurry of color-coded sticky notes. My garden is that same combination of orderliness and chaotic abundance, so I guess he's right.

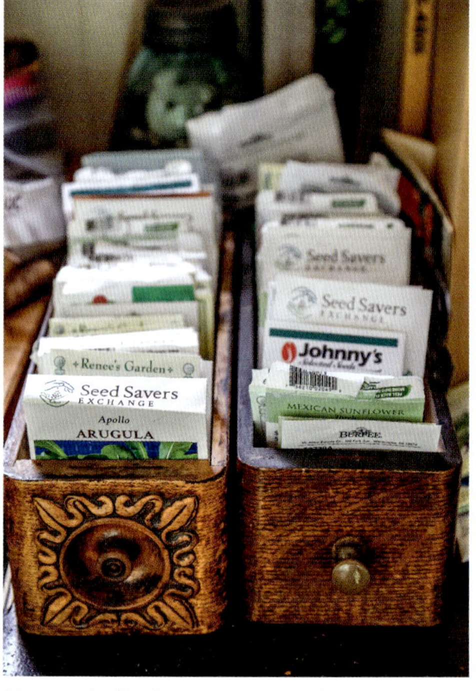

My seeds filed in sewing machine drawers.

As for organization, I keep my seeds in alphabetical order in antique sewing machine drawers. I plan my kitchen garden design on legal pads (I buy them by the dozens). I collect my plant tags in a plastic bag. I know, I must do better. Although I blogged about my horticultural adventures for almost a decade when we first moved to Minnesota, I wish I had kept a written journal of my gardening from the very, very beginning.

As you grow older, it's easy to think that the ship has sailed on adopting new behaviors. It's never too late to start.

When it comes to recordkeeping you might prefer pencil and paper, iPad, or some hybrid version of high- and low-tech. You can use a simple spiral notebook, a school binder, index cards, a beautifully bound journal, an online app. I remember interviewing a fellow Master Gardener who was an engineer. He showed me a detailed spreadsheet that contained every plant he had ever grown. The last column was lovingly devoted to plants that were "deceased." Another gardener I know uses Word documents to catalog her plants by Latin name.

The amount and depth of information you record is up to you. The possibilities are many:

- Seed varieties—sowing dates, seed viability, germination times, germination rates, transplant dates
- Plant purchase location, cost, size, availability

- Plant names—Latin and common, cultivar and variety
- Planting details—date, location, light exposure, moisture requirement, soil type and condition
- Individual plant issues—health, disease, pest damage, injury, survival status
- Pest emergent dates, pest generations, prevention methods used
- Disease issues—arrival dates, chronic cases, treatment
- Plant emergence dates, bloom time, fruiting dates, harvest windows
- Vegetable rotation schedules
- Weather conditions—first and last frost dates, daily temperatures and precipitation, weather events
- Seasonal chores, tasks completed, outside help
- Wildlife observations—birds, insects, other garden creatures
- Triumphs and challenges, changes to be made

What else can you think of?

Whatever method of recordkeeping you use, it has to be simple, accessible, easy to view, and convenient so that taking notes becomes routine. The reward is a treasure trove of information (and maybe a bit of garden memoir) for practical use as well as reflection.

Habits form when new behaviors become automatic. Tips for creating and maintaining good habits are usually geared toward healthy eating or exercise, but similar ideas can be adapted for tracking your garden. First, find the right form of journal, with templates suited for the kind of information you want to record. Most journals are inexpensive; maybe try a few at first. Then focus on one aspect or area, like the vegetable garden, and once you do that successfully, add another part of the garden.

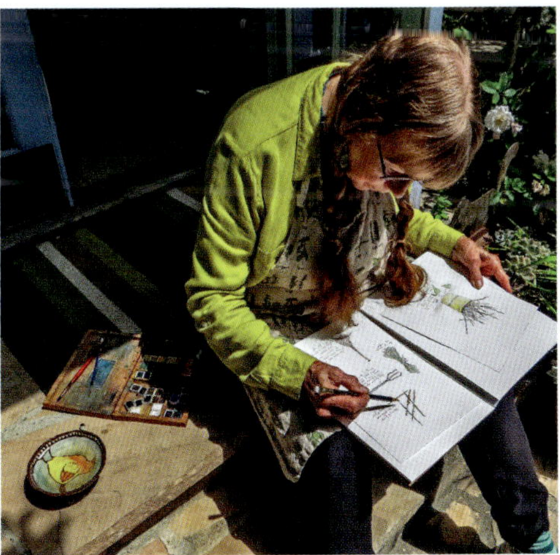

Sharon Lovejoy sketching in her garden.
Photo courtesy of Jeff Prostovich

Be patient with yourself. A widely cited 2010 study published in the *European Journal of Social Psychology* found that forming a habit takes an average of sixty-six days, with the time required varying significantly by individual and behavior type, ranging from a minimum of eighteen days to a maximum of 254 days.[1] Repetition, repetition.

Timing helps. Spring might work best for you, with the adrenaline rush

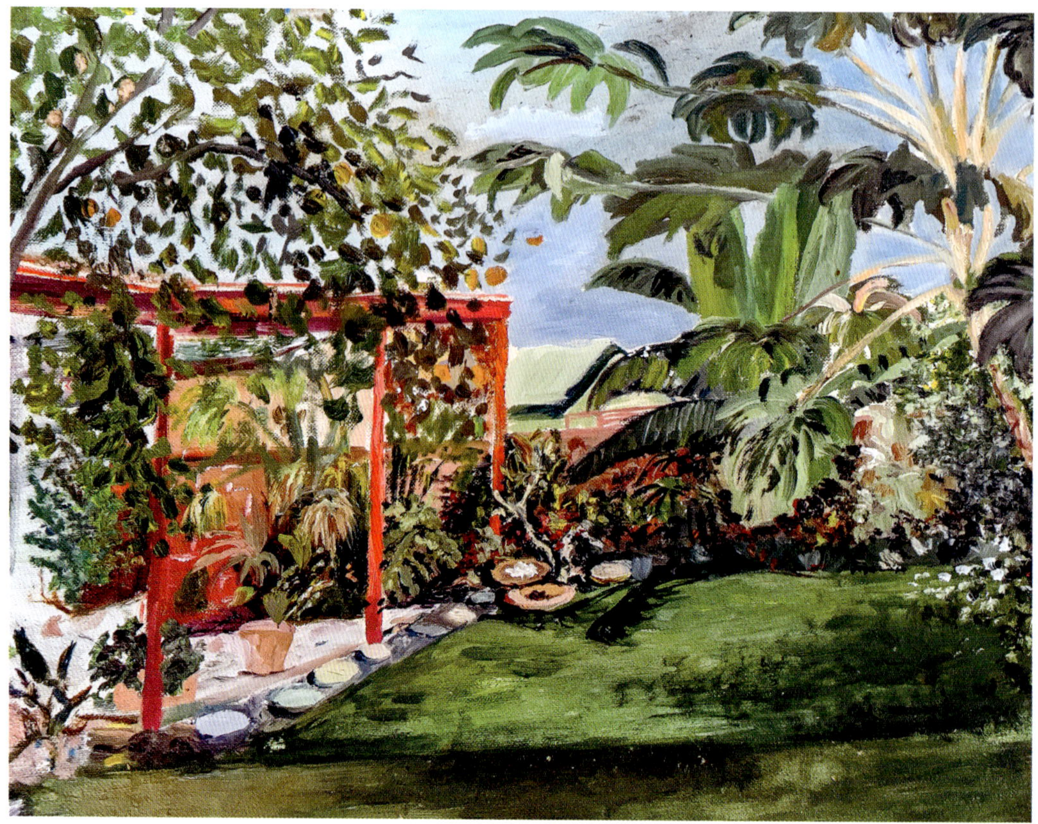

I cherish this painting of our garden from my early childhood.

of a new growing season. Or maybe it's autumn, when you find yourself with more spare time for evaluating the past season and feeling reflective. Your musings can be both practical and poetic.

Little incentives or rewards go a long way—a regular time with your journal and a cup of tea, or maybe a new plant.

And here are a few more thoughts for inspiration and motivation. The information in your garden journal might be a huge help to the young homeowners who one day live in your house and inherit your garden. It could be a teaching tool for a garden club or historical society. Or it might be a precious heirloom for your family members, a legacy of your love of gardening that lives on.

There's an App for That

So far, my written and online recordkeeping has been sporadic and sparse. I'll admit, I often fly by the seat of my gardening pants. I rely heavily on phone photos to remember the goings-on of my garden. I probably do take more garden pictures than the average person. I once got one of those scam emails threatening to share all of my "naughty" photos online; my husband laughed and said, "I hope they like hundreds of bee photos."

By searching for photos on my phone by month and year I can usually look back and find what I want in visual form. I advise you to photograph your garden through all seasons. This helps me to remember what blooms when and where so I can make adjustments accordingly. For example, I might add plants to reinforce a certain color scheme at a very specific time, or I might add more shrubs or evergreens for overall better structure. This makes me think I would like a journaling app on my phone that allows for lots of photos. One of the many I looked at recently was Day One. It includes a notes app, voice memo, automatic reminders, calendar synching, and the ability to incorporate Google Docs or Excel spreadsheets, among other features. That sounds like a good fit for me.

I encourage you to investigate Day One and these other garden journal apps to see if one is right for you:

Garden Manager is a good choice for the visual and auditory learner who loves to grow vegetables. It includes incredibly detailed crop tutorials for over fifty plants that you watch or listen to. It also gives you a heads-up for changing weather.

Smart Gardener is a planner and tracker. It helps you choose the right plants for your growing conditions and gives you specific advice for your garden layout. Its garden journal helps you maintain a current list of your plants, and it provides a weekly task list customized to your information.

Moon and Garden is a great resource for those interested in biodynamic gardening, the practice of gardening by the influence of the moon. This app helps you take notes, check lunar phases, take photos, add reminders, and check the weather forecast.

Gardenize describes itself as "A digital garden diary with photographic memory." According to reviews, it is best for smaller gardens. It allows you to keep detailed information about your plants and care activities and includes recipes for homegrown veggies, as well as useful articles and a gardening calendar for the US, UK, Australia, and New Zealand.

For those of you who remain tech-weary or tech-leery, most of the applications today are user-friendly and offer easy steps to start using and documenting immediately. It might open up a whole new world, or a new calling.

Journaling the Garden

I still have the dog-eared copy of *The Country Diary of an Edwardian Lady* I was given in 1977, the year it came out. An unlikely bestseller for sure. It was my first exposure to the art of journaling, and what a beautiful book it is—Lady Edith Holden sauntering through the gentle English countryside with her watercolors and her words. I was fascinated and wanted to do just that. Later, when I lived in England for a while and had the opportunity to walk those paths, I was too busy holding the hands of two toddlers and missed my chance. It's not too late to buy those watercolors and brushes now . . .

Journaling your garden's progress through the seasons, including your feelings and insights, can strengthen your connection to nature. Bonus points if you can illustrate them. Whether you're an accomplished artist or just a doodler, I encourage you to illustrate your garden in whatever medium you choose. Not only will you reap the stress-reducing benefits of handwork (as discussed in chapter 1), but you'll also find it's a good way to practice mindfulness while producing a lasting memory of a beautiful bloom or a broader landscape.

Pressing flowers and leaves is another way to add value to your journal experience. I love opening a book and finding a pressed leaf or wildflower, the delicate remnant of a someone's perfect summer day.

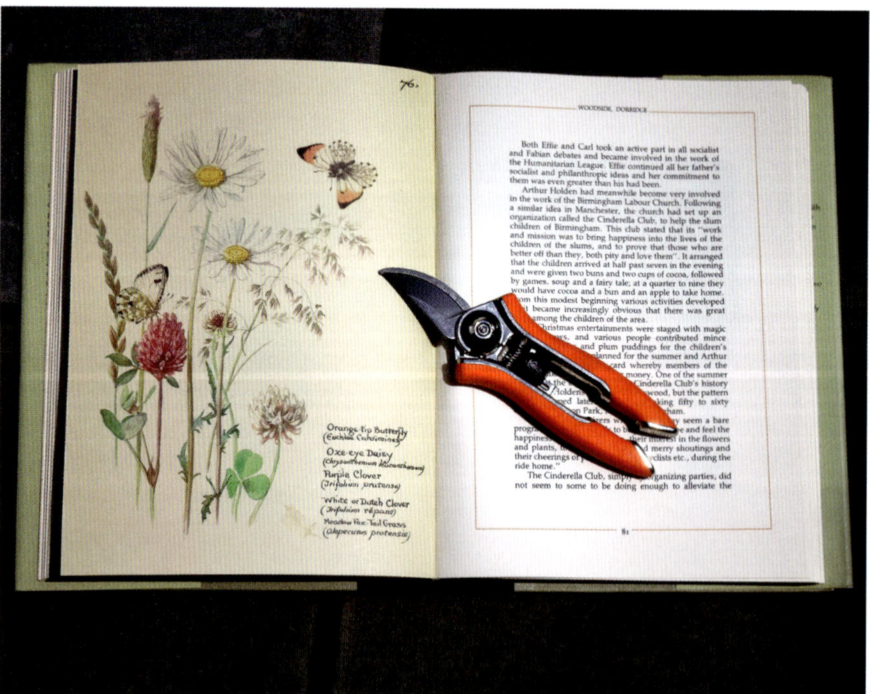

A page out of *The Country Diary of an Edwardian Lady*.

"And the May month flaps its glad green
leaves like wings." Thomas Hardy from
Afterwards. T.H. 1840-1928
All the Feijoas are flaunting their delicious
blossoms. I keep nibbling on their vanilla
petals. Roses all blooming. Lavender blooming.
The Oak titmouse is constantly flying
to the 'Forest Pansy' Redbud & then

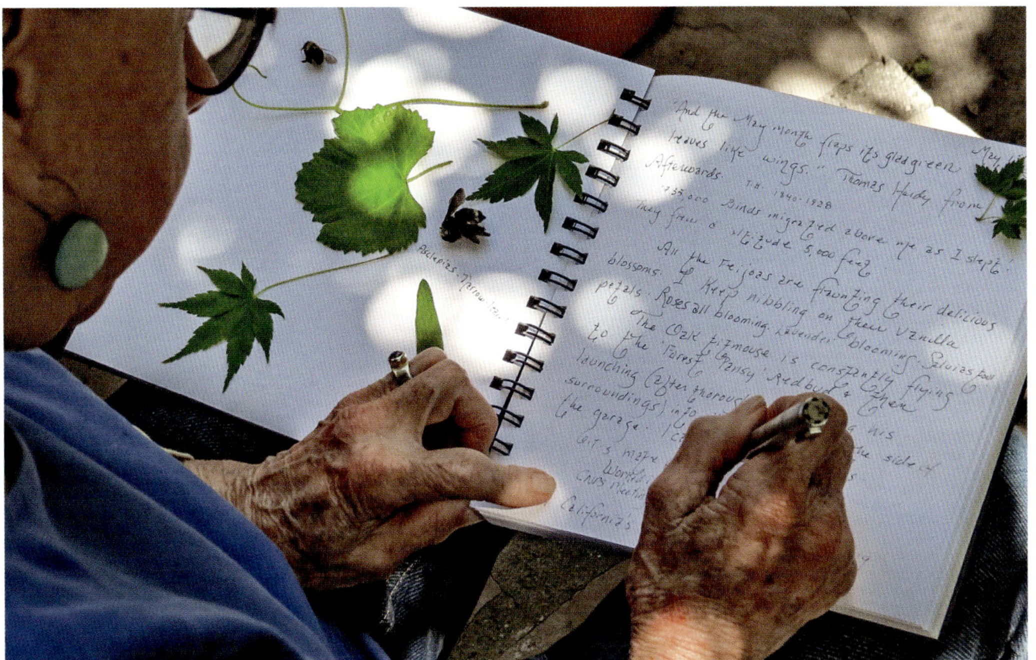

Sharon Lovejoy's journals include her observations and found treasures. *Photo courtesy of Jeff Prostovich*

Social media, for all its negatives, can be an affirming way to keep records of your garden. With its emphasis on the visual, Instagram (whether set to public or private) can provide a personal garden pictorial set in chronological order, with little effort. BlueSky has an active gardening feed. Blogging on any number of platforms is another way to share your garden with others. While more of an undertaking, making garden videos will capture that moment in time for another day.

Mapping and Marking Your Plants

Gardening amnesia is common to all gardeners, but is more troublesome for the seasoned gardener. It's annoying when you start to dig a hole and find your shovel has sliced through a dormant plant or a clump of bulbs. On the other hand, what a pleasant surprise when a plant emerges that you forgot about planting!

The lesson here is to mind your shovel, and be sure to watch out for these plants, which are slow to wake up come spring:

Balloon flower (*Platycodon grandiflorus*)
Black-eyed Susan (*Rudbeckia fulgida*)

Blue spirea (*Caryopteris* × *clandonensis*)
Butterfly weed (*Asclepias tuberosa*)
Culver's root (*Veronicastrum virginicum*)
Hardy hibiscus (*Hibiscus* hybrids)
Indian pink (*Spigelia marilandica*)
Joe-pye weed (*Eutrochium purpureum*)
Leadwort (*Ceratostigma plumbaginoides*)
Maiden grass (*Miscanthus sinensis*)
Montbretia (*Crocosmia* × *crocosmiiflora*)
Red-hot poker (*Kniphofia uvaria*)
Russian sage (*Perovskia atriplicifolia*)
Swamp milkweed (*Asclepias incarnata*)
Whirling butterflies (*Gaura lindheimeri*)

A simple garden map and strategically placed markers help you avoid double planting or accidental destruction. Better yet, they help you find unoccupied spaces for when you buy that gorgeous viburnum or other irresistible specimens with absolutely no idea where you'll plant them. And nature will still provide surprises.

Just as journaling jogs your memory about what you have planted, mapping and marking will provide the where. A map is also useful for knowing how many plants you might need for a new project, for calculating soil, compost, and fertilizer amounts, for maintaining rotation schedules for vegetable crops, and more. Once again, you can use pencil and paper or one of the many online garden tools and apps.

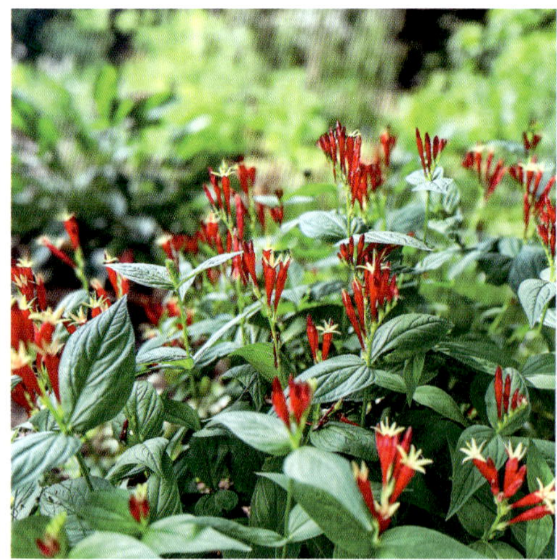
Indian pink is another latecomer in spring.

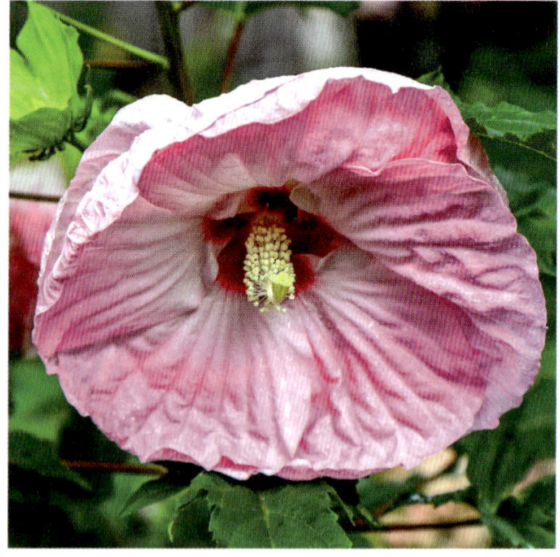
Be sure to mark hardy hibiscus; it is late to emerge in spring.

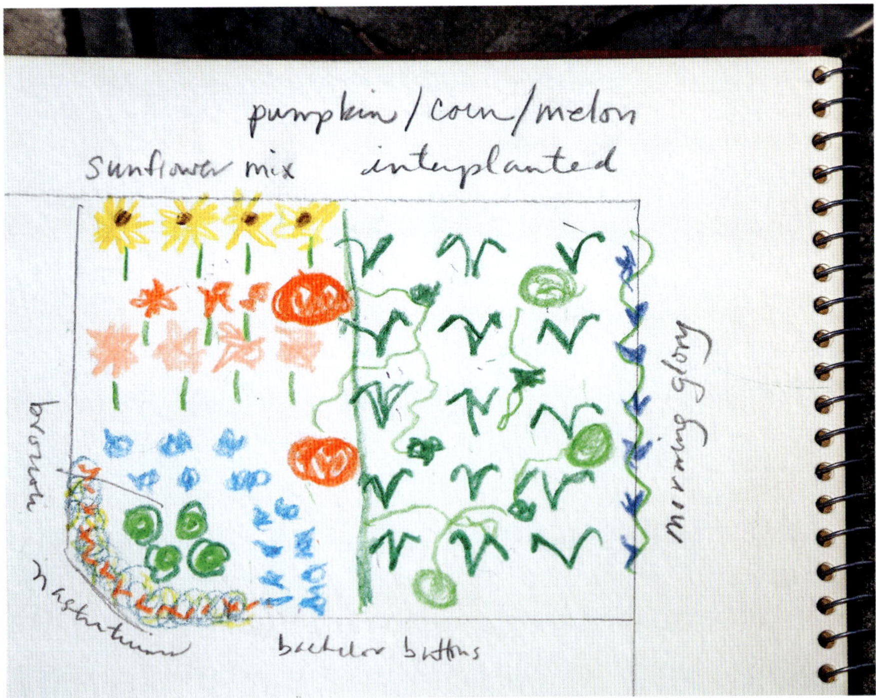

A simple plan I sketched for my Kansas kitchen garden many years ago.

HOW TO MAP YOUR GARDEN OR LANDSCAPE

There are a few different ways to create a map (or maps) of your property. If you're lucky enough to have existing blueprints of your home and property, or a previous professional landscape design, use them as is or piggyback off of those plans and add your own design or plant inventory. Another option is to do what the landscape maintenance and snow removal companies do when they estimate pricing for your lot: They don't bother to visit anymore; they use Google Earth to determine your square footage and landscape boundaries. There are detailed instructions online for how to do this; however, it doesn't always do a good job showing changes in elevation.

A third option is to go old-school and simply draw maps from scratch, using graph paper and a pencil. First determine an appropriate scale, based on the size of your property or garden. The grid on the graph paper will be made up of either ⅛″ (.3 cm) or ¼″ (.6 cm) squares. To turn this into a scale, you can say, for example, that one square on the paper equals 1′ (.3 m) of actual ground in the garden. So, a 10′ × 25′ (3 × 7.5 m) planted area will take up ten by twenty-five squares on the graph paper. To draw curves, plot points representing every few feet, then connect the dots to make the curve. You can measure the actual space by pacing off the different areas of your garden or, if they're not too large, using a measuring tape.

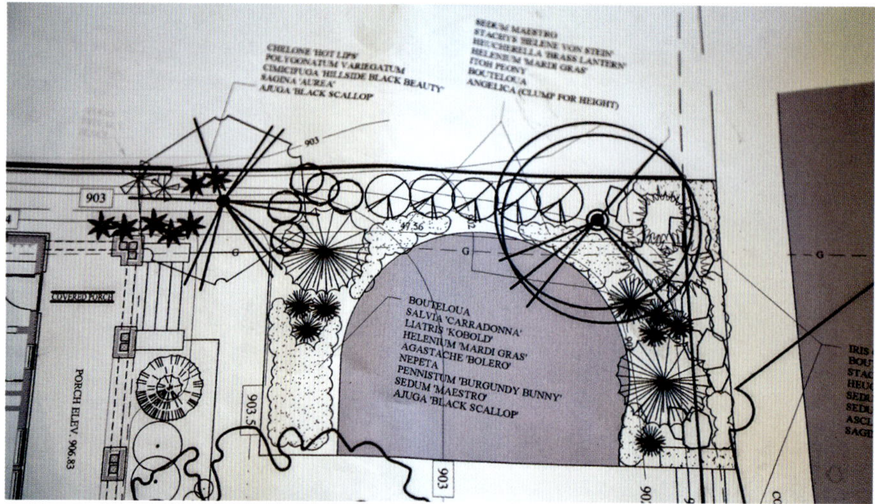

Existing landscape plans can be useful for updating your garden inventory and map.

Once you have a basic plan view (bird's-eye view) of your property, mark north on your map. This will help you later to determine where light and shadows fall as the season progresses.

The next step is to populate your map with plants. There are design kits for drawing your own landscape plan that include graph paper, colored pencils, and templates for flowers, grasses, vines, shrubs, and trees. You can use the same idea and find things around your house to represent plants. Or, you can simply draw various sizes of circles or buy stickers to denote plant locations. If you want it to look more professional, you can download icons online that show each plant's leaf shape, texture, and size. You might want to use only circles for larger plants, and bubbles for where there are drifts or mass plantings of one species. Finally, note the location of sheds, patios, and furniture for extra context.

Once you have the map, how should you use it? For starters, it can be a visual record for reminding you at the beginning of spring, when things look sparse, that, yes, the garden will fill out as the weeks pass. A map's overhead view also helps you make sense of all those plant icons and symbols representing your garden's plant population and features, and it could help identify a problem or solution you wouldn't see otherwise. For example, you might see opportunities to add more texture or definition in the form of bolder foliage shapes or variegation. If there are bare spots, it will help you calculate how many groundcover plants you need to create living mulch. To get the most from your map, try to update it with each season—because a garden is never finished.

Citizen Science

Maintaining detailed garden records can be a way of contributing to citizen science and community. The National Geographic Society defines citizen science as follows: "Citizen Science is the practice of public participation and collaboration in scientific research to increase scientific knowledge. Through citizen science, people share and contribute to data monitoring and collection programs." Usually, this participation is done as an unpaid volunteer.

One area of interest is phenology: the study of cyclic and seasonal natural phenomena, especially in relation to the climate and plant and animal life, such as bird counts and flowering times. Knowing that you should plant peas when forsythia flowers, beans when lilacs bloom, or tomatoes when apple blossoms fall is more than folklore. Your observations and recordkeeping might be helpful in growing a larger accumulation of data that can be used for research and problem solving.

Here are a few options for getting involved (see Resources, page 213):

Project Budburst: Gather local data observing trees, shrubs, and flowers and document first leaves, flowers, and fruits.

Audubon Christmas Bird Count: From December 14 to January 5 of each year, contribute to a wildlife census that will help scientists assess the health of bird populations.

Butterfly Census: Participate in a one-day butterfly count in your area for the North American Butterfly Association.

The Great Sunflower Project: Plant a Lemon Queen variety sunflower and help identify the effects of pesticides on pollinators.

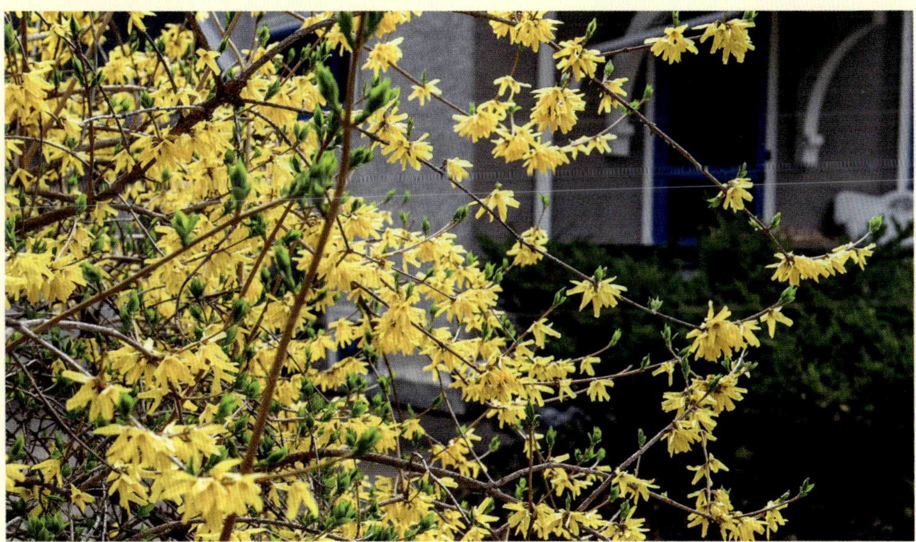

Forsythia blooming is a phenological sign telling you it's time to plant peas.

PLANT MARKERS

There are so many options for marking, tagging, and labeling your plants, and just as many reasons for doing so. These are small garden accessories that we ask a lot from: They should be informative, visually appealing, weather-resistant, legible, noticeable but discrete, and, sometimes, cute.

I have mixed feelings about plant markers. I love it when I can put a name to a face (a plant, that is) when I'm on a garden tour or visiting a public garden, especially when there's no one around to ask. But I hate it when markers get in the way of a great photograph, especially those black ones with the white lettering.

One question to ask yourself is whether the markers are there just for you or for visitors, too. Before I ever host another garden tour, I'm definitely going to label my katsura tree. Of all the questions I anticipated one summer when my garden was on back-to-back-to-back tours, I didn't think that it would be so popular, yet everyone wanted to know what it was. I guess I had grown accustomed to the charming fluttery heart-shaped leaves and silvery bark—and what's that interesting fragrance, is it cotton candy or caramel?

Marker materials vary, but the serious ones, the ones meant to inform and endure, are made of zinc, copper, anodized aluminum, or galvanized steel able to withstand harsh sunlight, heavy rain, and extreme cold. Plastic and wood labels are inexpensive but need replacing every few years. Those

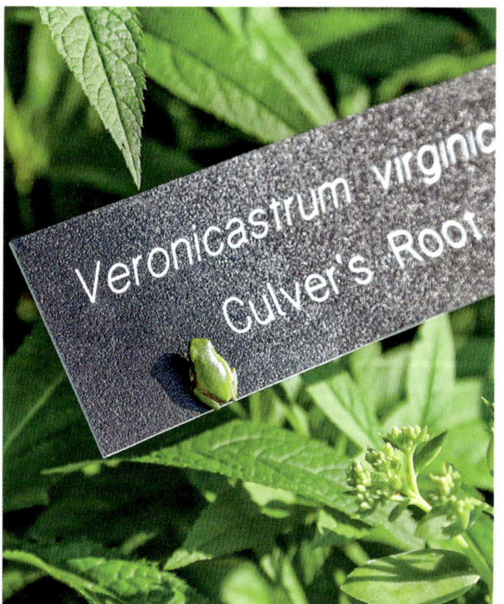

A little frog checking out this botanical marker at the Minnesota Landscape Arboretum.

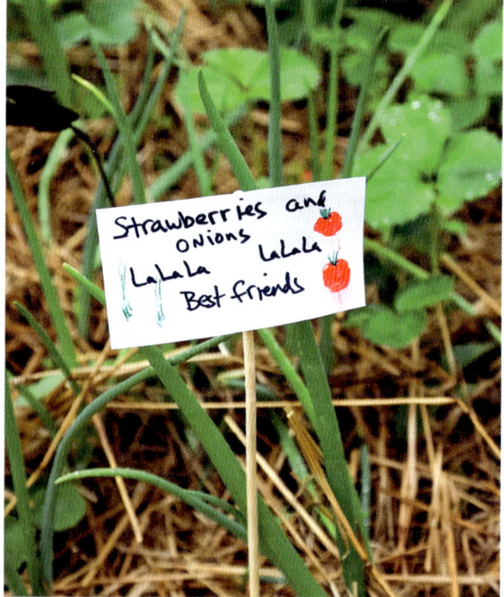

This drawing of strawberries and onions makes for a charming marker on a garden tour.

engraved black-and-white ones you see in botanical gardens are a laminated plastic that is UV-resistant and weatherproof. They are also pretty "spendy," as we say in Minnesota.

T-shaped markers are usually one piece, while cap-style and rose-style markers feature a small, horizontal plate for the plant name attached to hairpin-style legs. The legs might be made of another material that can rust eventually. The rose-style marker is tilted so it is easier to read without bending down—especially nice for those with dodgy knees or less-than-perfect vision.

Markers made of copper or other softer metals can be embossed with a ballpoint pen. Some markers are etched to make it easier to write on with a permanent marker or carbon marking pencil. In other cases, people simply make labels (with large print for people with visual limitations or impairments) and stick them to the tag. This is also helpful for those with arthritis in their hands who can't write as well as they once did.

If you want the markers to be more decorative, or even quirky, you can make them out of, or find, an array of natural materials: wood, clay, ceramic, bamboo, painted rocks, bricks, hewn twigs, and more. Upcycled objects, like spools, paint sticks, corks, silver spoons, skewers, and clothespins, might be better for showing sustainable style than displaying information. In any case, it's working if it helps you remember.

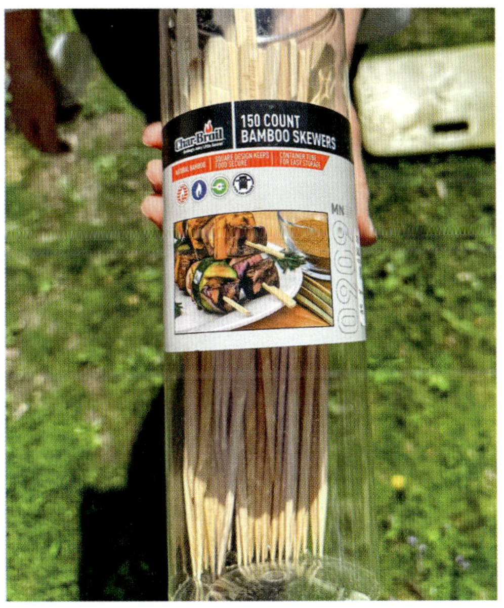

Skewers make handy temporary markers.

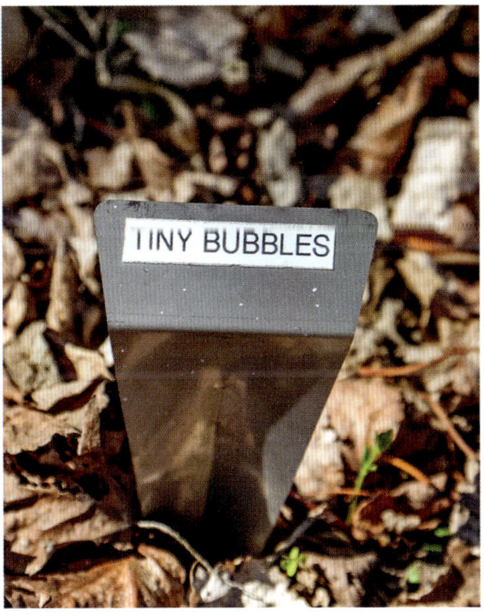

This variation of a rose-style marker reminds the gardener where hosta 'Tiny Bubbles' is planted.

GARDENER SPOTLIGHT
Sharon Lovejoy

Sharon Lovejoy's delightful column "Heart's Ease" ran in *Country Living Gardener* magazine between 1993 and 2006. During those same years, our family was moving all over the country and world for my husband's job. What little gardening I did was marked with fits and starts, and frustration. Yet, there was one constant: I looked forward to that column every month and, in a way, felt like I was gardening right along with Sharon; she seemed to know my gardening heart. Many others felt the same way. Her first book, *Sunflower Houses,* sold out over and over again.

Early on, Sharon combined her love for nature and art with paintings and drawings documenting her observations of the natural world. Since then, she has worked as an author, illustrator, speaker, and children's garden design consultant among her many endeavors. She owned and ran hugely successful garden-themed businesses that included public gardens of her own making.

An intuitive gardener, Sharon gives credit to her grandmother for instilling in her a love and wonder for nature. Her grandmother's tiny redwood cottage sat beneath apricot trees under a sycamore tree. As Sharon played outside, she fell in love with trapdoor spiders, lizards, gopher snakes, birds, and ladybird beetles. Her life's work is testimony to the importance of a grandparent's influence.

Sharon still feels that connection. She used to be super neat and pick up piles of leaves, but then she would see a legless lizard, a California glow worm, or an egg case in there, and she realized that what was incidental to her was their entire world, leading her to be very careful about disturbing this natural (dis)order.

A lot of Sharon's garden is in containers. "I could not imagine gardening without containers, for ease and because it's such an intimate relationship. It's up high and you're not contending with gophers or ground squirrels," she says.

Early every morning, Sharon goes out to her garden (still in her nightgown) and starts weeding, moving plants, planting seedlings, and filling birdbaths. She con-

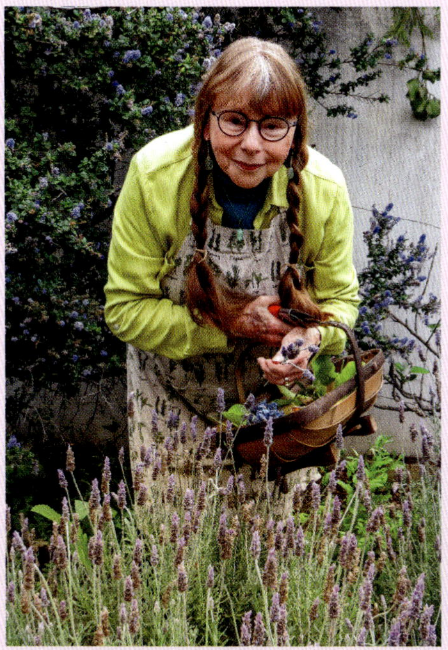
Photo courtesy of Jeff Prostovich

fides, "I do talk to everything." She cites a Stanford study on the benefits and observes, "They don't answer, but they do answer in flowers and fruit." Although she has arthritis, she says that once she's out there it's forgotten; she is bending over and picking up things and singing. "Gardens are the magical healers."

Sharon illustrates her garden journals with scenes and moments of the "riotous joy" she finds in her garden. She likes to be able to go back and remember a date from years before. "I know that in two weeks my beloved hermit thrush will leave, but I know that around March 22 the hooded orioles will arrive. So I'm always celebrating and anticipating and enjoying that moment."

SHARON'S TIPS FOR JOY IN THE GARDEN

- As she does every morning, go for a "discovery walk" and really look at things. She takes a magnifying glass or a jeweler's loupe. Always take time to see.
- Doing so much potting, she keeps four small garbage pails (with lids) containing topsoil, sand, fine soil, and pebbles for top dressing.
- She always carries a basket with her, to save trips and hold her harvest. She keeps a duplicate set of tools in the backyard in a big rural mailbox to avoid extra trips to the front yard.
- She advises: Don't do anything without the "joy factor."

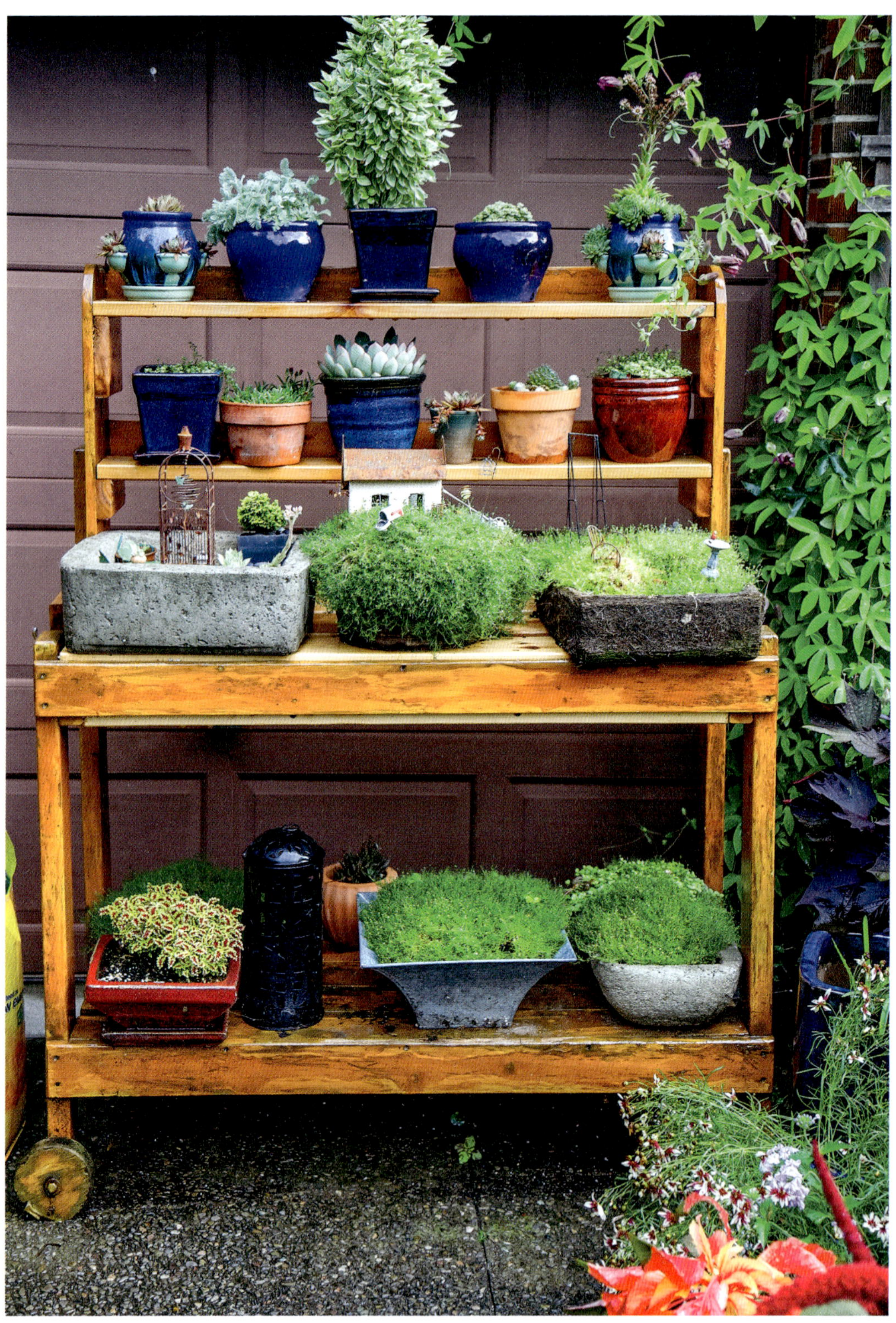

A potting bench filled with a variety of potted plants and containers can be a garden unto itself.

CHAPTER 10

Sit Down, Stand Up

Let's expand our idea of what it is to garden. The dictionary tells us, "A garden is a plot of ground where herbs, fruits, flowers, or vegetables are cultivated." But I believe a garden can be whatever and wherever you want, a place to tend a single plant or as many as you like. It doesn't necessarily require a piece of land or homeownership—or knees on the ground—just the desire to grow something.

Go beyond traditional gardening and there is still a whole world of planting possibilities. And most can be done easily while seated at the kitchen table or standing at the potting bench. Tabletop gardening is popular with people of all abilities, but is especially welcome for people with physical limitations or mobility issues. It takes a fraction of the strength and stamina of conventional growing methods, and you probably won't break a sweat.

Sitting or standing with a plant near to eye level, right at your fingertips, creates a special bond, a form of intimacy. It's a different relationship than appreciating trees from a distance or observing plants at your feet. You can see a plant's unique characteristics up close, note its behavior, and feel that interconnectedness to nature that is so important to emotional health. Tabletop or standup gardening can be a gateway to meeting new plants, cultivating plants in new ways, and finding calm and comfort for a few hours lost in another place. In this chapter we'll explore ideas, methods, and plant varieties for gardening at a closer, more intimate, range—both indoors and outside.

Terrariums

Our demographic remembers terrariums from way back when, in the same era when macrame plant hangers were trendy. Terrariums actually go back much further than the 1970s, but everything old is new again. And today, terrarium gardening is easier than ever before, thanks to an abundance of inexpensive containers, a wide variety of plants, and accessible materials. You can create a Lilliputian landscape in a bottle with little effort.

Closed terrarium or open terrarium? It depends upon what plants you want to grow. Do you want a tropical rainforest vibe or do you lean toward a sparse desert aesthetic? How much care can you provide? A closed terrarium creates a self-sustaining, humid, and moisture-rich environment by recycling water and maintaining high humidity levels. An open terrarium requires regular watering and monitoring, even with low-maintenance succulents.

Almost any kind of glass container can be made into a closed terrarium, but a glass cookie jar with straight sides, a wide mouth, and a sealable lid works best for a beginner. You'll need a planting medium (called a substrate), suitable plants, sheet moss, long tweezers or tongs, and a spray bottle. To make it interesting, add hardscape, like rocks, stones, driftwood, or simple twigs. Many garden centers sell tiny houseplants in 1–2″ (2.5–5 cm)

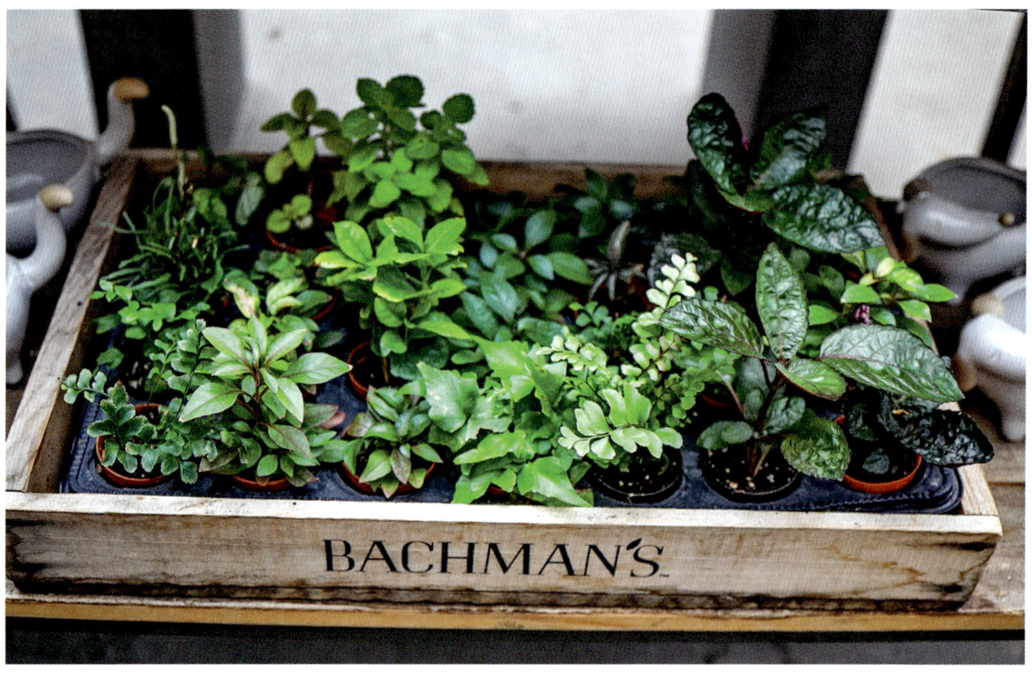

Tiny tropical plants are sold for making terrariums.

A Deeply Rooted Connection

Scientific studies have suggested that plants can smell humans and recognize their caretakers, even adjusting their growth to human interaction. It could be a particular scent they pick up or other chemical processes they experience; research is ongoing. While we can't prove that with our houseplants at home, we have all seen how the sensitive plant (*Mimosa pudica*) folds its leaves when touched, as one example.

Other studies claim that plants respond to music and sound, preferring classical and jazz, which actually increases their growth rate, while they get stressed by harsh rock and heavy metal. It might be that plants aren't actually "listening" to music but rather sensing vibrations; there is still much to be learned about this connection in the growing field of plant neurobiology. Meanwhile, crank up the Mozart.

Plants do communicate with one another, using volatile organic compounds (VOCs) released into the air and chemical signals sent through their root systems. There's so much going unknown and unnoticed when you repot a philodendron!

For humans, simply transplanting or repotting a plant requires mindfulness and attention to detail that redirect your thoughts from worry and stress. Caring for plants gives a sense of accomplishment and promotes self-esteem. Plants improve human well-being through reciprocity; they benefit from your care as much you benefit from their presence.

pots specifically for terrariums or other miniature landscapes. Here are some popular varieties:

Arrowhead plant (*Syngonium podophyllum*)
Asparagus fern (*Asparagus setaceus*)
Baby tears (*Pilea depressa*)
Mini orchids
Nerve plant (*Fittonia albivenis*)
Polka dot plant (*Hypoestes phyllostachya*)
Prayer plant (*Maranta leuconeura*)
Radiator plant (*Peperomia* spp.)
Small begonias
Small ferns
Strawberry begonia (*Saxifraga stolonifera*)

Don't use potting soil; it's too heavy, and it will sour and smell over time. You can make your own substrate or buy premade terrarium mix. The most popular substrate recipe, known as ABG mix for its Atlanta Botanical Garden origins, has been updated for sustainability reasons, substituting coconut coir for peat moss, and pumice or lava for hard-to-find tree fern fiber. You can find these materials at a garden center, pet store, or aquarium supply store:

1 part sphagnum moss
2 parts pumice or lava
2 parts orchid bark
1 part coconut coir
1 part activated charcoal

Some prefer to put a layer of pea gravel or lightweight expanded clay aggregate (LECA) at the bottom for better looks and drainage, separating it from the substrate with a piece of window screen or similar mesh, trimmed in a circle to fit.

HOW TO CREATE A TROPICAL TERRARIUM

1. Add your substrate material to the bottom of the terrarium jar or other container, using a layer of gravel or LECA below the substrate, if desired. Slope the substrate to give it some topography. The different levels will better highlight the plants and make this little green world more realistic.
2. Add any hardscape items you're using on top of the substrate.
3. Cut moss into pieces and layer them on top for a forest floor effect, leaving spaces to insert your plants.
4. Remove most of the soil from your plants' roots and gently plant each into the substrate.
5. Mist the plants—don't drench them—and put the lid on the container.
6. Place the terrarium in a location that receives adequate light but not direct sunlight. Open it for a moment every two weeks to air it out and let in oxygen. Without a lid, an open terrarium with tropical plants will need to be watered more often. With time you'll learn how much is enough, or too much.

HOW TO CREATE A DESERT OR XERIC TERRARIUM

If you'd like a drier mini-landscape rather than a rainforest, an open terrarium fits the bill. In addition to all the succulents and cacti available (there are so many nowadays), here are some reliable xeric plants to try:

Button fern (*Pellaea rotundifolia*)
Cushion aloe, pearl plant, zebra plant (*Haworthia* spp.)

Hens and chicks (*Echeveria* spp.)
Jade plant (*Crassula ovata*)
Stonecrop (*Sedum* spp.; smaller cultivars)

Now, all you need is a glass container with a wide opening, pebbles, charcoal, cactus potting soil (formulated for dry plantings), and a teaspoon. This one is almost too easy.

1. Spread a 1–2″ (2.5–5 cm) layer of pebbles on the bottom, then 1″ (2.5 cm) of charcoal, then 2–3″ (5–7.5 cm) of cactus potting soil on top of that.
2. Trim any dead leaves off the plants.
3. Use the teaspoon to make a small planting pocket for each plant, and insert the plant. Be sure to space them with room to grow. Tamp down the soil around each plant.
4. Give each plant a teaspoon of water to get established. Thereafter, water only once a month; a few teaspoons will do.

Cloches, Cases, and Mini-Greenhouses

Growing under glass harkens back to the golden age of botanical exploration when intrepid plant hunters traveled the world, seeking exotic specimens for a burgeoning group of plant enthusiasts back home and launching the world's live plant trade. Transporting plants was difficult until 1827, when amateur botanist and entomologist Nathaniel Ward noticed a fern growing in the wood-and-glass case in which he kept the caterpillars he studied. What became the Wardian case made all the difference.

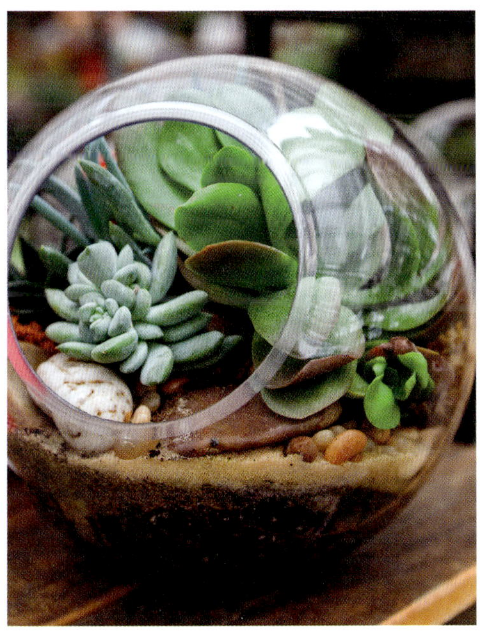
Open terrarium, desert-style.

I would have loved gardening in this era. Imagine the wonder of seeing these far-flung tropical plants for the first time and then growing them in your front parlor! Nowadays, glass cloches and containers give you the same Victorian vintage look, plus they have a practical side: They provide high humidity for plants. Think of them as a tropical vacation (or

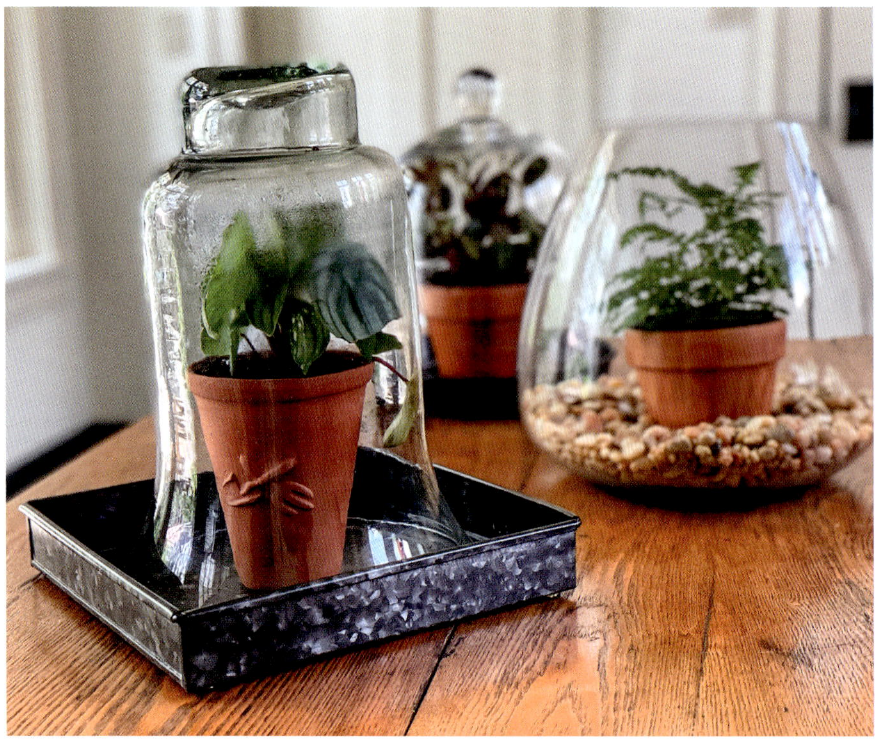

Houseplants under glass cloches in my garden room.

hospital) for your plants—especially helpful when the AC or heat can make the indoors dry as a desert. They also protect plants from drafts, dust, and pests.

Growing an indoor garden under glass can be as simple as a single plant covered with a cloche or a grouping of plants under cloches of various shapes and sizes. You can grow several plants at a time in a Wardian-style mini-greenhouse, as long as all of the plants are suited for the same microclimate. You'll want to avoid placing them in direct sun so as not to cook them. Ensure they have good drainage, and set the potted plants on a saucer or metal tray to catch condensation. Remove the cloche or greenhouse cover from time to time for ventilation, and check for signs of fungal disease. Make sure the size of the cloche or greenhouse cover can accommodate the plant as it grows; if it gets too big, prune it back or rotate out with a new plant.

Here are some good plants to grow under glass:

Begonia (*Begonia crispula*, *Begonia* 'Tiny Gem' (other begonias, like 'Rex' and 'Angel Wing,' are suitable but will require more trimming)

Chinese money plant (*Pilea peperomioides*)

Creeping fig (*Ficus pumila*)
Flame violet (*Episcia cupreata*)
Maidenhair fern (*Adiantum pedatum*)
Nerve plant (*Fittonia albivenis*)
Orchids (*Masdevallia, Dracula, Platystele, Angraecum,* and *Lepanthes* varieties are designated as suitable for terrariums)
Philodendron (*Philodendron micans*)
Radiator plant (*Peperomia*; among all the great cultivars, *Peperomia caperata,* with its intriguing purple foliage, is a looker)

Carnivorous Plants

Looking to go beyond the usual plant selection? Carnivorous plants make for meaty subject matter—an entirely new plant genre to collect, study, and observe, not to mention impress your fellow gardening friends. You can grow them year-round indoors in a terrarium. Otherwise, grow them inside a container sitting in a shallow tray of water, or a container with continuous moisture, taking them outside to a patio during the warmer months where they will enjoy the sunlight. Bring them indoors for the winter once frost is due, keeping them by a cool, sunny window or under lights.

These plants grow best in ericaceous compost, a planting medium for acid-loving plants that can be found in specialist nurseries and online, and occasionally in garden centers. Water with rainwater or filtered or distilled water only—never tap water. They don't need fertilizer because they catch their own food! No matter how tempting it is, don't poke the Venus fly trap; it depletes their energy. You can find carnivorous plants at specialist nurseries (see Resources) and occasionally at garden centers; for a wider selection, go online to find these species:

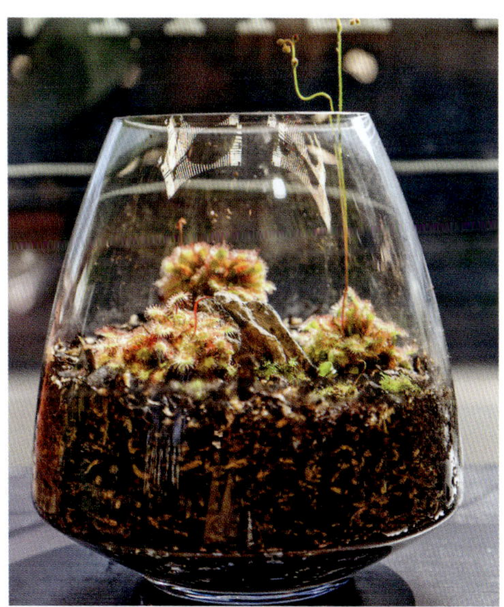

Carnivorous terrariums are a specialty at We Bite Rare & Unusual Plants in New Orleans.

Bladderwort (*Utricularia* spp.)
Butterwort (*Pinguicula* spp.)
Carnivorous bromeliad (*Brocchinia reducta*)
Cobra plant (*Darlingtonia californica*)

North American pitcher (*Sarracenia* spp.)
Sundew (*Drosera* spp.)
Tropical pitcher (*Nepenthes* spp.)
Venus flytrap (*Dionaea muscipula*)

Greenhouse Cabinets

Looking for more of a challenge? A statement piece for your plants? Then you should join the IKEA greenhouse community, the hundreds of clever and crafty people who repurpose IKEA shelving units into custom habitats for their prized plants. Online videos abound with instructions for how to fit DETOLF, FABRIKÖR, RUDSTA, and MILSBO cabinets with lights, fans, and even misters and automatic humidifiers to make a dream house for your tender plants. The level of sophistication depends upon your abilities, budget, skills, and commitment. This would make a great project to do with kids, combining their biology and STEM curricula. Or you could just sit your plants on the shelves, water them when needed, and enjoy.

Other IKEA greenhouse cabinet aficionados take it one step further and use the cabinet to make one big terrarium (look for instructional videos online). They seal and waterproof the cabinet interior. Then they fill the bottom with substrate for planting and nest plants into nooks and crannies of driftwood and fabricated natural-looking structures attached to the back side of the cabinet. The terrarium is equipped with misters to manage moisture levels. Some even make it a bioactive environment with small invertebrates. Think of it as a next-level science fair project, sure to keep your neural networks growing.

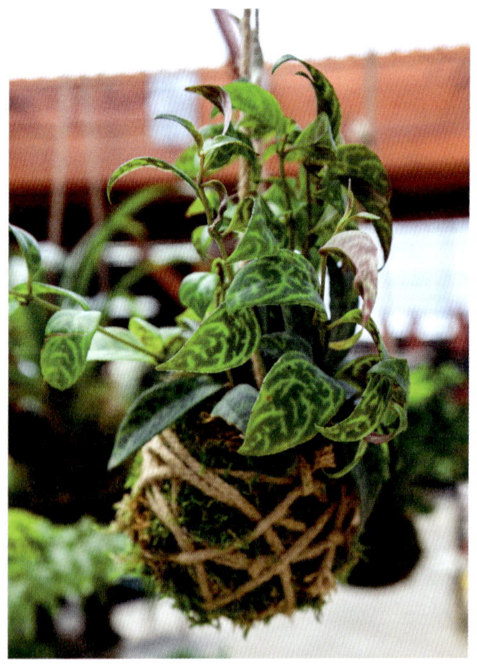

Kokedama radiator plant.

Kokedama

Looking for something a bit more Zen? Kokedama might be the answer. It's the Japanese art of planting in a moss ball; in fact, it means "moss ball." Sometimes called "poor man's bonsai," it's really more like instant gratification. You can make one or several in a single session at your potting table. The materials are easy to find at the garden center, but it's possible you might already have some of them on hand. The first thing to do is decide which method you want to try: the neat and tidy method or the "get your hands dirty" version. There's something therapeutic about both.

MESSY METHOD

You will need potting soil and peat moss; for a more eco-friendly solution, use coco coir instead of peat moss. You will also need sphagnum moss, twine, small scissors or clippers, and your plant.

1. Lay down some plastic on your work surface, and scoop equal parts of potting medium onto the surface.
2. Mix the media together and gradually add water until you have a stiff batter-like consistency and can form a ball of soil big enough for planting. Think back to making mud pies.
3. Using your hands, pack the ball tightly. If you're feeling confident, do the toss test: Toss the ball and catch it. Did it stick the landing?
4. Once you have a firm ball you will have to break it in half. I know! Take your plant and knock most of the soil from the root ball and sandwich it between the two halves and gently press them back together.
5. Swaddle the ball with pieces of moss and wrap the twine around it a couple of times to secure it onto the ball. Keep adding moss and twine until the soil ball is covered and the plant is secure. Tie off the twine, and trim off any loose moss.
6. Soak the plant ball in a small tub of water for 5–10 minutes. Remove the ball from the tub and let it drain.
7. Once it stops dripping, it's ready to display on a small plate or shallow container; choosing that is half the fun. Or you can affix a length of twine to hang it by a window with indirect sunlight. Hang several together at different heights and you have an aerial "plantscape."

QUICKER, TIDIER METHOD

Gather the same supplies used in the Messy Method, plus a nylon knee-high stocking

1. Remove your plant from its pot and break off some of the soil and roots until it is the right size for the finished ball.
2. Slip the plant into the foot of the stocking. Add moist potting medium inside the stocking around the roots, forming a ball shape.
3. Secure the stocking around the plant stem, using twine, but be careful not to strangle the plant. Trim any excess stocking.

4. Spray-mist sphagnum moss or sheet moss, and layer it around the ball until you can't see the nylon, wrapping it with thread or twine. You can choose the color of the twine to contrast with the moss or blend in; your call. Tie off the thread or twine.
5. Soak the plant ball and then display as described in steps 6 and 7 of the Messy Method.

Kokedama care is simple: Water it whenever it feels light; soak it until it feels heavy again. When the plant gets too big, trim it back or transplant to a conventional container and then, if you want, make a new kokedama. Depending upon the look you want, any small tropical houseplant will work. Here are some good options:

African violet (*Saintpaulia ionantha*)
Baby tears (*Pilea depressa*)
Corn plant (*Dracaena* spp.)
Creeping fig (*Ficus pumila*)
Cyclamen (*Cyclamen persicum*)
Fern (*Adiantum pedatum or* small houseplant cultivars)
Flamingo flower (*Anthurium* spp.)
Golden pothos (*Epipremnum aureum*)
Ivy (*Hedera helix*)
Nerve plant (*Fittonia albivenis*)
Prayer plant (*Maranta leuconeura*)
Radiator plant (*Peperomia* spp.)

Bonsai

People who practice the art of bonsai are playing the long game. That might lead you to believe that it's too late to begin such a hobby "at your age." But ten years down the road, will you look back and regret not pursuing any activity or passion, thinking you didn't have enough time? Bonsai is not for everyone, but it rewards those with patience and persistence.

The "how" of bonsai is too complicated to condense for quick instruction here, and that's part of its beauty. The best place to learn this ancient technique is through bonsai clubs, classes, and workshops, with the added gift of social interaction that is so important to seniors' well-being.

This contemplative practice of miniaturizing trees relies on certain aesthetic principles: proportion, balance, line, movement, rhythm, contrast, and unity. It's done by restricting growth through container size, pruning, wiring, and root pruning to obtain upright and cascading styles, often with a windswept appearance that suggests resilience and adaptability, something to which we older gardeners can relate.

As a means of artistic expression, bonsai can be part of a meditation process, prompting you to be present while also at one with the tree. In this way it can help to reduce stress, improve focus, give a sense of accomplishment, and provide a vital connection with nature.

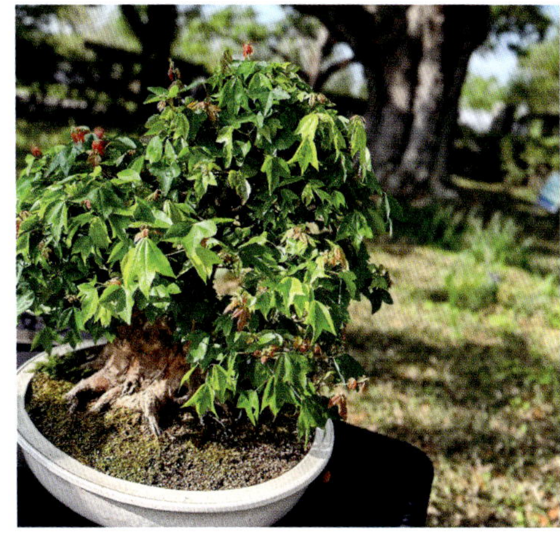

It's never too late to discover the art of bonsai.

Alpine Gardens

So far in this chapter we've discussed tabletop gardens that make for a snapshot of larger natural environments—from rainforest to bog to desert—that we can appreciate indoors. But maybe the mountains are more to your liking. Let's go back outside and make an alpine container garden. Alpine plants are tough and adorable all at once. They are resilient and cold-hardy; in their high-altitude home they grow in thin, rocky soil, called scree, and are exposed to harsh winds and thrive with scant rainfall. Many of these plants are endangered in their natural habitats, moving higher up the peak as climate change encroaches.

Alpine containers overwinter easily and can be stored in an unheated garage or under the deck, out of the wind, before you bring them out the next spring. They're also easy on the budget and low-maintenance, since you only have to plant them once.

You can design and create an alpine garden while seated or standing. Planted in lightweight "hypertufa" containers (bowls, basins, or troughs), many of these miniature mountainside plantings are easy to handle. They can sit on an outdoor table, pedestal, or other elevated surface; in fact, that's where they are best appreciated.

You can buy ready-made containers or make your own. Hypertufa is a mix of cement, peat moss, and perlite (some recipes add sand). Recipes and detailed instructions are available online. Do it with a friend to share materials and muscle, or if this seems daunting, check with local garden centers or botanical gardens to see if they offer classes on hypertufa. It's best to start with a bowl or basin shape, but some people go big and make them using fish boxes or coolers

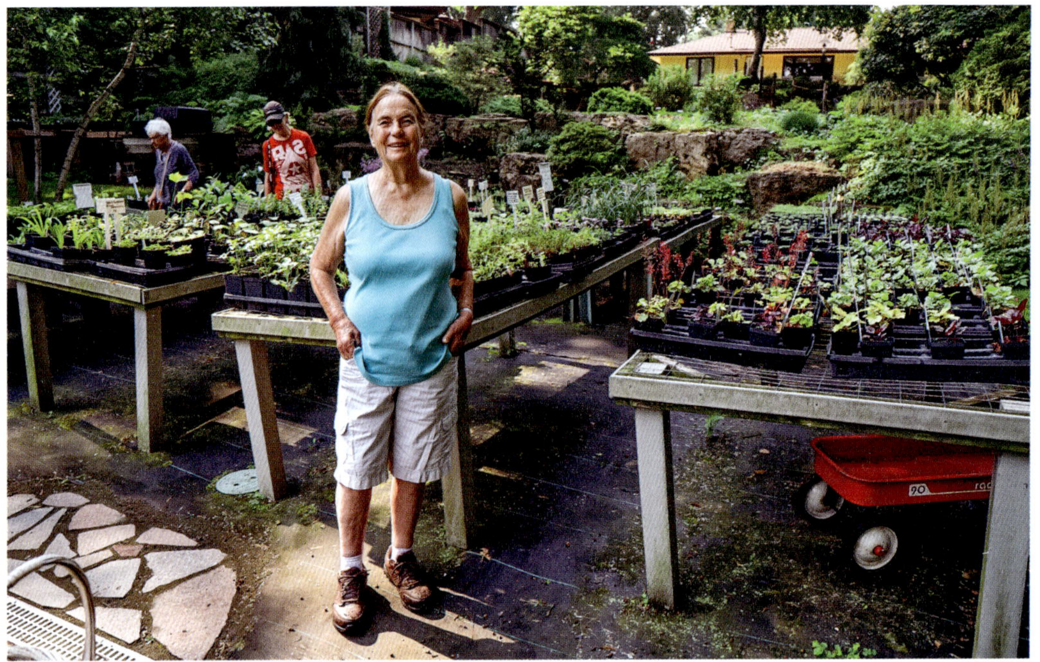

Betty Ann Addison, 89, sells hardy and rare plants suitable for alpine gardens; her nursery has been in business for fifty years.

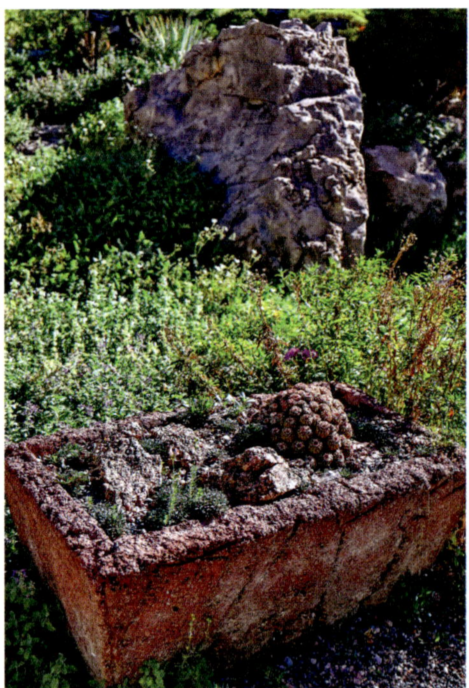

Alpine plants growing in a hypertufa trough. *Photo courtesy of Pam Penick*

for a mold. Be aware that a large container will get heavy and take you out of the tabletop realm.

Mimic alpine soil with a planting mix of one-third potting soil, one-third sand (you can use play sand), and one-third crushed gravel. You want a low-nutrient mix for these slow-growing plants. You can add rocks for hardscape and nestle plants among them. You don't want to crowd these plants since the negative space in the design is part of the charm. Just like with any container, pick plants with varying heights, growth habits, textures, colors, and bloom times for long-season interest. Top-dress with gravel for sharp drainage and a finished look.

Alpine gardens can be addictive; bet you can't stop at one. But this is no problem, as they look great grouped together. Consider joining the North American Rock Garden Society for expert advice and plant sources. The Alpine Garden Society, based in the UK, has a wealth of information as well. Many alpine plants are smaller, low-growing cousins of familiar perennials. Some hug the ground, forming cushion or mat shapes, but in spite of their size they have robust root systems.

Here are some great alpine plants to try:

Alpine lewisia (*Lewisia pygmaea*)
Campanula (*Campanula alpina*)
Creeping phlox (*Phlox subulata*)
Creeping thyme (*Thymus serpyllum*)
Dianthus (*Dianthus* spp.)
Pasque flower (*Pulsatilla vulgaris*)
Primrose (*Primula marginata*)
Saxifrage (*Saxifraga* spp.)
Sea pink (*Armeria maritima*)
Speedwell (*Veronica prostrata*)
Stonecrop (*Sedum* spp.)
Stork's bill (*Erodium*)

Garden Adjacent Activities

Use your horticultural curiosity to explore and discover new ways to celebrate and share your passion for plants. These ideas go a bit beyond the tabletop, but you can do them at whatever relaxed scale and pace you want. These suggestions are garden adjacent—think of your garden as a leaping-off point for new interests and adventures.

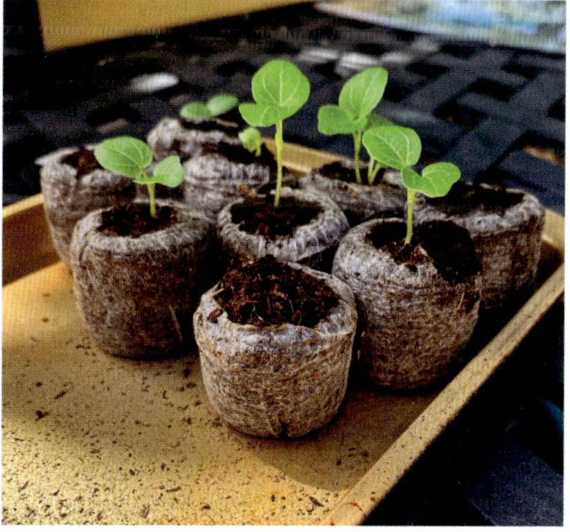
Start and tend seedlings for someone who's busy, then share the harvest.

Millennial "plant parents" and pandemic isolation brought about a big change in the houseplant world. Now there are more varieties available than ever. For a new take, you could do a deep dive into houseplants, discovering and growing multiple types of one plant family, such as Arums, which

GARDENER SPOTLIGHT

Shawna Coronado

I first met Shawna Coronado in 2010 at a garden writers conference in Dallas and was struck by her energy and enthusiasm for her work and her eagerness to share that knowledge with others. Since then, she has evolved from a hobby columnist to a multimedia producer with over two decades of experience. She's the author of many books, including *The Wellness Garden* and *101 Organic Gardening Hacks*.

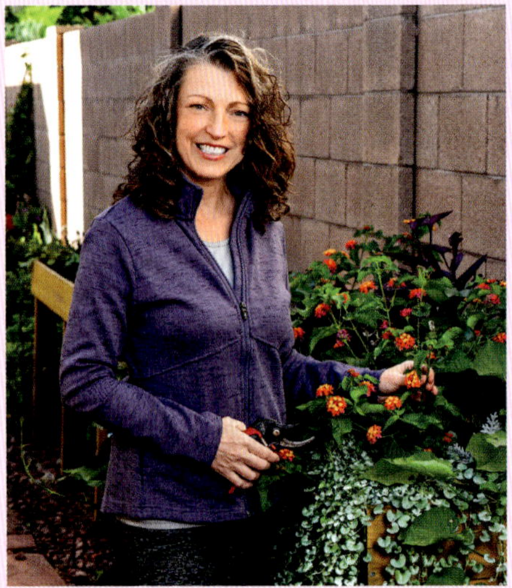

Photo courtesy of Cindy Dyer

Shawna's career pivoted, however, when she was diagnosed with severe degenerative osteoarthritis of the spine, prompting her to discover the therapeutic and healing benefits of gardening. She now focuses on teaching about low-maintenance food growing and health concerns that connect wellness, anti-inflammatory living, and sustainable growing practices.

Her gardening underwent a big change after moving from the Midwest to Mesa, Arizona, in Zone 9b. She now uses shade cloths and special soil combinations that prevent water waste, and she seeks out

contain the *Monstera deliciosa* and its cousins. Or you could see how many plants with pink variegation you can collect. Or maybe combine your existing houseplants in new ways to make captivating tablescapes or corner groupings using different containers and stands at various heights.

Here are some more ideas for garden adjacent fun:

- Start seeds for a busy but nimbler partner, family member, or friend, seeing the plants through until they are ready for planting out. Let the recipient of your gift do the bending and share in the bounty of this co-effort later.
- Source crafting materials straight from your garden, or a gardening buddy, to create dried flower arrangements, plant-based dyes, pressed flowers, collages, and more.

heat-tolerant plant varieties. She has high praise for raised beds: "They are for adapting to my osteoarthritis, but also they are such low-maintenance compared to a regular garden that I adore working with them."

Shawna integrates outdoor paintings and art pieces into her garden spaces, creating focal points that enhance the natural beauty while withstanding the harsh desert climate. In her side yard, an area that is often overlooked by other gardeners, Shawna has created an "art gallery garden," and the result is stunning. As she describes it, "I challenge traditional 'proper' gardening design rules, instead embracing creative, colorful approaches that bring me joy. I choose plants that are tough and provide beauty, flowers, and color—often native plants or shrubs that survive well in desert conditions."

Shawna's focus is on creating sustainable systems that work with climate challenges instead of against them. This includes water-wise plantings, protective structures like shade cloths, and container gardening that allows her flexibility during extreme weather.

SHAWNA'S TIPS FOR GARDENING MORE EASILY WITH HEALTH CHALLENGES

- "My favorite tool is the CobraHead, It's incredibly versatile and reduces stain on my joints by enabling me to have a good grip."
- "Flexible kink-resistant hoses reduce strain. Gardening during the optimal watering times, early morning and later evening, when it's cooler works best for both my plants and my comfort level. These cooler periods allow me to work in the garden without overexerting myself, while my plants get the water they need."
- Understanding the irrigation needs of various plants is crucial when moving to a new environment.

- Grow a unique blend of peppers to develop your own signature hot sauce.
- Paint, draw, sketch, model, or photograph your garden. Display, donate, or sell the resulting works of art at a plant sale, farmers market, or craft festival.
- Propagate small succulents, plant in funky containers, and sell them at your next community garage sale.

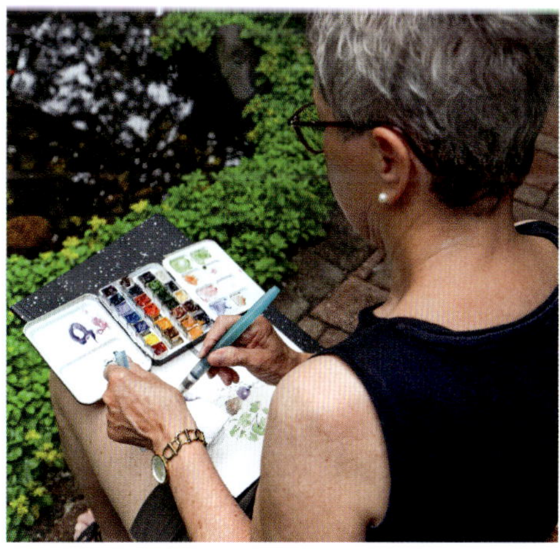

Paint your garden!

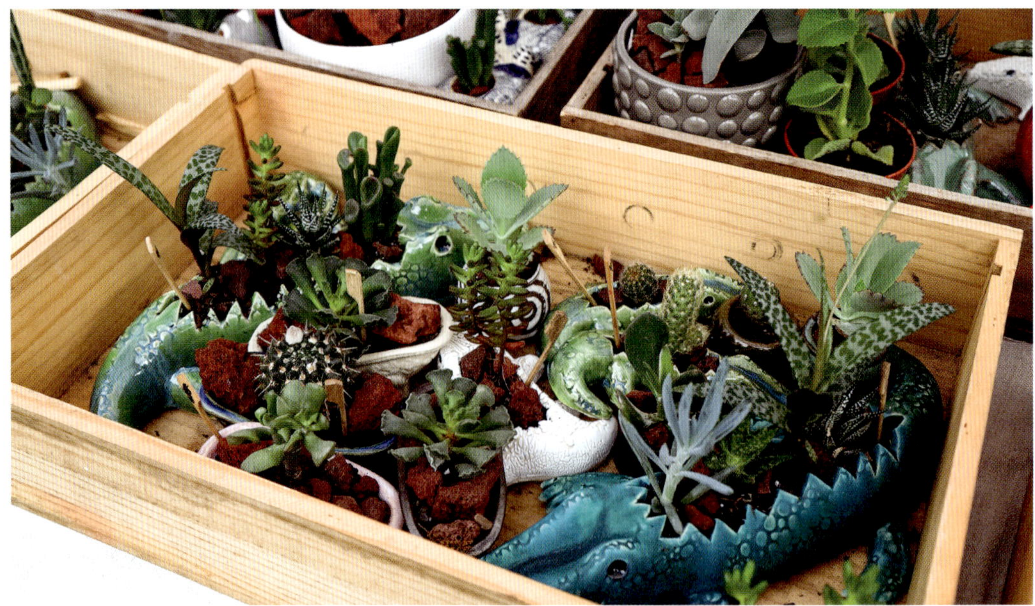

Have fun with succulents in funky pots.

- Go on a quest, thrifting with a friend or family member with your gardens in mind, seeking unusual objects to repurpose for containers and plant companions.
- Grow a cutting garden and make jam-jar bouquets for seniors at assisted living facilities. They will always be admired and appreciated more than you know. Take loose flowers with you and demonstrate how to do it, and let them help.

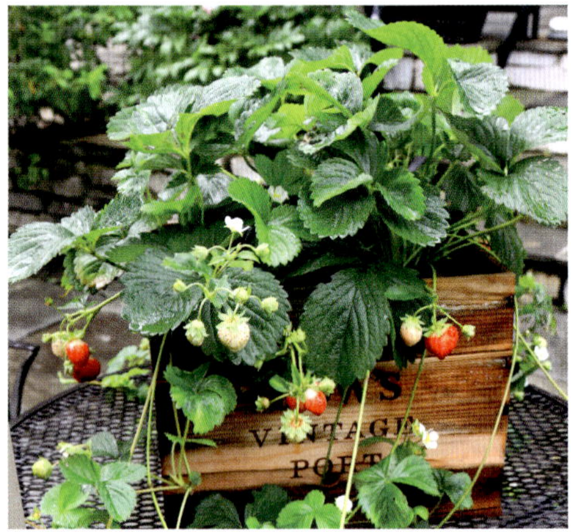

Look for unusual containers, like this wooden port box that these strawberries call home.

Or, you could write about gardening like I do!

CELEBRATING OLDER GARDENERS, GROWING NEW GARDENERS

Not many people publish their first book at the age of sixty, much less their second one as they are approaching seventy. But here I am. One more bit of proof that older people, older gardeners, still have so much to contribute.

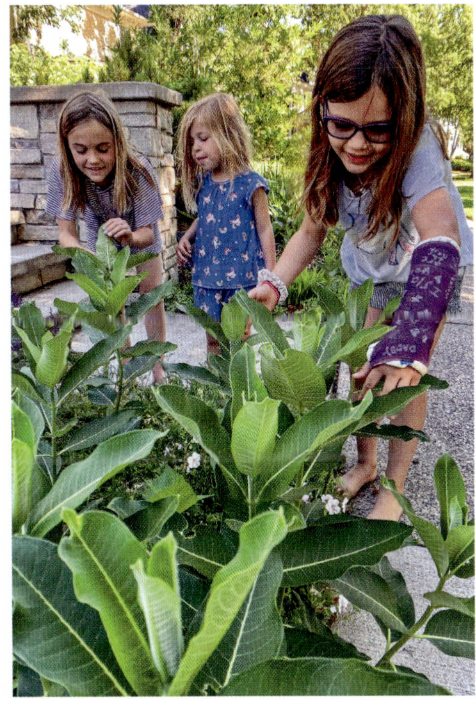

My young neighbors—Isla, Noe, and Cody—finding monarch eggs on our milkweed.

Collectively, we have killed a lot of plants. But we have planted and cared for far more that have flourished. During that time, we have acquired vast amounts of horticultural knowledge, some through formal training or higher education, and much more through life experience. Our passion for plants has grown stronger with every season, even if our stamina has waned. It is ours now to pass on to the next generation of gardeners.

There are countless ways to do this, including many that draw upon your strengths and feel natural to you. But sometimes the best way to feel alive is to step out of your comfort zone. You can join a group, or lead by quiet example;

it's up to you. Think back to the person or people who set you on your garden path, and how you might do the same for a child, a young adult beginning gardener, or even a late bloomer just retired and looking for a hobby, or greater purpose.

Volunteerism

Volunteering is a two-way street. It starts with helping other people, of course. Beyond that, the Mayo Clinic states that volunteering offers significant additional benefits, especially for older adults, including improved physical and mental health, greater life satisfaction, improved self-esteem, and potentially a longer life.[1] It also builds social connections and nurtures new and existing relationships.

For those who want to get their hands dirty, there are volunteer opportunities for individuals or groups, like planting containers on small-town main streets or creating colorful pockets on urban boulevards. You can find these activities through word of mouth and by checking with city hall, civic organizations, or garden clubs. If teaching is more your thing, summer camps, continuing education programs, and garden center workshops are always looking for personable, knowledgeable people to do this.

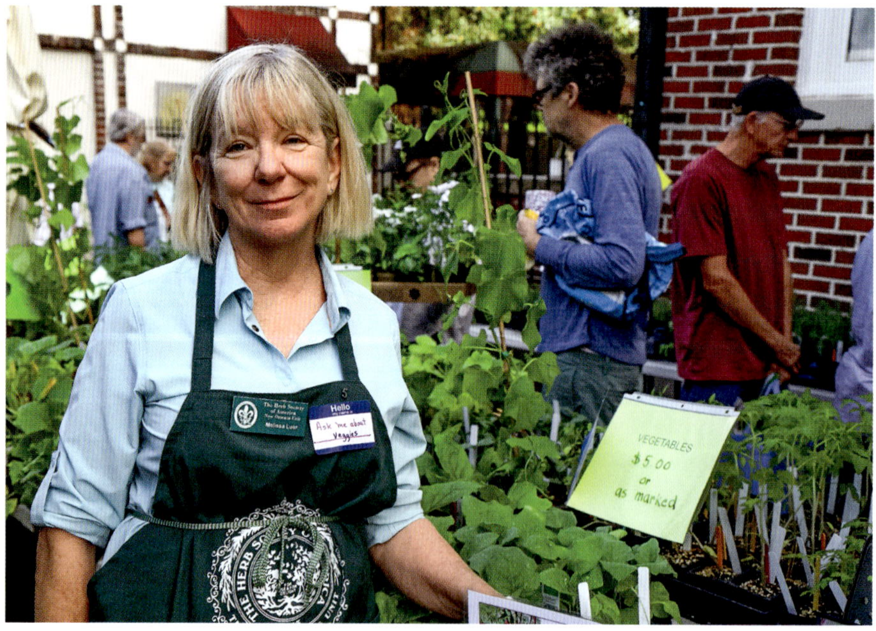

Melissa Luer helping at a plant sale—she volunteers with the Herb Society of America and Master Gardeners of Greater New Orleans.

Senior facilities are often understaffed and appreciate any type of gardening lessons you can provide, according to the residents' skill levels. For example, you could help them plant containers for their patio, or they might be content to look at a slide presentation of pretty gardens. Don't underestimate the power of plants to alleviate anxiety and depression and rekindle happy memories.

Garden Clubs and Plant Societies

I speak to a lot of garden clubs and I'm noticing a trend lately: more members and younger members. That's exciting news. These newcomers are looking for advice and plant-based camaraderie—you could be the one to help solve their problems with apple scab or pesky ground squirrels tunneling into their veggie beds. Or they might be looking to take some extra plants off your hands, or perhaps just find a new friend.

Plant societies that specialize in one type of plant, such as hostas, orchids, daylilies, or roses, are a great place to swap detailed information or rare plant varieties. They often hold tours or host sales where you find even more of your particular plant people.

Extension Master Gardeners

I've said it before, and I'll say it again: You'll get so much more than you expect from serving as a Master Gardener. Programs vary from state to state or even county to county, but generally they are the best places to find your tribe and find your calling if you want to share your gardening expertise with others. The opportunities for helping are many: answering gardening questions online and in booths at events like farmers markets or fairs, helping underserved groups learn to grow their own food, and teaching classes on tree care, to name just a few.

There are also lots of ways to help out at school gardens and with summer school programs. School gardens are especially in need of a consistent voice and helper, as students and parents cycle in and out of these gardens because their children change grades and move on. Intergenerational activities like this provide so many chances to mentor young kids who might not have someone else to spark an interest in gardening.

Mentoring as Elders and Grandparents

Imagine seeing your garden all over again through the eyes of a child! I'm not a grandparent but I still hope to be someday. So many of us count our grandparents or other close elders as the ones who had the time and patience to foster a love of gardening within us. They let us tag along and help and maybe even let us grow our own patch of flowers. Those small and seemingly ordinary moments had a big impact on our gardening futures. Amidst all the busyness that children experience today, don't forget to spend time with them and plant some seeds—and sow the gardening seed.

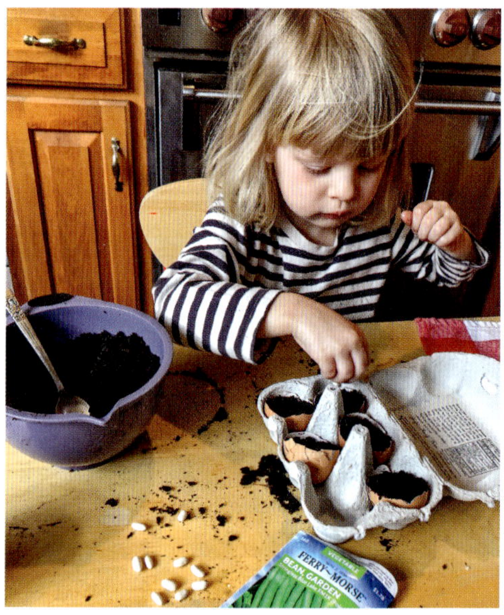

Our neighbors' granddaughter, Osla, carefully sowing her bean seeds.

A Final Thought

As older gardeners, we might never know how many people, even ones we've never met, have been cheered through a bad day or been inspired by our gardens as they walk or drive by without a word. I love the children's book *Miss Rumphius* by Barbara Cooney. It tells of a woman who traveled the world and then returned to a home by the sea where she sprinkled lupine seeds along the coast of Maine with a mission to "make the world more beautiful." With gardening, I have always hoped to do the same. And so have you.

ACKNOWLEDGMENTS

First thanks go to my editor, Anna Bliss, for her guidance and expertise, and for believing that a book about aging gardeners was ripe for writing. Thanks to all the rest of the Chelsea Green Publishing team for putting together and polishing the pieces of this project. It took a village to make this book.

Before it was a book it was a newspaper story. Thanks go to my dear friend, across-the-street neighbor and tireless gardener, Donna Hamilton, for inspiring me to write that story.

Thanks to my fellow gardeners, garden communicators, and advocates for providing their thoughts and advice on the joys and challenges of gardening as you age: Meleah Maynard, Kylee Baumle, Mary Yee, Mary Schier, Eric Johnson, Zach George, Larry Cipolla, Chris VanCleave, Dee Nash, Sharon Lovejoy, Shawna Coronado, Benjamin Vogt, and Thomas Kerby.

Thanks to all the gardeners who allowed me to photograph you or your gardens: Christine Scotillo and Doug Peine, Dean and Donna Erickson (and granddaughters Ida and Osla), Lara Lau-Schommer, Barb Gasterland, Bryce Hamilton, Broadus Miller, Flo Golod, Doris Wickstrom, Betty Ann Addison, Susan Warde, Sandra Mangel, Brian and Joyce Johannson, Janet and Janice Robidoux, Kurt Herke, Jeffrey Loesch, Mary Montgomery, Jeanne Morgan, and Melissa Luer. And thanks, Cory Barton, for your generous help with the story and the book and for going garden peeping with me.

For indulging me for photos, thank you to my sweet neighbor kids Isla, Noe, Cody, and Nora. Also fierce tomato picker, Violet.

Thanks to Vego Garden, Greenstalk, Gardener's Supply Company, Crescent Gardens, and Skidger for their generous offerings of sample products.

Thanks to my senior fitness trainer, Jacq Hauser, for keeping me fit to garden and giving me new perspectives on how movement makes it possible. Many thanks for starring in the photos demonstrating proper form for common gardening activities.

Thanks to talented photographer Tracy Walsh for making me look good on the cover.

For supporting my writing endeavors and all the dinners and grocery shopping done while I was working on the book, love to my husband, Tom. Love to my children, Hannah and Will, for their support; writing about gardening is great, but being your mom is still my favorite job.

RESOURCES

READ

Baumle, Kylee. 2017. *The Monarch, Saving Our Most-Loved Butterfly*. St. Lynn's Press.

Chapman, Karen. 2019. *Deer-Resistant Design: Fence-free Gardens That Thrive Despite the Deer*. Timber Press.

Cipolla, Larry. 2018. *Hydroponic Gardening: The Very Easy Way*. CreateSpace Independent Publishing Platform.

Cooney, Barbara. 1985. *Miss Rumphius*. Puffin Books.

Coronado, Shawna. 2017. *101 Organic Gardening Hacks: Eco-friendly Solutions to Improve Any Garden*. Cool Springs Press.

Coronado, Shawna. 2017. *The Wellness Garden: Grow, Eat, and Walk Your Way to Better Health*. Cool Springs Press.

Gattone, Toni. 2019. *The Lifelong Gardener: Garden with Ease and Joy at Any Age*. Timber Press.

Hayes, Rhonda Fleming. 2016. *Pollinator Friendly Gardening: Gardening for Bees, Butterflies, and Other Pollinators*. Voyageur Press.

Holden, Edith. 1977. 2001. *The Country Diary of an Edwardian Lady*. Friedman.

Jentz, Kathy. 2023. *Groundcover Revolution: How to use sustainable, low-maintenance, low-water groundcovers to replace your turf.* Cool Springs Press.

Kondo, Marie. 2014. *The Life-Changing Magic of Tidying Up: The Japanese Art of Decluttering*. Ten Speed Press.

Levy, Becca. 2022. *Breaking the Age Code: How Your Beliefs About Aging Determine How Long and Well You Live*. William Morrow.

Lovejoy, Sharon. 1999. *Roots, Shoots, Buckets and Boots: Gardening Together with Children*. Workman Publishing

Maynard, Meleah, and Gilman, Jeff. 2011. *Decoding Gardening Advice: The Science Behind the 100 Most Common Recommendations*. Timber Press.

Penick, Pam. 2013. *Lawn Gone! Low Maintenance, Sustainable, Attractive Alternatives for Your Yard*. Ten Speed Press.

Rooney, Theresa. 2017. *Guide to Humane Critter Control: Natural, Nontoxic Pest Solutions to Protect Your Yard and Garden*. Cool Springs Press.

Schier, Mary. 2017. *The Northern Gardener: From Apples to Zinnias, 150 Years of Garden Wisdom*. Minnesota Historical Society Press.

Vogt, Benjamin. 2023. *Prairie Up: An Introduction to Natural Garden Design*. 3 Fields Press.

LISTEN

Nash, Dee. Michel, Carol. *The Gardenangelists: Flowers, Veggies, and All the Best Dirt*. Apple Podcasts. thegardenangelists.buzzsprout.com

VanCleave, Chris. Byington, Teresa. ROSE CHAT. *The Rose Chat Podcast: Exploring the World of Roses*. VanCleave Media Group. ROSECHATPODCAST.COM

SHOP

A.M. Leonard. www.amleo.com for gardening tools and supplies

Birdies Raised Beds. www.epicgardening.com for garden beds and planters

Burpee. www.burpee.com for seed varieties suited to containers and small spaces

CobraHead. www.cobrahead.com for garden weeding and cultivation tools

Corona Tools. www.coronatools.com for pruners, loppers, hand tools, and more

Crescent Garden. www.crescentgarden.com for planters, self-watering systems, and more

DeWit Garden Tools. www.gardentoolcompany.com for garden tools

Dramm Corporation. www.dramm.com for garden and watering tools, watering wands

Faytra Grow Bags. www.faytra.com for potato grow bags

Felco. www.felco.com for pruning and cutting tools

Fiskars. www.fiskars.com for gardening tools

Flexilla. www.flexilla.com for lightweight garden hoses

Gardenize. www.gardenize.com app for plant care gardening journal and database

Garden Manager. Google Play. App for journaling and tracking the garden

Gardener's Supply Company. www.gardeners.com for gardening tools and supplies

Gardens of Rice Creek. www.gardensofricecreek.com for rare, hardy plants

Gorilla Cart. www.gorillamade.com for garden and utility carts

Greenstalk. www.greenstalkgarden.com for vertical planters

Gronomics. www.gronomics.com for handcrafted cedar raised beds

IKEA. www.ikea.com for planters and glass-front cabinets (suitable for plants)

Johnny's Seeds. www.johnnyseeds.com for 'Cipolla's Pride' organic tomato seed

Melnor. www.melnor.com for RelaxGrip watering tools, nozzles and wands

Merlin Bird ID. www.merlin.allaboutbirds.org for bird ID. Shop at the App Store.

Moon and Garden. App Store. App for moon gardening

Original Soil Scoop™. www.gardenworksusa.com for the original tool

Peta Easi-grip. www.arthritissupplies.com, www.amazon.com for adaptive garden tools

Potwheelz. www.potwheelz.com for garden dollies

Proven Winners. www.provenwinners.com for annuals, perennials, and shrubs, native cultivars

Rachio. www.rachio.com for smart watering systems

Radius. www.radiusgarden.com for ergonomic watering, digging, cutting, and hand garden tools

Renee's Garden. www.reneesgarden.com for seed varieties suited for containers and small spaces

ROCKr. https://www.thexceptional.com/collections/rockr for TheXceptional Garden Rocker Seat

Skidger. www.skidger.com for Xtreme Weeder, Wicked Little Weeder

Shawna Coronado. www.shawnacoronado.com for patio art, fountains, umbrellas, and more

Smart Gardener. www.smartgardener.com for garden planning app

Stihl. www.stihlusa.com for cordless gardening tools

The Farmer's Almanac. www.gardenplanner.almanac.com for vegetable garden planner

The Garden Grid™. www.gardeninminutes.com for raised bed watering systems

The Tick Suit. www.theticksuit.com for protection from ticks while you garden

Toni Gattone, The Resilient Gardener Online Store. www.tonigattone.com for ergonomic tools

Vego Garden. www.vegogarden.com for garden beds and planters

Walensee. www.walenseecollections.com for stand-up weeders

WallyGrow. www.wallygrow.com for wall planters and Wooly Pocket planters

We Bite Rare and Unusual Plants. www.webitenola.com for carnivorous plants and guidance

LEARN

American Academy of Dermatology. www.aad.org for more information on skin protection

Americans with Disabilities Act. www.ada.gov for more information on ADA regulations, technical assistance, and accessibility standards.

Arthritis Foundation. www.arthritis.org for support, resources, and research

Blue Zones. www.bluezones.com for longevity information and research

Centers for Disease Control. www.cdc.gov to find diseases and conditions; healthy living; workplace safety; environmental health; injury, violence and safety; global health; travelers' health and more.

Cleveland Clinic. www.clevelandclinic.org for research, education and health information.

Ecoregions. www.epa.gov/eco-research/ecoregions for maps and further information

Heather Holm. www.pollinatorsnativeplants.com for more information on soft landings

Heat-Zone Map. www.usbg.gov/blog/heat-zones-plant-health-and-ahs-heat-zone-map

Mayo Clinic. www.mayoclinic.org for more information on health and wellness

Missouri Plant Finder. www.missouribotanicalgarden.org for native plant information and database

North American Rock Garden Society. www.nargs.org for more publications, meetings, and events.

Sunset Zones. www.sunsetplantcollection.com/climate-zones for maps

University of Maryland Extension. www.extension.umd.edu for science-based home gardening information

University of Minnesota Extension. www.extension.umn.edu for science-based home gardening information

USDA Hardiness Zones. www.planthardiness.ars.usda.gov for maps

U.S. Department of Agriculture. www.usda.gov for more information on poisonous plants

ACT

Monarch Waystations. www.monarchwatch.org to help create and certify your monarch waystation

National Wildlife Federation. www.certifiedwildlifehabitat.nwf.org to create and certify your backyard habitat

Pollinator Pathways. www.pollinator-pathway.org to start a pathway in your town

NOTES

Preface: Pour Some Tea, and Walk with Me

1. Lisa Wimmer, “Dig Into the Benefits of Gardening,” Speaking of Health, Mayo Clinic Health System, July 12, 2022, https://www.mayoclinichealthsystem.org/hometown-health/speaking-of-health/dig-into-the-benefits-of-gardening.

Chapter 1: Changes and Positive Aging

1. Tuo-Yu Chen and Megan C. Janke, “Gardening as a Potential Activity to Reduce Falls in Older Adults,” *Journal of Aging and Physical Activity* 20, no. 1 (2012): 15–31, https://doi.org/10.1123/japa.20.1.15.
2. Jon Traunfeld, “Pollination of Vegetable Crops in a Changing Climate,” University of Maryland Extension, May 2022, https://extension.umd.edu/resource/pollination-vegetable-crops-changing-climate.

Chapter 2: Evaluating Your Garden

1. “Older Adult Fall Prevention,” U.S. Centers for Disease Control and Prevention, September 2024, https://www.cdc.gov/falls/pdf/CDC-DIP_At-a-Glance_Falls_508.pdf.

Chapter 5: Reimagining Your Garden

1. “Energy-Efficient Landscaping,” U.S. Department of Energy, https://www.energy.gov/energysaver/energy-efficient-landscaping.
2. Regan Davis Hopper, “Mentally and Physically, Trees Make a Difference,” USDA (blog), May 16, 2024, https://www.usda.gov/about-usda/news/blog/mentally-and-physically-trees-make-difference.

Chapter 7: Tools of the Trade

1. Joaquín L. Sancho-Bru, D.J. Giurintano, A. Pérez-González, and M. Vergara, “Optimum Tool Handle Diameter for a Cylinder Grip,” *Journal of Hand Therapy* 16, no. 4 (2003): 337–42, https://doi.org/10.1197s0894-1130(03)00160-1.
2. “Sunscreen,” Sunscreen FAQS, American Academy of Dermatology Association, https://www.aad.org/media/stats-sunscreen.

Chapter 8: When and How to Get Help

1. “The Best Investment for Increasing Home Value: Landscape Architecture,” Greening Your Home, American Society of Landscape Architects, https://www.asla.org/residentialinfo/1pager.html?mf_ct_campaign=tribune-synd-feed.

Chapter 9: Remembering, Forgetting, and Recordkeeping

1. “How Long Does It Take to Form a Habit?,” UCL News, University College London, August 4, 2009, https://www.ucl.ac.uk/news/2009/aug/how-long-does-it-take-form-habit.

Celebrating Older Gardeners, Growing New Gardeners

1. Angela Thoreson, “Helping People, Changing Lives: 3 Health Benefits of Volunteering,” Hometown Health/Speaking of Health (blog), *Mayo Clinic Health System*, August 1, 2023, https://www.mayoclinichealthsystem.org/hometown-health/speaking-of-health/3-health-benefits-of-volunteering

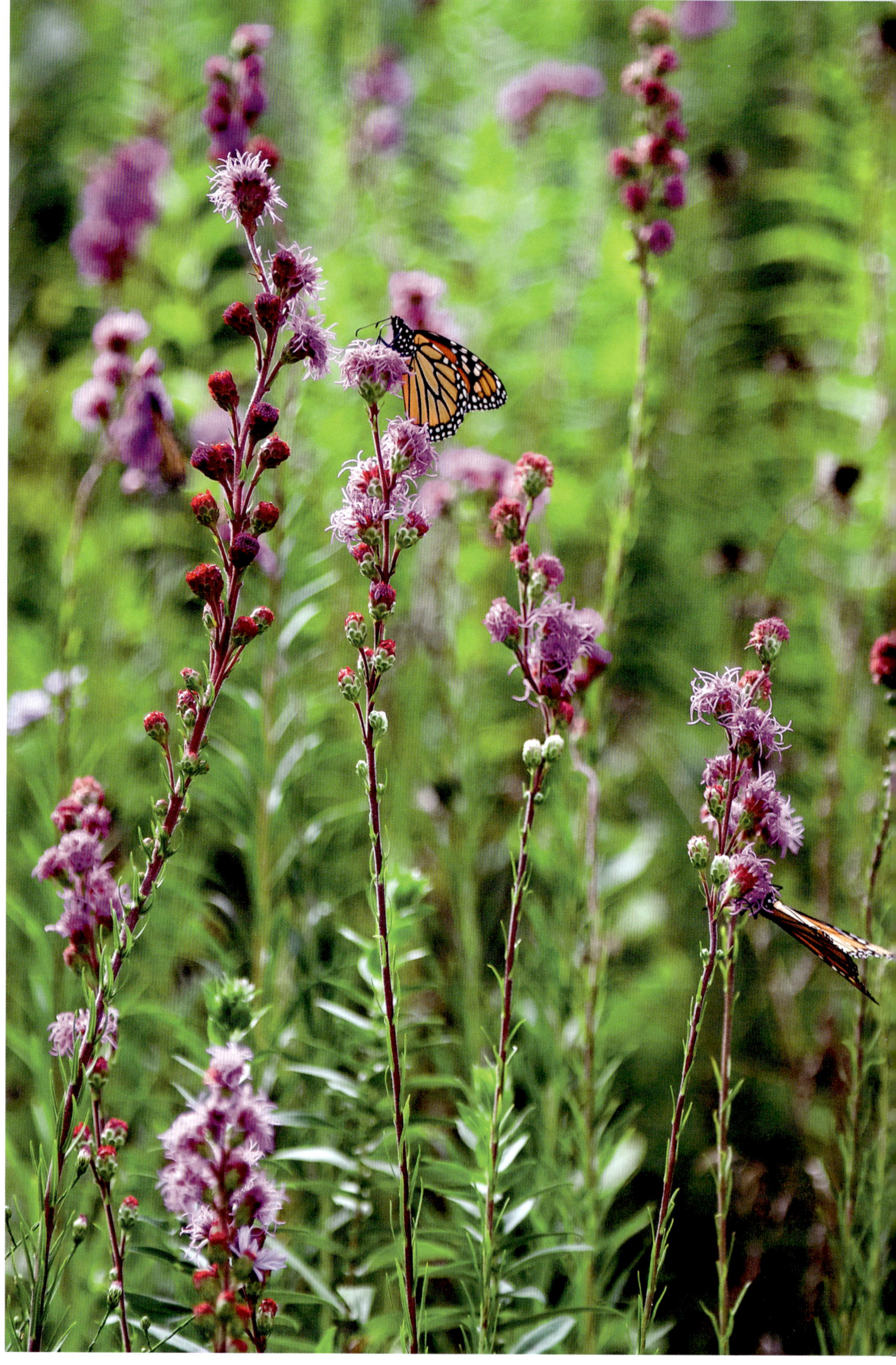

INDEX

A

B

C

D

H

N

ABOUT THE AUTHOR

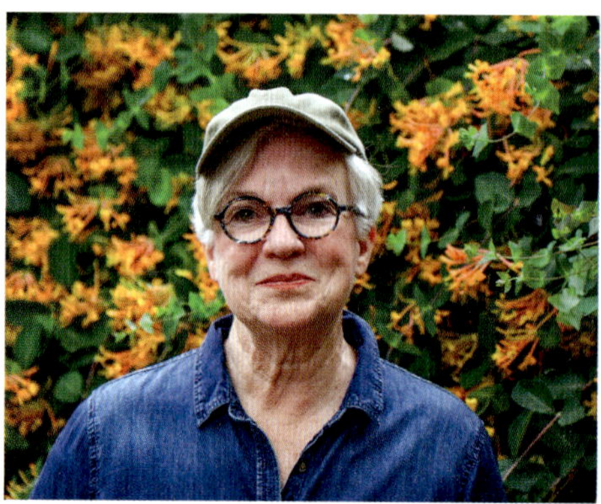
Tom Hayes

Rhonda Fleming Hayes is an award-winning writer and photographer applying her passion to all things plant related. Combining a lifetime of gardening experience with wit and solid research-based advice, her stories can be found in the *Minnesota Star Tribune*, *Northern Gardener*, and *Mpls.St.Paul Magazine*. She has also been published in *Southern Living*, *Midwest Living*, and *Savannah Magazine*. Her first book was *Pollinator Friendly Gardening: Gardening for Bees, Butterflies, and Other Pollinators*.

Rhonda has volunteered as an Extension Master Gardener since 2000. She is a member of GardenComm, Minnesota State Horticultural Society, and Herb Society of America, as well as an emeritus trustee of the Minnesota Landscape Arboretum. She's a popular speaker for garden clubs and other groups, presenting on pollinators, butterfly gardening, native plants, and the art of kitchen gardening, among other topics.

Rhonda gardens in Minneapolis in an urban neighborhood surrounded by woods and water. The abundant plot is home to many bees, butterflies, birds, and beneficial insects. Nowadays, she and her husband spend the winter in New Orleans, where she delights in growing her own Meyer lemons. Regardless of location, she has learned to bloom where she's planted. She loves to share the fruits (and veggies) of her garden with friends, family, and wildlife.